An Alternative History
of Hyperactivity

Critical Issues in Health and Medicine

Edited by Rima D. Apple, University of Wisconsin–Madison,
and Janet Golden, Rutgers University, Camden

Growing criticism of the U.S. health care system is coming from consumers, politicians, the media, activists, and healthcare professionals. Critical Issues in Health and Medicine is a collection of books that explores these contemporary dilemmas from a variety of perspectives, among them political, legal, historical, sociological, and comparative, and with attention to crucial dimensions such as race, gender, ethnicity, sexuality, and culture.

For a list of titles in the series, see the last page of the book.

An Alternative History of Hyperactivity

Food Additives and the Feingold Diet

Matthew Smith

Rutgers University Press

New Brunswick, New Jersey, and London

Library of Congress Cataloging-in-Publication Data

Smith, Matthew, 1973–

An alternative history of hyperactivity : food additives and the Feingold diet / Matthew Smith.

p. ; cm. — (Critical issues in health and medicine)

Includes bibliographical references and index.

ISBN 978-0-8135-5016-9 (hardcover : alk. paper) — ISBN 978-0-8135-5017-6 (pbk. : alk. paper)

1. Feingold, Ben F.   2. Attention-deficit hyperactivity disorder—Nutritional aspects. 3. Attention-deficit hyperactivity disorder—Diet therapy.   4. Attention-deficit hyperactivity disorder—History.   5. Food additives—Toxicology.   I. Title.   II. Series: Critical issues in health and medicine.

[DNLM: 1. Feingold, Ben F.   2. Attention Deficit Disorder with Hyperactivity—diet therapy.   3. Attention Deficit Disorder with Hyperactivity—history.   4. Child.   5. Diet Fads—psychology.   6. Food Additives—adverse effects. 7.   Food Hypersensitivity. 8. Research Design—standards. WS 350.8.A8]

RJ506.H9S643   2011

618.92′8589—dc22

2010042034

A British Cataloging-in-Publication record for this book is available from the British Library.

Visit our Web site: http://rutgerspress.rutgers.edu

Manufactured in the United States of America

This is for my dad, who taught me about taking risks.

Contents

Acknowledgments

As with new medical ideas, the success of a book is often directly proportional to the number of debts accrued during its development. This project would not have been possible without the financial support of the Wellcome Trust and the Social Sciences and Humanities Council of Canada. The Wellcome Trust has also provided me with indispensable training, especially its oral history course. I am grateful for the support and encouragement of Tony Woods, Liz Shaw, Nils Fietje, and Ross MacFarlane, in particular, as well as the members of the Wellcome Trust's History of Medicine funding committees. I am humbled by the prizes awarded to me by the Society for the Social History of Medicine, the British Society for the History of Paediatrics and Child Health, and the American Association for the History of Medicine. Oral history has been a crucial component in my project, and I would like to thank warmly all of my interviewees, as well as the Feingold Association of the United States for connecting me with families who had employed the Feingold diet. Your contribution was invaluable and I hope you all enjoy the book. The staff at the Francis A. Countway Library of Medicine (Harvard University), the Howard Gotlieb Archival Research Center (Boston University), the Archives of the Academy of Allergy, Asthma and Immunology (University of Wisconsin–Milwaukee), the Wellcome Library, and the British Library were all helpful and also deserve thanks.

I am grateful for the suggestions and advice provided by Gregg Mitman, Rima Apple, Jo Melling, Kate Fisher, Matthias Reiss, Michelle Smith, Court Smith, and Sandra Smith for reading this at various stages, and I am thankful for the fulsome support of the Centre for Medical History, the Department of History, and all of my friends and colleagues at the University of Exeter. My PhD and postdoctoral supervisor Mark Jackson deserves enormous credit for his encouragement, attention to detail, sharp analytical skills, diligence, and humor. I have enjoyed putting this book together with the staff at Rutgers University Press and am particularly thankful to Rima Apple for suggesting the Critical Issues in Health and Medicine series and all of her enthusiasm during the last few years. I am also grateful to Marlie Wasserman, Peter Mickulas, and Ann Youmans for their editorial expertise and support.

Finally, I would like to thank my family and friends for giving me the confidence to pursue my academic goals. I am forever indebted to Michelle, Mom, Dad, Liz, Jeremy, Addison, Kellan, the Burkes and, of course, Alice.

List of Abbreviations

AAA   American Academy of Allergy
AAAAI   American Academy of Allergy, Asthma, and Immunology
AAP   American Academy of Pediatrics
AASA   American Association for the Study of Allergy
ACSH   American Council on Science and Health
ADD   Attention-Deficit Disorder
ADHD   Attention-Deficit/Hyperactivity Disorder
ADI   Allowable Daily Intake
AJP   *American Journal of Psychiatry*
AMA   American Medical Association
APA   American Psychiatric Association
BBC   British Broadcasting Corporation
BHA   butylated hydroxyanisole
BHT   butylated hydroxytoluene
BMJ   *British Medical Journal*
BSE   Bovine spongiform encephalopathy
CBC   Canadian Broadcasting Corporation
CJD   Creutzfeldt-Jakob disease
CMA   California Medical Association
CNN   Cable News Network
CSPI   Center for Science in the Public Interest
DES   diethylstilbestrol
DSM   *Diagnostic and Statistical Manual of Disorders*
FAUS   Feingold Association of the United States
FDA   Food and Drug Administration (United States)
FSA   Foods Standards Agency (United Kingdom)
IgE   immunoglobulin E
IJSP   *International Journal of Social Psychiatry*
IUD   intrauterine device
JAACP *Journal of the American Academy of Child Psychiatry*
JAMA   *Journal of the American Medical Association*
K-P   Kaiser-Permanente
LSD   lysergic acid diethylamide
MBD   minimal brain dysfunction

MMR   measles, mumps, and rubella vaccine
MSG   monosodium glutamate
NACHFA   National Advisory Committee on Hyperkinesis and Food Additives
NDEA   National Defense Education Act
NIH   National Institutes of Health
PTA   Parent-Teacher Association
SSAAC   Society for the Study of Asthma and Allied Conditions
USDA   United States Department of Agriculture

An Alternative History
of Hyperactivity

Chapter 1

Food for Thought

In 1974, a self-help book written by Ben F. Feingold (1899–1982) entitled *Why Your Child Is Hyperactive* arrived on the shelves of bookstores across North America.[1] On the surface, the Random House publication was not particularly exceptional. By the mid-1970s, hyperactivity, a disorder characterized by hyperactive, impulsive, inattentive, aggressive, and defiant behavior, was the most commonly diagnosed childhood psychiatric disorder in the United States.[2] Many other books, including primers, self-help books, and medical textbooks, had also been written about the disorder. Medical journals such as the *American Journal of Psychiatry (AJP)*, the *Journal of the American Academy of Child Psychiatry (JAACP)* and *Pediatrics* had published hundreds of articles on the disorder and the pharmaceutical companies that advertised on their pages made millions on the sales of hyperactivity drugs such as methylphenidate, better known as Ritalin. The popular magazine *Life* had published a seven-page article on hyperactivity in October 1972. Perhaps most indicative of the emergence of hyperactivity as a disorder of both medical and social significance was the publication of two books, Peter Schrag and Diane Divoky's *The Myth of the Hyperactive Child: And Other Means of Child Control* (1975) and Peter Conrad's *Identifying Hyperactive Children: The Medicalization of Deviant Behavior* (1976), which questioned the very existence of the disorder.[3]

Feingold's *Why Your Child Is Hyperactive* was also contentious but in a completely different way. Unlike psychiatrists who blamed the disorder on unresolved family conflict, socioeconomic problems, or, increasingly, neurological dysfunction, Feingold, a well-known San Francisco allergist, argued that the ingestion of food additives triggered hyperactivity. Basing his hypothesis on his clinical observations of hyperactive children as well as decades of experience researching and treating allergy, Feingold announced that hyperactivity could be alleviated with a diet free of these substances, a diet soon dubbed the Feingold diet. Almost immediately Feingold's hypothesis attracted attention. Spurred by media reports, Feingold's books, and word of mouth, thousands of parents tried the diet and discovered that it appeared to ease the symptoms experienced by their children. Some were so convinced of the Feingold diet's efficacy that they founded the Feingold Association of the United States (FAUS), which developed lists of "Feingold-friendly" foods and provided support to member families.

The media also picked up on Feingold's story. He and his diet were featured on popular television programs such as *Today* and the *Phil Donahue Show*, in influential newspapers such as the *New York Times* and the *Washington Post*, and in widely circulated magazines such as *Newsweek*, making the allergist a media celebrity.[4] Shortly before the publication of *Why Your Child Is Hyperactive*, Senator Glen Beall of Maryland included Feingold's findings about the perils of food additives in the U.S. Congressional Record. Due in part to this attention, *Why Your Child Is Hyperactive*, as well as Feingold's sequel, *The Feingold Cookbook for Hyperactive Children*, which was co-written by Feingold's wife, Helene Feingold, became best sellers, the latter reaching fourth place on the *New York Times* nonfiction best seller list. The proceeds from *The Feingold Cookbook* were used as an endowment for FAUS.[5]

Along with media coverage and popular interest, however, came controversy. That the Feingold diet was a matter for heated debate is not particularly surprising, given some of the implications of Feingold's theory. Feingold's hypothesis raised alarming questions about the adverse neurological effects of consuming the synthetic colors, flavors, and preservatives found in everything from sodas and candy to cheese and luncheon meat. Hyperactivity was believed to affect anywhere from 5 to 20 percent of American children, depending on how one interpreted the diagnostic criteria, and was thought to prevent children from reaching their educational and vocational potentials. Many psychiatrists also saw hyperactivity as a precursor to subsequent mental health problems and suggested that children who suffered from it were more likely to get involved in crime and drug abuse. More extreme commentators such as Camilla Anderson, who had served in California as chief psychiatrist for the world's largest women's prison, believed that the disorder was so pernicious that it warranted eugenic solutions, including the "need for selective population control," "changing age-old laws and values regarding abortion," and forced "family limitation" through "'the pill,' intrauterine devices (IUD), sterilization, or whatever techniques were reliable and nonmorbid."[6] Feingold's hypothesis, if correct, could be used to justify similarly severe measures to rid the food supply of troublesome additives.

The association of food additives and behavioral problems implied that hyperactive children were the proverbial canaries in the coal mine, presenting obvious and immediate effects of eating substances that could be harming the entire population in slower, more surreptitious ways.[7] If eating an artificially colored popsicle could render a child uncontrollable after a few minutes, some observers wondered about the long-term and less noticeable effects of consuming large amounts of additives over a period of years or decades. In many ways, such views fitted neatly into the "negative nutrition" mantra of the period, whereby specific nutrients, particularly cholesterol, saturated fat, sugar, and salt, were seen to be causative factors in chronic diseases such as heart disease, cancer, and diabetes.[8] As such, Feingold's theory threatened to have momentous and expensive ramifications for a food industry that increasingly used chemicals to add color, flavor, and shelf life to food. Not only would food and chemical manufacturers be pressured or compelled by the Food and Drug Administration (FDA) to stop selling certain additives, they, and food retailers ranging from supermarkets to restaurants, would have to find different and more natural ways of processing, flavoring, and preserving the food to which Americans had grown accustomed. Nutritionists, many of whom supported the use of chemicals in the food supply, would also have to change the way in which they assessed the safety and nutritional content of foods that had been heavily processed. As *Business Week* contributor Geraldine Pluenneke warned in a review of *Why Your Child Is Hyperactive*, Feingold's "hypothesis spells bad press for food men."[9]

The Feingold diet also destabilized recently established paradigms about how to understand and treat hyperactive children. During the 1960s, different factions within American psychiatry argued about what caused hyperactive behavior; while psychoanalysts implicated unresolved family issues, social psychiatrists blamed social problems such as poverty, crime, and overcrowding, and biological psychiatrists stated that hyperactivity was a genetic neurological disorder. By the early 1970s, however, these disagreements had largely been resolved and the biological explanation for the disorder dominated, meaning that stimulant drug therapy was the most commonly offered treatment to children diagnosed with hyperactivity.[10] Not only did Feingold undermine these neurological explanations and pharmaceutical solutions by claiming that food additives were responsible for rising rates of hyperactivity, but he suggested that chemicals in food could be a factor in other social disorders, such as juvenile delinquency and violence, and condemned the use of drugs to treat childhood behavioral problems. To the pharmaceutical companies who manufactured hyperactivity drugs and to psychiatrists who believed that the debates about hyperactivity had finally ended, Feingold's hypothesis complicated what was already a problematic and contentious, but also profitable, disorder.

Given the implications of Feingold's theory, and because physicians were often highly skeptical of "cure by diet," most of Feingold's colleagues, including psychiatrists, pediatricians, and allergists, did not echo the public's enthusiasm for his diet. Instead, they designed dozens of trials to put the Feingold diet to the test, most occurring between the publication of *Why Your Child Is Hyperactive* in 1974 and Feingold's death in 1982. The majority of physicians believed that the findings of these trials disproved Feingold's hypothesis and refused to recommend his diet to treat hyperactive children. As a result, by the mid-1980s, both Feingold's hypothesis and his diet were marginalized to the fringes of medical practice, and the media had ceased reporting on what had been one of the most discussed children's health stories of the 1970s. Although FAUS continued to promote Feingold's theory and to attract parents, the Feingold diet was perceived by most to be nothing more than another food fad. Today, most physicians concur that the Feingold diet was never proven to be effective and consider it a regrettable, yet persistent, aberration in the progression of treatment for hyperactivity.[11]

Historical analysis, however, reveals that the status of the hypothesis was not so clear-cut. Close examination of the trials intended to test Feingold's hypothesis, including the ways in which they were interpreted, demonstrates that they yielded neither uniformly positive nor negative findings. While some trials were supportive of Feingold's conclusions, others were negative and still others reported mixed results. Most researchers concluded their discussion of the results with the suggestion that more research into Feingold's claims was necessary, and the small numbers of trials conducted in the last twenty years have been more supportive of Feingold's thesis. Many of the original trials were funded and at least partially designed by the Nutrition Foundation, a lobby group for the food, chemical, and pharmaceutical industries. Feingold's hypothesis had not been scientifically proven to be correct, but it had also not been adequately tested or assessed, and many lingering questions about the effects of additives on health remained. Why then, were most physicians so quick to reject the Feingold diet? Conversely, why were thousands of families willing to discount official medical opinion regarding Feingold's hypothesis and try the diet for themselves? What explains the rise and fall of the Feingold diet?

In order to answer these questions, *An Alternative History of Hyperactivity* investigates the history of the Feingold diet, addressing why it became so popular and controversial and how the media, physicians, and parents made decisions about whether it was a valid treatment for hyperactivity. To understand the fortunes of the Feingold diet, it is essential to analyze the historical context into which his diet had to exist and, ideally, thrive. The fate of Feingold's hypothesis, in other words, was dependent upon a great deal more than the scientific trials designed to test it. Instead, an array of specific socioeconomic, cultural, and political factors, rather than the rigors of scientific testing, were paramount in determining how Feingold depicted his theory, how he presented it to his medical peers and the public, and whether or not physicians and patients would implement his diet.

Such factors touched upon every aspect of the origins, popularization, and assessment of the Feingold diet. For instance, Feingold's methods, personality, and, particularly, the manner in which he described the genesis of his theory and subsequently promoted it, had a great impact on how both his medical peers and the American public perceived his theory. Physicians may have found Feingold's positive, authoritative style grating and suspicious, but many parents were attracted by his confidence and charm. Similarly, while Feingold's careful balance of science and anecdote in *Why Your Child Is Hyperactive* made the book comprehensible and convincing for a nonscientific audience, many scientists were frustrated by its lack of evidence. Feingold's early attempts to balance the medical and the popular spheres ran the risk of alienating both audiences.

Although it might be expected or hoped that the clinical trials of the Feingold diet were free of subjectivity, detailed analysis suggests that their results were also affected considerably by external forces. With a handful of exceptions, most of which were carried out after the debate had petered out, the trials that tested the Feingold diet were riddled with problems related to design, methodology, and interpretation. While the researchers could be forgiven for certain flaws in their trials—creating a double-blind clinical trial to test the effects of diet on a complex behavioral disorder was a difficult task in itself—it is harder to overlook the manner in which they interpreted their results and the results of others. For instance, both critics and supporters of the Feingold diet either ignored or exaggerated flaws in trial design in the tests they evaluated in order to support their own positions. For some reviewers, finding that only 10 percent of children reacted to synthetic colors amounted to unconvincing evidence and a clear reason for rejecting the Feingold diet, whereas others argued that the identical results demonstrated that Feingold's idea had to be treated seriously. Such differing interpretations suggest that economic, political, and ideological factors, such as ties to pharmaceutical and chemical companies, the threat Feingold's hypothesis posed to prevailing hyperactivity theories and treatments, and prevailing beliefs about the links between nutrition, allergy, and behavior, influenced physicians more than the actual results of the trials.

Finally, the families who contemplated employing the Feingold diet were also swayed by social, domestic, and economic pressures, as well as their particular beliefs about the danger of chemicals in the environment and the wisdom of prescribing psychoactive drugs to children. These issues often outweighed the advice provided by their physicians and were much more important than the results of clinical trials, about which parents learned little. For those who attempted the diet, practical barriers, including accessing and preparing food-additive-free meals, preventing violations of the diet, and accurately recording reactions to various foods, meant that even if the Feingold diet was proven to be effective in theory, it was often onerous to implement in practice. Whether or not the Feingold diet worked for a particular family was determined in large part by how they were able to cope with its imposition upon their lives rather than its scientific validity. At all stages, therefore, the most crucial tests faced by Feingold's hypothesis were not those devised by medical researchers but rather those posed by cultural expectations, ideological trends, and political and economic interests.

These arguments are based upon evidence mined from a wide range of sources, reflecting the views of physicians, patients, and the media from the early 1970s to the present day.[12] It is apparent from the depictions of the Feingold diet made by Feingold's supporters and detractors that its history can be viewed in many different ways, leading to dissimilar judgments about Feingold's hypothesis. To some, Feingold's story has been merely the history of a food fad, albeit one that gained an enormous amount of popularity, which was shown scientifically to be nothing more than quackery. To others, it has signified a case in which powerful industrial and professional interests quashed a promising idea because it had dire financial and political implications for them. These approaches, though they are the most common popular perceptions of the Feingold diet, do not appreciate the complexity of the issues Feingold's hypothesis raised and, because of this, provide few helpful lessons as to how historical analysis may help to resolve similarly intractable medical controversies. In order to avoid such pitfalls, I have attempted to present as many sides of the debate as possible and, in so doing, hope that the history of the Feingold diet offers insights into how history has a role to play in informing medical debate and, by extension, improving health policy.[13]

The History of Hyperactivity

The story of the Feingold diet is a compelling chapter in the broader history of hyperactivity, a topic that historians are just beginning to explore. Although much work has been done on sociological aspects of hyperactivity, historical interest in the disorder is lacking, and tends to focus on the first half of the twentieth century, when hyperactivity was not commonly diagnosed or treated.[14] This means that many questions still remain about why hyperactive children became cause for such concern during the late 1950s.[15] Nevertheless, a few points can be made about why hyperactivity went from being not even mentioned medical textbooks, such as Leo Kanner's *Child Psychiatry* (1935, 1949, 1957), to becoming the most commonly diagnosed children's psychiatric disorder by the late 1960s, a topic "guaranteed to stir up vigorous discussion in medical, psychological, social work, and educational circles."[16] First, it is important to acknowledge that the first hyperactive children were of the baby boom generation, the 75 million children born between 1946 and 1964 who would make up the largest cohort in American history.[17] It is difficult to overestimate the impact of child and adolescent baby boomers on American society during the 1950s and 1960s. As historians Steven Mintz and Susan Kellogg have argued, American society during this period can be described as "filiarchal," that is, dominated by and greatly concerned with American children.[18] Mintz and Kellogg's observations echo the views of many contemporary educators and physicians, some of whom feared that American culture was becoming too "child centered."[19]

Although preoccupation with the baby boom generation fed into many aspects of American life, from what was shown on prime-time television to the founding of new medical journals such as *JAACP*, the sector most impacted was education. Pressure exerted on the education system from the millions of baby boomers, however, was not simply due to their sheer numbers. Against the background of the Cold War competition with the Soviets for ideological, intellectual, physical (the Olympics), and technological (especially military) superiority, the academic success of the baby boom generation was believed to be particularly crucial to American security and future prosperity.[20] Such concerns were made manifest in the elevated expectations of academic achievement that accompanied the baby boomers into the classroom. Not only were more students expected to complete high school and go onto postsecondary education, a trend that had started during the early part of the century, but there were demands that students should achieve higher standards in order to graduate.[21] Students who in previous decades would have left school in their early teens for unskilled labor were now expected to attain higher levels of education. These standards applied not only to middle-class students in the burgeoning suburbs but also to poorer students in the slums of the American cities.[22] The pressure to attain high levels of schooling was also due to the perception that workers would require more education to cope with technological advances in the workplace. According to research presented to the American Psychopathological Association in the late 1960s, "As a result of increasing emphasis on academic credentials as prerequisite to occupational success, years of schooling have been continuously prolonged . . . current pathways of vocational development are encumbered with hurdles that make the transition to work seem more like an obstacle course than a choice of desirable alternatives."[23]

The Soviet launch of two Sputnik satellites in 1957 made matters even more pressing. Sputnik signaled to many American politicians, educators, and scientists that they might be losing the so-called brain race with the Soviets and that, if they did not improve matters, they might lose the Cold War altogether.[24] According to physicist Asa S. Knowles (1909–1990), "This sphere [Sputnik] tells not of the desirability but of the URGENT NECESSITY of the highest quality and expanded dimensions of the educational effort . . . the future of the twentieth century lies in the hands of those who have placed education and its Siamese twin, research, in the position of first priority."[25] Admiral Hyman Rickover (1900–1986), father of the American nuclear navy, echoed these views, charging that "the schools are letting us down at a time when the nation is in great peril. To be undereducated in this trigger-happy world is to invite catastrophe."[26] The alarm of Rickover and Knowles did not go unheeded. In 1958, the National Defense Education Act (NDEA) was passed and invested $1 billion to improve the teaching of science, mathematics, English, and foreign languages at all levels of schooling, to hire guidance counselors, and to encourage student achievement. Despite or perhaps because of such investment, schools remained under great pressure. As Dorothy Barclay (1918–2009), parent and child editor for the *New York Times*, described:

> The school picture . . . in 1958, reflected almost entirely a tightening-up. But in some classrooms or communities, unfortunately, it was more like a cracking down. Concern about college admissions and general anxiety about America's technical ability, as highlighted by the space race, combined to produce demands for higher standards of achievement

in the upper elementary grades and in high schools. The switch has given new incentive to some youngsters, but, where misapplied, its sudden severity has put a strain on others who have been unable, thorough lack of adequate preparation, to meet the new demands. . . . Even more significant to the average family, however, is the amount of attention being given to smoking out and stimulating the efforts of the underachievers. These youngsters of varying abilities who are not working up to their potential.[27]

Writing two years prior to when Ritalin was first marketed to children, Barclay was not aware of the irony inherent in her phrase "smoking out and stimulating the efforts of the underachievers." Nevertheless the behaviors most often associated with underachieving youngsters during the post-Sputnik period were those connected with hyperactivity which, in turn, would increasingly be treated with stimulant drugs.

Concern about impulsivity and hyperactivity echoed a shift regarding which behavioral characteristics were deemed to be most pernicious by American educators, physicians, and politicians. Whereas shy, withdrawn, and neurotic children who tended to be inactive were of greatest concern prior to the late 1950s, the increased premium on intellectual achievement following the launch of Sputnik meant that the most acute apprehension swung to excessively active children. As child psychiatrist Gregory Rochlin commented on the previous trend to pathologize neurotic children, "motor activity in the young child, even if excessive, is more favorably regarded than its opposite. Although the child who is hyperactive may be as emotionally disturbed as the shy inhibited child, the latter is apt to receive more attention than the former."[28] Or as Katherine Reeves described in her column "The Children We Teach" series in the education periodical *Grade Teacher*, teachers shifted from concentrating on shy, withdrawn children to addressing children like "Charles" who "slips from one interest to another, intense in his preoccupation of the moment, absorbing the essence of each, but moving insatiably from one activity to the next."[29] The hyperactive child had become symbolic of American educational shortcomings and the target of both educational and medical intervention.

While understanding the social, cultural, and political context enveloping the emergence of hyperactivity is an essential part of determining why the disorder became the most commonly diagnosed childhood psychiatric condition, the very creation of the label, hyperactivity, was an equally important development. Physicians, parent groups, and even some historians have looked to the past to search for precursors to hyperactivity in medical journals, or in the behavior of historical figures ranging from Mozart and Lord Byron to Oliver Cromwell and Winston Churchill.[30] One of the many problems with retrospective diagnoses is that they assume that behavior deemed to be pathological today would be seen as problematic in the past. When the accounts of so-called hyperactive behavior found in the writings of Thomas Clouston (1840–1915), George Still (1868–1941), and Charles Bradley (1902–1979) are analyzed closely, it quickly becomes clear that their descriptions do not bear much resemblance to the children diagnosed with hyperactivity during the second half of the twentieth century. In short, the children they described tended to be severely disturbed children whose behavior was marked more by violent, criminal, and sexually inappropriate behavior than hyperactivity and inattentiveness. These children often suffered from the aftereffects of brain trauma and were typically institutionalized or bound for such a fate.[31] The number of children matching such criteria was far smaller than the enormous numbers of children diagnosed with hyperactivity during the late 1950s and onward.

In 1957, however, a pair of articles made it much easier for a large number of children to be diagnosed with hyperactivity. The authors, Maurice Laufer (1914–1978), Eric Denhoff (1913–1982), and Gerald Solomons, all of whom worked at Charles Bradley's children's psychiatric institute in Rhode Island, outlined a condition they called "hyperkinetic impulse disorder."[32] Their description has served as the blueprint for how hyperactivity has been defined ever since. The condition they described had hyperactivity at its core, as its name suggested, although "short attention span and poor powers of concentration; irritability; impulsiveness; variability [of behavior and school performance]; and poor school work" were also mentioned.[33] As pediatrician Howard Fischer noted recently in the *Journal of Pediatrics*, there are only minor differences between Laufer and his colleagues' conception, description, and understanding of hyperkinetic impulse disorder in 1957 and what is believed about hyperactivity or ADHD today.[34]

The specific, yet easily applicable, constellation of behaviors that they highlighted amount to what historian of science Ilana Löwy has called a "loose concept," one with fluid or indeterminate elements that is easily applied by members of disparate groups.[35] Described in another way by contemporary child psychiatrist Justin M. Call, the "label of hyperactivity owes its popularity to the soothing effect such simple conceptions have upon issues of great cognitive complexity."[36] Unlike the severe and correspondingly rare symptoms Still and others described, the characteristics found in hyperkinetic impulse disorder were "to some extent normally found in the course of development of children."[37] Hyperkinetic children were usually of "normal intelligence," and were to be found in mainstream classrooms; the disorder would not be restricted to children in a psychiatric hospital.[38] Along with the fact that Laufer and his colleagues left the question of what caused hyperkinetic impulse disorder open for debate, unlike previous researchers who suspected that brain trauma was usually responsible, the disorder they described had the potential to reach epidemic proportions.[39] Hyperkinetic impulse disorder could be applied not just to a small number of severely disturbed children but to a large percentage of the child population. After 1957, hundreds of researchers began studying the disorder.

In 1957, when deepening concerns about the scholastic achievement of American children were combined with a label that succinctly encapsulated and pathologized the behaviors believed to contribute to such shortcomings, the conditions were set for hyperactivity to become not only a medical but a cultural phenomenon. As interest in the disorder grew, other factors were seen to have contributed to the proliferation of hyperactivity diagnoses. These included everything from the marketing of the disorder by pharmaceutical companies intent on selling hyperactivity drugs to changes in how children spent their leisure time and, as Feingold suggested, increased consumption of food additives.[40] At the root of the story, however, remains the profound changes in what was expected scholastically of American children during the late 1950s and early 1960s, and the willingness and ability of medical professionals to respond to such concerns with labels such as hyperactivity. To a considerable degree, the history of the Feingold diet reflects what happened when the manner in which psychiatrists and pediatricians came to explain and treat hyperactivity began to be questioned and criticized.

Food Fears

As much as the history of the Feingold diet is a key aspect of the history of hyperactivity, it is also part of a story about how Americans have perceived the relationship between the food additives and health. Following World War II, farming and food production was revolutionized by the use of chemicals in the form of pesticides, fertilizers, synthetic hormones, antibiotics, emulsifiers, stabilizers, colors, flavors, preservatives, and a long list of other agents. These chemicals were intended to increase yields; protect against spoilage, pests, and disease; and make food more attractive, easier to prepare, and marketable. But alongside agriculture's "Green Revolution" came another green revolution, connected instead with the preservation of the environment and the effect of pollutants upon health. Almost as soon as the food industry began to rely on chemistry, concern arose about the effects such substances could have on health. During the 1950s, for instance, the longest ever series of Senate hearings, chaired by Congressman James Delaney (1901–1987), were held to discuss how to determine what chemicals posed a risk to human health. The Delaney Clause, which was passed in 1958, highlighted not only the concern Americans had about food chemicals but the difficulty in proving definitively whether a particular chemical was harmful. As a result, the Delaney Clause, which focused primarily on cancer, was criticized not only for being draconian by supporters of the food industry such as Frederick Stare (1910–2002) and Thomas Jukes (1906–1999), but it was also bemoaned by consumer advocates such as Ralph Nader (b. 1934) and Beatrice Trum Hunter (b. 1918) for not going far enough.

Most effectively and poignantly illustrated by Rachel Carson (1907–1964) with respect to pesticides in *Silent Spring*, by the 1960s and 1970s, the health effects of food chemicals became an important concern of political activists. As historian Warren Belasco has argued, the counterculture merged with counter-cuisine to help give rise to the organic food movement.[41] While this served to increase awareness about the possible dangers found in food additives, it also dichotomized the debates about such chemicals. Whether the issue was pesticides such as DDT, artificial sweeteners such as cyclamates, synthetic hormones such as diethylstilbestrol (DES), or the colors and flavors that concerned Feingold, those involved in the debates tended to line up on one side of the issue or another.

Despite Feingold's efforts to situate his theory outside of these debates, the assessment of his hypothesis similarly divided opinion before it had even been tested. Many of the issues raised about Feingold's hypothesis mirrored themes in the debates surrounding other food chemicals. While those in favor of the use of food additives argued that the cost of food would skyrocket if producers had to stop using colors, flavors, and preservatives, those against their use contended that the only individuals benefiting from the chemicalization of the food supply were food and chemical manufacturers. Arguments in support of scientific advancement and technological development in the food industry were levied against calls for food that was natural and organic. The Feingold diet was either a clear sign that food additives had to be removed from the food supply or another instance of food faddism getting in the way of progress. Caught between these competing ideologies were families, often with little interest in food politics or the environment, who were desperate for solutions to their child's behavioral problems.

Although the history of the Feingold diet provides insight into many aspects of how Americans experienced and understood food and health during the late twentieth century, it is also a story about the development of medical knowledge and how decisions are made about unconventional medical ideas. It demonstrates the obstacles involved in attempting to transform a novel and unorthodox medical idea into authoritative medical knowledge. For Feingold, this process proved to be frustrating; despite his efforts to associate his theory with those of other respected researchers and to submit it to scientific scrutiny, his hypothesis jarred with many established medical paradigms and vested interests, and was viewed by most physicians as being close to quackery. To a certain degree, however, physicians were not to be the final judge of Feingold's theory. While most of Feingold's medical peers rejected his theory, many thousands of parents found his argument to be convincing and attained success with his diet. This makes it difficult to determine who, in fact, were the experts judging Feingold's idea. In the case of the Feingold diet, it could be that Feingold families, some employing the diet for thirty-five years over multiple generations, have been correct and that medical researchers have been wrong.

If the medical assessment is indeed wrong, then it is possible that millions of children have been denied an effective treatment for their hyperactive behavior and have been diagnosed powerful amphetamines instead. Although this is a sobering thought in itself, there are broader implications for how medical researchers, clinicians, health policy makers, and patients and their families understand medical knowledge and judge new medical hypotheses. It is not enough to simply state, as many historians have, that medical knowledge is complicated and contingent on social factors that transcend the laboratory. It is easy to make this claim, and to provide good evidence to support it, but the critique does not provide any constructive guidance as to how those involved in determining health policy should proceed. In this book, I hope to go a step further and make two suggestions that would change the way in which medical ideas are evaluated, particularly when such ideas clash with prevailing medical ideologies or affect a wide variety of financial and political interests.

First, the history of the Feingold diet indicates that the assessment of novel medical ideas, especially those that divide opinion, should not only involve clinical trials but should include the experiences and observations of patients, parents, and the health professionals who treat them. Second, historical analysis should be regarded as a tool to help in the resolution of medical debates. In other words, there should be more proactive and constructive communication between medical historians and those who make health policy in order to improve the decisions made about difficult medical issues. Taking up these suggestions would not make difficult decisions about health policy any easier to achieve, but it would lead to more informed and honest decision making and, ultimately, better decisions. It would empower those involved in receiving medical treatment, as well as those providing it, and encourage a more nuanced understanding of health, disease, and the complexities of medical treatment and expertise.

Chapter 2

Why Your Child Is Hyperactive

How have scientists depicted the origins of their discoveries? In order to understand how new medical hypotheses are perceived by physicians and the public, it is helpful to explore how their authors present such ideas. We often learn first about medical advancements such as vaccination, pasteurization, and penicillin by way of captivating tales, often featuring heroic physicians succeeding despite difficult circumstances. Such accounts can be entertaining and even inspiring, but, as many historians have demonstrated, they do not always present an accurate picture of how medical knowledge has developed over time.[1] Reflecting on how pioneering immunologists have described their own history, historians Warwick Anderson, Miles Jackson, and Barbara Gutmann Rosenkrantz have cautioned against relying on "the memory of the discipline" and working within the historical boundaries imposed by those involved in medical discovery.[2] If such accounts are analyzed critically, however, with a view to understanding how and why they were written, historians can uncover more about not only the nuances of medical discovery but about why scientists decide to portray themselves and their findings in particular ways.

Superficially, the origins of the Feingold diet are easy to trace. In *Why Your Child Is Hyperactive*, Feingold dedicated the first three chapters and several subsequent passages to outlining the laboratory and clinical origins of his theory. According to Feingold, his hyperactivity hypothesis had its roots in research he had done into flea bite allergy during the 1950s but was also influenced by Feingold's early medical experiences as a pediatric resident in Austria and his interpretation of the studies conducted by a number of leading scientists. By depicting how he discovered the link between food additives and hyperactivity, Feingold wrote the first history of his diet. His purpose in doing so appears to have been the achievement of three goals: to depict a plausible narrative for his discovery; to show that his theory was the result of years of cumulative, yet often disparate, research; and, finally, to link his findings with those of prominent immunologists and allergists. The achievement of these objectives would presumably help convince both parents and physicians that Feingold's hypothesis was the product of legitimate scientific investigation and was in accordance with research conducted by other respected scientists. Feingold depicted his story of as one of perseverance, Sherlock Holmes–like induction, and heroism, depicting himself as a diligent, talented, and dedicated clinician and researcher, a physician that parents trusted and colleagues admired.

When viewed, however, in the light of other available evidence, including Feingold's other writings, medical literature about food allergies, and the opinions expressed by Feingold's colleagues, a different story emerges. Inconsistencies and gaps appear. These do not necessarily cast doubt on his depiction of events; rather, they reveal that the origins of his theory were not only more complicated than Feingold admitted but involved more and differ-ent actors. Specifically, Feingold took great pains to associate his work with that done by leading scientists, including many Nobel laureates, rather than his fellow allergists. Notably, he separated his work from that of food allergists who had been linking allergy and behavioral problems since the early twentieth century. Why was this the case?

The answer to this question involves exploring the turbulent history of food allergy in the United States and, in particular, engaging with how aller-gists debated the definition, prevalence, and treatment of the condition.[3] In describing the history of his hypothesis, Feingold attempted to negotiate a posi-tion between orthodox allergists, who limited the definition of food allergy to those in which an immune response, such as eczema or hives, could be demon-strated, and unorthodox food allergists, who believed that food allergy could result not only in a proven immunological response, demonstrated, for example, by skin-prick tests, but also a wide range of other reactions, including behavioral problems. Although Feingold's theory fitted those of more unorthodox food allergists, he himself had always been an orthodox allergist and resisted being perceived as an unorthodox food allergist. Feingold also recognized that the theories of food allergists were increasingly vilified by the broader medical community; if his hypothesis was to become authoritative medical knowledge, he needed to associate himself with respectable allergists and immunologists and distance himself from those whose theories were controversial. The potential benefits but also inherent difficulties involved in striking such a balance help to explain why the Feingold diet became, and has remained, such a divisive issue. Feingold's version of the origins of his diet provides an example of a manicured history, a story tweaked and teased to emphasize some aspects and to downplay others. There is nothing inherently incorrect about the story Feingold describes, but it is an incomplete story, one that fails to describe fully a long history of associating food allergies and intolerances with behavioral problems. When the absent aspects are reintroduced, the reasons for Feingold's omissions become clear, as do the dilemmas he faced in deciding how to present his theory to the medical community and the public.

From Fleas to Food Additives

In writing *Why Your Child Is Hyperactive*, one of Feingold's chief objectives appears to have been the creation of an account of the origins of his hypothesis in a compelling yet plausible manner that would appeal not only to parents, to whom the book was primarily directed, but also to physicians, whose support would be needed if the diet was to become accepted medical practice. As such, Feingold narrated the story in a friendly, familiar style that would engage parents but also included technical details and citations that were intended to impress a medical audience. The book began with the unusual account of an Oakland woman who in the summer of 1965 entered the Kaiser Permanente Medical Center where Feingold was chief of allergy, seeking treatment for a serious case of hives. Feingold overviewed the patient's medical history, examined her, and conducted allergy tests that yielded negative results or, in other words, no obvious allergies. Stating that "food additives had been a causative factor in previous cases of hives that I had seen," he placed the woman on a diet eliminating these substances and, within seventy-two hours, her skin had improved.[4] Ten days later, Feingold received a surprising call from the center's chief of psychiatry who stated that not only had the woman's hives vanished, but her aggressive and hostile behavior, for which she had undergone two years of psychotherapy, had also disappeared. After confirming these changes with the patient, Feingold alerted his staff to make note of similar cases but cautioned that what he had witnessed might have been a coincidence.

Having captured the attention of his readers with this perplexing case, Feingold took them in a completely different direction by describing his considerable experience researching allergies to flea bites. As Feingold would relate, the woman with hives represented the decisive link between his theory linking food additives and hyperactivity and his nearly fifteen years of studying flea bite allergies in the San Francisco Bay area. In connecting these seemingly disparate investigations, Feingold sought to establish at the outset that his theory was not only the culmination of years of serious scientific investigation but was akin to piecing together a complex jigsaw puzzle, in which the picture emerged gradually as each dissimilar piece was set into place. Or, in his words, "not only in medicine, but in many fields of science, one important observation can lead to another, although they do not, on the surface, appear to be related."[5]

Feingold proceeded to describe his flea bite allergy research in detail. In 1951, he left his private allergy practice in Los Angeles to join the Kaiser Permanente Medical Care Program in northern California as chief of its department of allergy, believing that Kaiser Permanente's system of private medical insurance was "a new trend in medicine," and hoping to engage in research, "a lifelong personal ambition."[6] As Feingold set up allergy clinics at several area hospitals and established a laboratory for the preparation of allergens, he noticed that allergies to flea bites were a common complaint in the local area. As flea allergen, the protein found in the flea's saliva that induced the allergic reaction, was difficult to acquire, Feingold applied to the National Institutes of Health (NIH) for a grant to procure "a million of the pests," in the hopes that he could manufacture a solution that could desensitize patients against their allergy. He received the grant, and soon the newly founded Laboratory of Medical Entomology, directed by Feingold and mandated to investigate how certain insects cause disease, was "the proud father of a million fleas per week."[7]

The key finding from Feingold's flea bite allergy research relative to hyperactivity was that "the reaction to the flea bite was induced by a low (molecular weight) chemical present in the saliva of the insect," otherwise known as a hapten, which combined with proteins of larger molecular weight in order to induce an allergic response. This phenomenon, Feingold added, had been recently demonstrated by two prominent American immunologists, Nobel laureate Karl Landsteiner (1868–1943) and Merrill Chase (1905–2004) of the Rockefeller Institute.[8] What struck Feingold about the haptenic mechanism in immune responses was the fact that *the chemicals man uses as drugs and chemicals used as food additives are both low-molecular compounds subject to the same behavior as the hapten demonstrated in flea saliva.*[9] In other words, there was a relationship between how the immune system responded to flea saliva and the way in which it responded to ingested chemicals.

At this point in *Why Your Child Is Hyperactive*, Feingold reported shifting from researching flea bite allergies to studying the impact of other low-molecular-weight chemicals, particularly those found in drugs and food additives. Although it is likely that this abrupt transition was precipitated by Feingold's failure to manufacture an effective allergen to desensitize patients to flea bites, he did not mention this in his book, and instead proceeded to discussing the research of leading scientists into the immunologic effects of dyes such as Yellow Number 5 (tartrazine) and drugs such as aspirin (acetylsalicylic acid).[10] After reading a report by leading American dermatologist W. B. Shelley in the *Journal of the American Medical Association (JAMA)* that emphasized how many foods contained a chemical, called a salicylate, that had a structure similar to aspirin, Feingold realized that his aspirin-sensitive patients could also react to these foods. In response, he designed a diet that placed such foods, including grapes, oranges, and tomatoes as well as additives that contained the salicylate radical, in "dietary prison."[11] Feingold described being influenced by the research conducted by a number of important allergists, including Max Samter (1908–1999), a former president of the American Academy of Allergy (AAA), Frederic Speer, who in 1958 coined the term "allergic tension-fatigue syndrome," and prolific allergy researcher Guy Settipane (1930–2004), as well as London pharmacologist and future Nobel laureate in physiology and medicine, Sir John Vane (1927–2004) and his associate Sergio Ferreira (b. 1934), which all suggested that other artificial dyes and additives could also induce reactions. Feingold "redesigned the diet once again to include *all foods* and *all drugs* that were artificially dyed; *all foods* and *all drugs* that were artificially flavored, as well as those containing nature's salicylates."[12] Feingold called this revised diet the Kaiser Permanente (K-P) diet, a name he preferred to "Feingold diet." Although Feingold's use of "K-P diet" was in part an homage to Kaiser Permanente, who remained broadly supportive of his research, despite its controversial nature, he also joked that K-P also stood for "kitchen police, of which a certain amount is required."[13] The K-P diet was the one Feingold prescribed to the Oakland woman with hives and many other patients suffering from itching, skin rashes, and asthma. Although Feingold stated that he had heard reports about improvements in the behavior of children on the diet, he stressed that he was "an allergist, not a behaviorist" and had not focused on these aspects, adding that he was "unaware of the critical situation in hyperkinesis [hyperactivity] and learning disability that was developing throughout the country."[14]

As an allergist, however, Feingold was concerned with the nature of the reactions he observed. Initially he believed he was witnessing an allergic response, an example of "the defense processes of the body" and not just "any form of intolerance or even dislike." Soon, however, Feingold "became a convert to the non-allergenic concept" after reading about how allergists Max Samter and Richard Farr (1922–1997) had "convincingly demonstrated that the adverse reactions to aspirin were nonallergic."[15] In his book, Feingold elaborated about the differences between allergic and nonallergic reactions. In a telling passage, Feingold stated,

> Allergy is concerned with the defense processes of the body, but the term has wandered far astray from its scientific interpretation. In common speech, allergy has now become synonymous with any form of intolerance or dislike. "Allergic" is frequently used when an individual doesn't care for a food, though he may tolerate it easily. "I'm allergic to onions, plastic pillows and Sam" usually means that the person simply detests onions, plastic pillows and poor Sam. Even in medicine, the general practitioner or the specialist outside the allergy field sometimes forgets that everything that looks or acts like allergy may not be allergy.[16]

Elsewhere, in his 1973 textbook, *Introduction to Clinical Allergy*, Feingold criticized the failure of food allergists "to appreciate that nonimmunologic as well as immunologic mechanisms operate to produce unfavorable food responses," and that this shortcoming helped to explain "the great variety of symptoms and diseases which are arbitrarily attributed to allergic mechanisms, often without supporting evidence."[17] Feingold's words indicate his belief that the true meaning of the term *allergy* had been obscured and, more specifically, that many supposed instances of food allergy were merely food intolerance. Feingold argued that enzymatic deficiencies, chemical irritation, toxic reactions to tainted foods, bacterial contamination, and food additives were all examples of nonimmunologic adverse food reactions.[18]

That Feingold stressed the "nonallergic theory" in his conception of the adverse reaction to food additives and salicylate-laden foods suggests that he condoned a considerably more limited and conservative definition of allergy than that employed by many of his contemporaries, particularly food allergists such as the controversial Chicago clinician Theron Randolph (1906–1995). By doing so, Feingold demarcated himself as a conservative allergist whose views were distinct from those of food allergists. While most parents reading *Why Your Child Is Hyperactive* might not have recognized the importance of this distinction, allergists would have interpreted Feingold's discussion of allergic versus nonallergic reactions to food as a clear message that Feingold viewed his theory as fitting in with those of conservative allergists. In other words, the history of the Feingold diet according to Feingold was not connected to the broader history of food allergy.

Defining allergy had been problematic and controversial ever since Clemens von Pirquet (1874–1929) coined allergy as "any form of altered biological reactivity."[19] As historian Mark Jackson has observed, such debates about the definition of allergy reflected deeper "disputes about the meaning or evolutionary purpose of allergic reactions."[20] Similarly, science writer and alternative medicine advocate Ralph W. Moss, who coauthored *An Alternative Approach to Allergies* (1980) with Theron Randolph, observed that during the 1920s, "allergists ruled out many bizarre and puzzling reactions which formerly had been a valid subject for inquiry. From this point forward, allergists were divided into two camps, the 'orthodox,' who accepted the antigen-antibody definition and worked within its boundaries, and the 'unorthodox,' who continued to investigate reactions in which such immunological reactions could not necessarily be demonstrated."[21] Randolph also added an ecological dimension to the debates about how to define the condition, arguing, according to Jackson, that "allergy constituted an entirely appropriate protective response to dangers posed by widespread environmental and ecological damage."[22]

From the 1920s onwards, food allergists almost always fitted into the unorthodox camp. This was partly because they tended to define allergy broadly, but also because of the inherent difficulties in identifying, diagnosing, and treating food allergy. Food allergists had to treat patients differently than other allergists. As New York City allergist and 1947 AAA president Will C. Spain explained:

> Of all the problems in clinical sensitization which face the investigator, that of food allergy is the most difficult to resolve. There are three potent reasons for this: first, the patient lacks objectivity in presenting his problem because of his whims, fancies, and aversions relating to various viands, ideas which are often construed by him as proofs of specific food allergy; second, the physician, shorn in at least half of his cases of the benefit of positive food reactions by skin test, tends to be influenced unduly by the description made by the patient of his untoward behavior with certain comestibles; and third, thanks to the ability of food allergy to mimic many other nonallergic complaints, the actual allergic nature of the particular problem remains debatable and unsettled.[23]

Despite the difficulties in determining whether a reaction was caused by a food or not, many prominent food allergists believed that food allergy was a widespread condition, and they diagnosed it frequently. Employing an expansive definition of allergy, food allergists were quick to blame a wide range of disparate, yet unexplained, symptoms to reactions to food. Such practices raised the ire of orthodox allergists, some of whom went as far as describing food allergy as a form of "quackery."[24] Given these tensions, this assessment in

1954 by Boston allergists Irving W. Schiller and Francis C. Lowell is not surprising: "controversy rages around the clinical importance and frequency of food allergy in a more lively manner than around any other subject in the field of allergy."[25] Such controversy also helps to explain why Feingold was so careful to delineate his definition of allergy and why he resisted associating himself with food allergists.

Debates about the definition of allergy, food allergy, and environmental risks to the immune system became even more schismatic during the 1960s, partly because of increasing concern about the environment following the publication of *Silent Spring* but also because of important developments in the field of immunology. Feingold's hyperactivity theory emerged soon after Kimishege Ishizaka (b. 1925) and Teruko Ishizaka (b. 1926) discovered the antibody IgE (immunoglobulin E) in 1967. The Ishizakas determined that IgE played a central role in immediate allergic reactions, and allergists believed that the antibody might provide a novel way to test for the presence of "true allergy."[26] IgE provided evidence for orthodox allergists that there were key immunological differences between what they described as true allergy, which could be proven by the presence of the antibody, and mere intolerance, in which IgE would be absent. In contrast, Randolph and other food allergists, such as William G. Crook (1917–2002), downplayed the importance of the antibody.[27]

It is important to note that such disagreements were not merely academic. Debates about the definition of allergy struck at the heart of what it meant to be an allergist, in terms of theoretical grounding, professional standing, and clinical practice, and the debates about how to define allergy could become heated. In discussing the relevance of IgE, for example, Randolph argued, "The allergists are stuck in a trap of their own making. There are numerous mechanisms in allergy. It's ridiculous to limit the concept of hypersensitivity to the one mechanism of IgE. They're trying to make it an exclusive practice. They won't give up. Why? Because they are blockheads."[28]

Although Feingold didn't mention IgE in *Why Your Child Is Hyperactive*, his careful differentiation between allergic and nonallergic reactions suggested that he wanted to be perceived as an orthodox allergist and distinguish himself from those who employed a wide definition of allergy. It also implies that the audience Feingold envisioned when describing his hypothesis was represented by orthodox allergists, rather than food allergists such as Crook and Randolph, who might have been more inclined to support his views. Feingold's conservative stance on the definition of allergy was also evident in a 1962 article about psychological factors and allergy in which his team of researchers assessed whether there was a relationship between skin reactivity and personality in patients being treated for allergy. In this study, Feingold emphasized the distinction between allergy patients with "true allergic disease," those who had pronounced skin test reactions to allergens, and "nonreactive allergic" patients, those whose skin test reactions were weak or nonexistent.[29] He argued that patients who did not have "true allergic disease" were more likely to have psychological problems, suggesting that their symptoms might have been psychosomatic.

Two relevant implications arose out of this study. First, Feingold based his investigation into psychosomatic factors in allergy on his contention that allergy sufferers consisted of two distinct groups: the "nonreactive allergic" and those with "true allergic disease." This distinction foreshadowed how he would distinguish between allergic and nonallergic symptoms in *Why Your Child Is Hyperactive*, in which he claimed that hyperactivity triggered by food additives was a nonallergic phenomenon. Second, by implying that the symptoms of the nonreactive patients might be psychosomatic and, more specifically, hypochondriacal, Feingold underscored his belief, shared by other orthodox allergists, that for symptoms to be truly allergic, they had to be rooted in an immunologic response. Although Feingold might have reconsidered this opinion following his food additive research—perhaps some of these patients were sensitive to food additives—this article reinforced Feingold's position as an orthodox allergist who employed a conservative, restricted notion of allergy.

The restricted definition of allergy that Feingold employed, which led him to emphasize the nonallergic nature of salicylate reactions, had an additional, paradoxical effect of expanding the potential scope of the threat posed by food additives. By stressing that the reactions were nonallergic, Feingold implied that individuals who reacted to food additives were not idiosyncratic or immunologically abnormal but simply more sensitive to substances that were harmful to all people. In his words, "whether the patient is an adult or a hyperkinetic child, there is no natural body defense against the synthetic additives."[30] In contemplating the potential threat to the unprotected human body from ingesting food additives over time, Feingold expanded on the ideas of Nobel laureate and founder of ethology (animal behavior studies) Konrad Lorenz (1903–1989) with respect to aggressive behavior. According to Feingold, "Lorenz's concept of 'overrapid change' applies to the intentional introduction of synthetics into what man eats and drinks; the chemical by-products in the air he breathes; the synthetic pollution of the soil in which his food is grown; the chemical wastes in his lakes, rivers and oceans." Such "overrapid change" was also responsible for "*man's steadily growing tendencies toward unprovoked aggression and violence.*"[31] Feingold contended that the "time is now long overdue to look at these chemicals, not only in regard to the H-LDs [children with hyperactivity and learning disability] but in regard to the human species as a whole. It is time to coldly question whether or not some of them have the possibility of disrupting the normal neurological pathways."[32]

Feingold's description of food additives as a potentially universal problem echoed views of allergists whose expansive definitions of allergy Feingold rejected. In particular, Feingold's portent about food additives and other types of chemical exposure was reminiscent of allergist Warren T. Vaughan's (1893–1944) alarming portrayal of the scope of allergic disease. Vaughan estimated in the 1930s that up to 60 percent of the American population suffered from some form of allergic disease, leading him to contend that "allergy 'is no longer the exception; it is the rule.'"[33] Vaughan's views were supported by allergists such as Arthur Coca (1875–1959), the founder of the *Journal of Immunology* and past president of Society for the Study of Asthma and Allied Conditions (SSAAC), who in 1943 considered "Vaughan's figure as essentially correct if it is not possibly somewhat conservative."[34] Feingold's belief that chemical exposure was the root of so many societal problems linked his thinking to that of Theron Randolph, who also emphasized the role of environmental pollutants in causing many chronic physical and mental illnesses.[35]

A key difference remained, however; while Vaughan, Coca, and Randolph believed that the reactions they witnessed were allergic, Feingold argued that they were not. From a patient's perspective, such a difference might have been moot, since the root cause of the reaction was the same, as was the solution of avoiding exposure to such noxious agents. That Feingold repeatedly emphasized the distinction highlights how questions about the nature, definition, and extent of allergy persisted into the 1970s, despite the discovery of IgE, and that these questions divided practitioners. It also underlines Feingold's desire to be perceived as a traditional allergist who was not only clinically astute but current with developments in immunological research. The mechanism behind the reaction to food additives might not have mattered to patients, but it certainly had political implications within the allergy community.

In the midst of his realization of the potential problems associated with food additives, Feingold's own health deteriorated. He described being "struck down" by serious illness in the late 1960s and having to cede his duties as chief of allergy and take up the title of chief emeritus of the department. But while Feingold was recuperating and contemplating retiring to a life of orchids and travel, something unexpected happened: he discovered the hyperactivity epidemic.[36] The next few pages of his book were used to provide an overview of the epidemic, stating that "from the serenity and safety of my apartment study high over the Golden Gate, I was alarmed, if not shocked, by the depth of the problem, the soaring incidence, the frightening but often necessary drug management, the despair noted by both parent and teacher." Retirement no longer an option, Feingold "launched into educating my self on the problems surrounding the hyperkinetic child."[37]

As he studied the disorder, Feingold described being bemused about why he never came across such high frequencies of hyperactivity while working as a pediatrician during the first half of his career (1924–1945). Trying to make sense of the controversy surrounding the disorder, Feingold thought of the curious case of the Oakland woman, but also recalled an experience in 1928, when he was a pediatric resident in Vienna at the Pirquet Clinic.[38] One of his colleagues, psychiatrist and neurologist Bernard Dattner, ran a seizure clinic and required that his patients maintain a strict food diary, believing that there was a correlation between foods ingested and the frequency and severity of seizures. Dattner's use of diet diaries spurred Feingold to consider if something hyperactive children were eating was causing the epidemic. His ideas about haptens, food additives, elimination diets, and unexplained behavior changes coalesced into a theory about hyperactivity when he recognized that the use of food additives and the meteoric rise in hyperactivity were postwar phenomena. In his words, "a Standard & Poor's graph projecting the dollar-value increase in artificial flavors looked much like a graph indicating the rising trend of H-LD for the same period."[39] Believing that the elimination diet he used for his other patients might help hyperactive children and at least do no harm, Feingold began prescribing it in late 1972 and was soon confident that his theory was correct.[40]

Feingold described how he developed his hyperactivity hypothesis and elimination diet as a story of routine and even tedious medical research, notably fifteen years of flea experiments, punctuated by serendipitous events such as the case of the Oakland hives patient and his recollection of Dattner's seizure clinic. The account is reminiscent of many stories of medical discovery, but as with many such accounts, a number of factors, individuals, and circumstances are also omitted.[41] Feingold's selectivity is particularly similar to how Hungarian-Canadian immunologist Hans Selye (1907–1982) depicted the origin of his theories on the physiological impact of social stressors in *Stress without Distress* (1974).[42] As Mark Jackson has argued, Selye failed to cite the influence of E. O. Wilson (b. 1929) and Robert Trivers (b. 1943) despite the fact that they were researching similar questions.[43] While some of the aspects left out of *Why Your Child Is Hyperactive* were fairly trivial, many relevant details were also excluded from the book. These unmentioned details demonstrate how Feingold's theory fitted neatly into over a half century of research by food allergists dealing with the link between food allergy and behavioral problems. Analysis of this history not only discloses that the context in which the Feingold diet emerged was more complex than Feingold allowed but also suggests that Feingold endeavored to assert the originality of his idea while at the same time distancing himself from controversial food allergists.

Food Allergy and Behavior

Although Feingold was careful to mention the influence of certain leading immunology and allergy researchers, the impression given to the reader was that Feingold's theory linking food and behavior was a groundbreaking, novel, and isolated epiphany. This impression was created by Feingold's bafflement, in the first pages of his book, over the improvement in his Oakland hives patient's behavior and reinforced when he had to refer to a forty-year-old memory of Bernard Dattner's Vienna seizure clinic in order to convince himself that there could be a link between nutrition and behavior.[44] A close look at the history of food allergy research in the United States, however, makes it difficult to trust Feingold's apparent surprise at this link. In contrast to Feingold's depiction of events, allergists had been observing behavioral reactions to foods for decades.

Indeed, ever since food allergy research began in earnest during the late 1910s, physicians such as Detroit pediatrician B. Raymond Hoobler (d. 1943) had linked food allergy and nervous system disturbances including irritability, fretfulness, restlessness, and sleeplessness.[45] In a frequently cited article, Minnesota pediatrician W. Ray Shannon claimed in 1922 that "food proteins to which the patient has become sensitized" could cause "extremely restless," "introspective," "nervous," "high-strung," "cruel," and "out-of-sorts" behavior, as well as poor school performance.[46] Children were often the subject of researchers studying the link between allergy and behavior; children, who in Shannon's case study, "could not sit still" and were "very hard to manage."[47] Both Shannon and other 1920s researchers, including George Piness (1891– 1970) and Hyman Miller, advised that "exclusion of foods has been found far more advisable than attempted immunization" and, therefore, advised individualized elimination diets that foreshadowed the Feingold diet.[48]

Allergists often described the effect of allergens on behavior as cerebral allergy. It was generally believed that allergic reactions to foods and other substances could trigger cerebral edema (swelling) or impaired vascular function in the brain, which could cause migraine headaches, epilepsy, and abnormal behavior.[49] Support for the theory that allergy could cause psychological problems, though controversial, was quite common among mainstream allergists.[50] For example, in T. Wood Clarke's (1878–1959) 1950 survey of 171 North American allergists, 95 "assured me that they had noticed personality changes due to allergy which corrected themselves when the allergic element was eliminated."[51] Clarke, a consulting allergist at the Marcy State Hospital in Utica, New York, had been introduced to the idea in 1945 when Richard H. Hutchings (1869–1947), past president of the American Psychiatric Society and editor of *Psychiatric Quarterly*, referred to him a fifteen-year-old boy whose "attacks of acute excitement in which he would rage around the house smashing china and furniture" had him bound for institutionalization.[52] Hutchings knew Clarke from Marcy State Hospital, had read some of his work, and referred the boy to him in a final attempt to prevent him from being placed in a state hospital for mental disorders. Clarke administered a full range of skin tests for various allergens and found that the boy reacted strongly to oat and wheat, as well as certain animals, pollens, and dusts. He eliminated oat and wheat from his diet and provided desensitizing inoculations for the inhalant allergens. According to Clarke, "the results of removing the oat and wheat from his diet were dramatic in the extreme. Almost overnight the boy's entire character changed. From being unhappy and apprehensive he became, in a very few days, happy and co-operative. He has had no outbreaks of temper for five years. He is friendly and full of fun. He is now doing well in college."[53] Curious as to whether other allergists had experienced similar cases, Clarke discussed the matter at the 1949 meeting of the American College of Allergists (ACA) where the officers of the college "were unanimously of the opinion that it was a subject worthy of systematic study" and encouraged him to investigate it and report back the following year.[54]

Clarke's survey included quotations and case studies from a number of leading American allergists, including Arthur Coca, Louis Tuft (1898–1989), who like Coca was a past president of the SSAAC, and Philip M. Gottlieb (d. 2002), a past president of the ACA.[55] The case study presented by Coca is particularly interesting in that it described a child who had many symptoms that would later be associated with hyperactive children, including an above average IQ, poor attention to detail, and trouble making friends: "Despite an I.Q. of 140, her schoolwork was not entirely satisfactory. She made frequent mistakes in copying. She was 'difficult' for her teachers, had a chip-on-shoulder attitude and imagined her classmates did not like her." After "tomato, cheese, pork, banana, mint and licorice" were removed from her diet, "her schoolwork improved and her attitude toward teachers and classmates ... [became] normal."[56] The reviewer chosen by the *Annals of Allergy* to review Clarke's article was Hal M. Davison, an allergist who had also written articles about cerebral allergy. Davison enthused that "Dr. Clarke's paper removes any possible doubt that these symptoms must be considered the direct result of allergic reactions in the central nervous system" and that "children, without the foods in their diet and with the foods in their diet, are literally Dr. Jekyll and Mr. Hyde."[57]

It is unknown whether Feingold had read or responded to Clarke's survey. It is probable that he had a subscription to *Annals of Allergy* in 1950, since he published an article in the journal that year and published there on three subsequent occasions.[58] Strong evidence exists nonetheless that suggests that Feingold was well aware that the link between food allergy and behavior had already been established by many allergists. A likely source of information was Albert H. Rowe (1889–1970), one of the leading food allergists in the United States. Rowe operated a "huge food allergy clinic in Oakland," just across the Bay Bridge from Feingold, which reportedly earned him $193,000 after taxes in 1963.[59] According to Richard Mackarness (1916–1996), British psychiatrist and ardent supporter of the link between food allergy and mental health, Rowe "pioneered the elimination diet in the treatment of food allergy symptoms, and did more than anyone else to bring to world medical attention the wide scope of this dietary treatment, and the variety of chronic symptoms – including mental ones - it could alleviate."[60]

Rowe, whose career spanned the late 1910s to the early 1960s and who was president of the American Association for the Study of Allergy (AASA) in 1929, began prescribing elimination diets for food allergies in the late 1920s and wrote dozens of articles and three textbooks on allergy, usually emphasizing the role of food allergy.[61] He believed that "psychological and emotional deviations from normal frequently arise from cerebral allergy to foods," causing symptoms such as "drowsiness, impaired ability to concentrate, confusion, depression, tenseness, and emotional instability."[62] Rowe was convinced that elimination diets could help "irritable, fussy, restless, unhappy, stubborn, unfriendly, uncooperative, antagonistic, at times angry, inattentive, tense, crying, recessive, somnolent, disliked, and at times enuretic [bed-wetting] children." Rowe described a child whose "teachers reported that the children were afraid of him, as he had such a desire to fight. He would injure his classmates. He was a spoil-sport and took joy in ruining one game after another. His excuse for fighting was that they were trying to push him around." After a few months on the elimination diet, the boy "adjusted so well his teacher has nothing but praise, and his cry has changed from: 'I hate them, they are always pushing me around,' to a happy shout of: 'They like me, Ma, I'm the leader.'"[63]

Feingold was well aware of Rowe. Feingold's resident Alice Friedman noted in a 1986 interview that Feingold's allergy clinics in the mid-1960s used Rowe's "extremely restrictive" elimination diets to treat "all sorts of allergies."[64] In a chapter she contributed to Feingold's 1973 textbook *Introduction to Clinical Allergy*, titled "Management with the Elimination Diet," Friedman mentioned Rowe's diets, albeit suggesting that they should only be used as a last resort.[65] The fact that Feingold and Rowe had met each other is substantiated in a 1951 edition of *JAMA*, which included a paper Feingold presented in San Francisco to the AMA's Joint Meeting on General Practice and Pediatrics. One of the speakers who commented on Feingold's paper, "Treatment of Allergic Disease of the Bronchi," was none other than Rowe. While Feingold downplayed the role of food allergies in causing "bronchial allergy disease," Rowe emphasized that the role of food allergies in such conditions was paramount and that elimination diets were the best treatment.[66] Others who worked for Feingold during the 1960s have stated that Feingold did know Rowe, but that the two did not get along.[67]

The exchange between the two Bay Area allergists at the AMA meeting also reveals Feingold's awareness that there were connections between allergy and behavior, although not of the type Rowe emphasized. Feingold described how "one so frequently observes children with a history of recurrent attacks of asthma or recurring attacks of bronchial allergy who will show complete adjustment in their behavior problems when their allergy is under control."[68] This interest in the psychological aspects of allergy would later lead Feingold to participate in writing a series of articles about psychosomatic allergy, the theory that symptoms of allergy were often psychogenic, or had their origin in emotional disturbance rather than immunological malfunction.[69] The research, which was funded by Kaiser Permanente during the 1960s, critiqued the methodologies employed in investigating psychosomatic allergy, describing how "few substantive statements can be made in the field because of the many critical weaknesses in the vast bulk of research performed."[70] Feingold and his colleagues concluded that "the allergy population is far from homogeneous either physiologically or psychologically."[71] He similarly downplayed the role of psychogenic factors as a primary factor in allergic disease in his textbook *Introduction to Clinical Allergy.*[72]

Feingold's investigation into the psychosomatic aspects of allergy is relevant not only because it indicates his interest in the relationship between allergy and mental health, but also because clinicians who believed that allergies could cause mental illness were, understandably, some of the most vocal opponents of psychogenic allergy, believing that psychosomatic theories replaced cause with effect. Although psychosomatic theories of allergy were popular following World War II, allergists who were keen to pinpoint certain substances as being particularly allergenic, such as Rowe's identification of food or Randolph's concentration on chemicals, were highly critical of such theories.[73] W. Ray Shannon, for instance, stressed in the 1920s that the behavioral symptoms he witnessed were neither psychosomatic nor an emotional response to the distress of experiencing allergic symptoms such as asthma or eczema, but instead "the result of irritation of the nervous system resulting from anaphylactic reactions to food proteins to which the patient has become sensitized."[74] Rowe complained that psychogenic factors were mistakenly attributed in many cases of diarrhea and that "in one case entirely controlled by the elimination of allergenic foods, hostility to the patient's husband had been blamed!"[75] Not only did the title of Richard Mackarness's *Not All in the Mind* reflect his contention that allergies could cause mental health problems, but he questioned "emotionally determined" or psychosomatic theories of allergy.[76] Feingold's suspicion of psychosomatic allergy did not mean that he agreed with the theories of Shannon, Rowe, and Mackarness, but it does suggest that he was well aware of the debates raging about what caused allergic reactions and the relationship between the immune system and mental health.

Other allergists who were resistant to the notion that allergy could be psychosomatic looked towards other factors to explain the perceived rise in allergy. Frustrated by the popularity of psychogenic allergy theories, Ethan Allan Brown (1906–1979), president of the AAA in 1957, decried that "in present-day journals (the editors of which should know better) there are papers (by physicians who should also know better) stating that not only asthma, but all allergy as such is 'psychosomatic.'" Brown continued, "The less one knows of any aspect of medicine, the more likely one is to believe that it is all psychosomatic"; "much of this literature is excellent fiction."[77] What is especially interesting about Brown's criticism is his contention that food additives, not neuroses, were causing the rise in allergy. Specifically, Brown stated that "in this age of chemicals and synthetics there is truly no limit as to what substances may be discovered as causes of allergy . . . it is not too much to expect that one or several new ubiquitous allergens may be discovered at any time. This would, of course, change overnight the present practice of allergy. Among these might be the more than 1,000 'additives' now ingested with foods and now certified for safety but not to allergenicity."[78]

Although Feingold would eventually echo Brown's concerns about "the pollutants we ingest," he never mentioned Brown and was reluctant to associate his theory about hyperactivity with those of other clinicians who were concerned about chemical exposure.[79] The best example of this was Feingold's relationship, or lack thereof, with Theron Randolph, who was a food allergist, a friend of Rachel Carson, and the founder of the clinical ecology movement in the United States. Although some of the previously mentioned allergists had retired or died by the time Feingold became interested in hyperactivity, Randolph was active and well-known during this period for his work on multiple chemical sensitivity and food allergies, including how allergies could adversely affect the behavior of children.[80] The fact that Feingold never discussed Randolph in any of his publications despite the fact that both of them believed that food additives could cause behavioral problems vividly highlights Feingold's unwillingness to associate himself with unconventional allergists.

In some ways, the two physicians lived parallel lives; they were born within six years of one another, spent time teaching medicine at Northwestern University in Chicago early in their careers (though at different times), underwent significant midcareer changes and midlife divorces, courted controversy with their theories, and inspired their adherents to carry on with their work after they died. Aspects of both allergists' theories were influenced by the notion that industrial progress, and specifically the increased use of synthetic chemicals, was hazardous to human health in a variety of ways. As early as the 1940s, Randolph had begun to link chronic illness, including mental health problems, to various pollutants in the air, water, and food supply and to prescribe elimination diets to his clients.[81] Although his 1951 book *Food Allergy*, cowritten with Herbert Rinkel (1896–1963) and Michael Zeller, focused on allergic reactions to common, natural foods such as corn, wheat, milk, and eggs, by 1961 he had written a series of four articles for the *Annals of Allergy*'s "Progress in Allergy" feature on the topic of "Human Ecology and Susceptibility to the Chemical Environment."[82] It is likely that Feingold knew about Randolph's series of articles, since he published a paper on his flea bite allergy research in the same volume.[83]

The question Randolph addressed in these articles was "how much do we know about the long-term effects of such by-products of 'progress' as the chemical pollutants in the air of our homes and cities; chemical additives and contaminants in our foods, water and biological drugs, as well as our synthetic drugs, cosmetics, and many other personal exposures to and occupational contacts with man-made chemicals?"[84] Feingold was concerned with similar questions, arguing that "in the evolution of man, a hundred-plus years of technology torrent are as insignificant as a polyp on a coral reef. But applied to living in the last half of the twentieth century, they are cataclysmic to behavior. Man has not had adequate time to adapt to the changes and new environment, physically or mentally. All of the changes, mechanical and chemical, have twisted the physical environment as well as the social environment out of all recognition."[85] Feingold's interest in the ecological aspects of his theory increased during the 1970s, as is evident by his final publication in the inaugural volume of *Ecology of Disease* in which he warned that "in recent years the alterations in the biological profile have been accelerated by thousands of mutagenic agents provided by the increased concentration of pollutants in the atmosphere, water, soil and food."[86]

Despite their shared interests in food allergy, children's behavior problems, and exposure to environmental pollutants, Feingold never listed Randolph as an influence or even mentioned his work in passing.[87] Feingold never cited the work of allergists such as Rowe, Clarke, or Brown, despite his interest in the psychological aspects of allergy, his proximity to Rowe and use of his elimination diets, and the fact that his observations of hyperactive children bore a resemblance to those made by other allergists. Not only did Feingold fail to mention whether earlier allergists such as Shannon, Piness, Coca, or Vaughan had influenced his work, but he omitted research that linked food allergy and hyperactivity even more directly. These included a 1945 article by Wilmot Schneider, which contended that elimination diets could improve the behavior of hyperactive children, and Fred Kittler and Deane Baldwin's highly relevant 1970 paper on the role of allergic factors in hyperactivity.[88] It is particularly striking that Feingold did not mention Kittler and Baldwin's paper in any of his publications, since he would have been formulating his hyperactivity thesis contemporaneously with their paper's publication in *Annals of Allergy*. Instead, Feingold presented the history of his diet as a development distinct from the larger history of food allergy and the long association of food allergy and mental illness.

Conclusion

Why was this the case? What explains Feingold's decision to ignore food allergists and their theories in his description of the origins of his diet? Why did he stress the influence of some immunologists and allergists and not others? The answers to these questions clarify why Feingold's diet was not overly popular or groundbreaking for food allergists and clinical ecologists, but they also reveal insights into the controversial world of food allergy research and clinical practice before and after World War II. Specifically, Feingold's careful omission of the larger history of food allergy in the construction of his diet disassociated his theory from those of food allergists and clinical ecologists whose ideas, though popular, were also highly divisive. By ignoring the history of food allergy and focusing on more respectable research initiatives in *Why Your Child Is Hyperactive*, Feingold attempted to appeal to a broader spectrum of physicians, not just to food allergists who often operated on the fringes of medical practice.

Although it is clear that Feingold's hyperactivity hypothesis fitted neatly into the history of food allergy and, especially, the tradition of linking food allergy with psychological problems, it is likely that, had Feingold chosen to stress these associations, he would have effectively severed his ties with the orthodox allergy community. Indeed, this was what happened to Arthur Coca, one of the most important allergists of the interwar period, whose reputation suffered greatly when he began theorizing about food allergy late in his career.[89] Although in retrospect the historian might see many similarities in the career trajectories of Coca and Feingold, it seems apparent that Feingold's intention was to avoid Coca's fate by stressing his traditional background and orthodox beliefs about allergy. From this perspective, Feingold's choice to shun food allergists and attempt to retain his ties to traditional allergists made strategic sense.

Feingold's decision to describe the origins of his diet as distinct from the history of food allergy was not, however, merely strategic. The articles and books Feingold wrote on bronchial allergic disease, flea bite allergies, psychosomatic factors in allergy, and clinical allergy reflected the views of an orthodox allergist and the restricted definition of allergy that such a perspective presupposed. Feingold's traditional outlook predisposed him to interpret his observations of the effects of food additives on children's behavior in a markedly different manner than the food allergists who had been claiming for decades that food allergies could cause mental health problems. He simply held different beliefs about allergy than most food allergists. It is likely that, having employed a restricted definition of allergy for decades, Feingold was unwilling to compromise his principles merely to link his theory to those of food allergists for whom he had little respect.

Feingold, it should be said, was not alone in this outcome. Other allergists also had difficulties reconciling their clinical observations with their theoretical understanding of allergy. Doris J. Rapp, a pediatrician who turned to an environmental theory of hyperactivity during the mid-1970s, was eventually more willing than Feingold to show how her ideas were linked to those of earlier food allergists, but she was not keen to do this at first. She was "ashamed to admit that from 1960 to 1975 while in practice as a pediatric-allergist, I seldom recognized or diagnosed this problem. Then, as often happens in medicine, my patients taught me."[90] Feingold was similarly willing to learn from his patients but was unwilling to change his core beliefs about allergy. It may have been more surprising if Feingold had abandoned the allergy paradigm within which he had operated successfully for decades and embraced the radically different one espoused by food allergists.

Despite Feingold's efforts to convince the allergy community about the legitimacy of his discovery, his hypothesis was actually discussed more often in psychiatry, pediatric, and psychological journals rather than those dedicated to allergy. It is likely that, regardless of Feingold's careful elucidation of the origins of his diet, most allergists saw his work as an extension of similar observations made by food allergists for sixty years and, thus, dismissed it or ignored it altogether. Feingold was understandably hurt by this reception. According to an associate, "Dr. Feingold was somewhat naïve [and] thought that he would be applauded as a benefactor of human well-being. I think that he was shocked by the rejection and criticism. From my viewpoint, he had been a traditional allergist who veered off the conventional path, and experienced what all iconoclasts experience: they are ignored, dismissed, scorned or ridiculed."[91]

Feingold's naïveté may indeed have inflated his sense of how palatable his theory would be to his colleagues in allergy. He often expressed to colleagues that his peers misunderstood his hypothesis, describing how he was "confident they do not appreciate the complexity of the problem."[92] Other aspects of Feingold's personality might also explain why he was reluctant to acknowledge the influence food allergists. Alice Friedman, who assisted Feingold during the 1960s, described him as "an extraordinarily autocratic gent" who did not suffer his critics particularly well.[93] Friedman suggested that Feingold tended to take sole credit for accomplishments and discoveries that should have been shared among others: according to Feingold, "No matter what anybody else does, it's the chief of the clinic who gets the credit for it . . . It's always the chief."[94] Friedman also claimed that she was responsible for alerting Feingold to the diet designed by Stephen D. Lockey at the Mayo Clinic that served as the model for the Feingold diet.[95] Another one of Feingold's researchers described Feingold as being "despotic" and "a bit full of himself," and that he was prone to disagree with other allergists, most notably the food allergists and clinical ecologists who might have sympathized with his ideas about hyperactivity.[96] Albert Rowe, for example, was only mentioned by Feingold "in a denigrating way."[97] Another colleague of Feingold's went further, stating that he "despised" food allergists and clinical ecologists such as Rowe, Randolph, and Mackarness as well as the work that they did.[98] The picture painted by Feingold's associates is not a particularly endearing one and is far removed from the charismatic, grandfatherly persona shown to the public when he was promoting his diet.

Feingold is presented in these testimonials as a rigid, egotistical autocrat whose contempt for food allergy and thirst for scientific acclaim clouded his judgment.

That said, the choices Feingold had before him upon writing *Why Your Child Is Hyperactive* were not easy ones. In many ways, he was caught between his observations of hyperactive children and his long-held perceptions about food allergy and its proponents, perceptions shared by most of his colleagues. The compromise reached by Feingold in *Why Your Child Is Hyperactive*, therefore, can be interpreted as an attempt to reconcile his clinical impressions and his theoretical underpinnings as a traditional allergist. While this compromise did not ultimately succeed in convincing allergists and other physicians that there was a link between food additives and hyperactivity, it did underlie Feingold's strong desire to have his hypothesis regarded as a legitimate medical theory and himself perceived as a respectable allergist.

On one level it is easy to criticize Feingold, and other scientists, for providing a misleading account of how his theory came to be. We can question his motives, his personality, his character, and, given the fact that his quest for scientific legitimacy went unfulfilled, argue that his approach was misguided all along. But we should perhaps also remember something that Feingold recognized, that scientific ideas never exist in a vacuum. They intersect and interact with other ideas that have their own histories and connections. Just as the new kid has to be wary about who to have lunch with on the first day of school, scientists have to determine which allegiances are in the best interests of their hypothesis. By emphasizing some of the connections to his theory and not others, however, Feingold was not only ascertaining what was most beneficial for his idea but, as the next chapter suggests, he was also concerned about what was best for his patients.

Chapter 3

Feingold Goes Public

Given Feingold's desire to make his theory respectable, it seems strange that he chose to publicize his idea not through articles in leading medical journals, such as *JAMA* or *Pediatrics*, but in a popular book aimed at parents. Prior to his work on hyperactivity, Feingold had published regularly in medical journals. Feingold's flea bite allergy research in the 1960s, for example, was accompanied by ten articles he wrote or coauthored in scientific journals ranging from *Experimental Parasitology* to the *Journal of Immunology*. Feingold's initial observations about the reactions triggered by food additives were also published in *Annals of Allergy* in 1968.[1] Moreover, Feingold was keen to submit his hypothesis about food additives and hyperactivity to the scrutiny of his peers, and proceeded to do so at the 1973 and 1974 meetings of the AMA in New York. Why then, did Feingold compromise the respectability of his theory, not to mention that of his public identity, by publishing his ideas in *Why Your Child Is Hyperactive*?

Feingold's decision to write for a popular audience was not entirely his own. Instead, it was a reaction to circumstances thrust upon him between 1973 and 1975 by an ambivalent medical community, by parents of hyperactive children who were frustrated with current explanations and treatments for hyperactivity, and by a media alarmed about the safety of the food supply, industrial threats to the environment, and the manner in which most physicians treated hyperactive children. Feingold's choice would have significant repercussions on the reception to his diet. While physicians were unimpressed by Feingold's decision to write a popular book instead of publishing a series of academic articles and were unmoved by, if not resentful of, his emerging celebrity,

parents and the media were captivated. *Why Your Child Is Hyperactive* introduced Feingold's ideas to millions of parents not only through book sales
but through television and radio interviews and hundreds of newspaper and
magazine articles that discussed his new theory during the 1970s.

Although *Why Your Child Is Hyperactive* was aimed partially at convincing physicians that Feingold's theory was accurate, it was essentially a popular
book published by a major publisher for a broad audience consisting largely of
parents. By the time of its publication, it was evident to Feingold that the path
to legitimizing his hypothesis did not necessarily involve running the gauntlet
of the medical approval process, consisting of double-blind trials and peer-
reviewed articles, but instead meant connecting with families via newspaper
articles and television interviews, helping to launch Feingold Associations
across North America, and consulting with individual parents. Feingold would
eventually exhibit little discrimination with regards to which newspapers and
magazines he would give interviews; parents would read about the Feingold
diet not only in respected newspapers such as the *New York Times* and the
Washington Post but also tabloids such as the *National Enquirer* and even the
pornographic men's magazine *Penthouse*.[2] He had come a long way from trying
to convince his medical peers.

Mixed Messages from the AMA

One of the striking aspects of how the Feingold diet spread across the United
States is how quickly this process took place. Feingold began treating hyperactive children in San Francisco with his elimination diet in the middle of 1972,
and by the autumn of that year he had prescribed the diet to a mere twenty-five
children, only fifteen of whom experienced improvements in their behavior.[3]
A year later, however, Feingold had reported his clinical findings about hyperactivity and food additives to the AMA and the Royal Institute in London, had
spoken to the international media about his hypothesis, had the manuscript of
his London presentation submitted into the U.S. Congressional Record, and
was the subject of numerous magazine and newspaper articles.[4] The explosion
of interest in 1973 was not so much due to Feingold's active promotion of
himself or his diet, however, but rather the public's and, initially, the medical
community's receptivity to his theory.

Although Feingold would become a willing and eager participant in such
publicity and media attention, he was not the instigator of it. Instead, Feingold
proceeded cautiously with regards to his thesis and attempted to gain the support of his medical colleagues prior to making conclusive claims. Feingold's
hesitation was reflected in the language he used initially to describe his

hypothesis to his fellow physicians, the AMA, the U.S. Congress, and the media, and suggests that Feingold's role in attracting media attention was largely passive, at least at first. In *Why Your Child Is Hyperactive*, Feingold stated that by 1972 he had begun discussing his observations about food additives and hyperactivity to "other doctors and with friends," and that the media in San Francisco were alerted simply because "word got around that I had a theory about the hyperkinetic-learning disabled child." The result of such rumors was that by "late October 1972 I found myself before the cameras of KPIX-TV, San Francisco, discussing what I had learned of the H-LD [hyperkinesis and learning disability] and talking about my slowly hardening hypothesis."[5]

It is possible that this television appearance prompted the AMA to invite Feingold to make a presentation at their June 1973 meeting in New York, and Feingold did recall being invited to the meeting in late 1972, shortly after his first television appearance.[6] That Feingold described his hypothesis as "slowly hardening" also suggested that he desired the opportunity to test his theory more thoroughly before submitting it to the scrutiny of his peers, let alone the media. Elsewhere in *Why Your Child Is Hyperactive*, Feingold mentioned "casually" discussing his observations in April 1973 with colleagues Alice Friedman and Don German, who had taken over from Feingold as chief of allergy for Kaiser Permanente when Feingold was fighting cancer during the late 1960s. Both physicians were "skeptical" and thought that the positive responses of children prescribed the elimination diet "might have been a psychological reaction to the diet program and to the constant attention and vigilance of the parents." Admitting that he had these suspicions himself, Feingold added, "As a very conventional medical doctor, I have always been leery of 'cure' by diet."[7]

Feingold's apprehensiveness spurred him to take advantage of his opportunities in 1973 to discuss his theory with his medical peers. He described these conferences, specifically his invitation to speak at the allergy section of the June 1973 AMA meeting in New York, as "an excellent forum for peer evaluation of our observations on behavior and dietary intervention."[8] In other words, Feingold was not so much looking for publicity as for feedback from other allergists and pediatricians. Feingold insisted that he was never responsible for making overtures to organizations such as the AMA or the media; it was the AMA that invited him to speak at their annual meetings and not the other way around.[9] The only organization Feingold did contact about his theory prior to his AMA presentation was the FDA, to whom he began writing in May 1973, urging that they market more additive-free foods and require fuller and clearer disclosures of additives on food product ingredient labels.[10]

Feingold's letters to the FDA notwithstanding, reports in the media of his June 1973 presentation to the AMA suggested that the San Francisco allergist still held some reservations about the validity of his theory and he desired more time to test it and discuss it with other physicians. An article in the *Hartford Courant*, for example, reported that "Dr. Ben F. Feingold says he has no solid evidence yet for this suspicion," but Feingold believed his "clinical observations call for a look into what effects on child behavior there may be from various of the thousands of chemicals added to foods."[11] Such sentiments were also reflected in a *Chicago Tribune* article that covered the AMA meeting and reported that, while Feingold was unclear about the physiological process by which additives caused hyperactive behavior, he believed that his observations warranted thorough investigation.[12] A *Newsweek* article in July 1973 stated that "because he has not yet done a controlled study, Feingold cautions that his observations must be regarded as preliminary."[13] Further evidence of Feingold's caution can be found in his 1973 *Introduction to Clinical Allergy* in which he refrained from making definitive statements about food additives and hyperactivity. Instead, he simply posed the question, "Is it possible that some cases of so-called MBD [minimal brain dysfunction, a contemporary term for hyperactivity] may be manifestations of neuro-physiologic disturbances induced by certain chemicals such as the food additives?"[14] In many of Feingold's other early media interviews, he similarly preferred to pose questions such as this rather than giving definitive comments. For example, in Morton Mintz's October 1973 story, which made the front page of the *Washington Post*, he asked, "Is it possible to attribute the increase in hyperkinesis and learning difficulty to the increased consumption of these chemicals in our foodstuffs? Do the additives ingested by the mother during pregnancy affect the unborn child?" In this story Feingold also mentioned that, since other causes of hyperactivity were possible, his diet did not work for all of his patients.[15]

Although Feingold believed his clinical observations, consisting of only twenty-five hyperactive patients in June 1973, to be preliminary, the AMA was much more enthusiastic. After Feingold submitted his manuscript for his presentation, they asked him if he would be willing to participate in a news conference on the day before his presentation. Feingold "accepted and met with between 75 and 80 correspondents from around the world, following which the report that hyperkinesis responded to a diet eliminating artificial food colors and flavors was covered by practically all the news media."[16] Reacting later to such media interest, Feingold stated, "Since I am not a behaviorist nor a psychiatrist, but rather an allergist and immunologist, I was not prepared for this response."[17]

Despite such media interest, Feingold endeavored in the autumn of 1973 to present his ideas to medical colleagues at scientific conferences and in medical journals rather than in the press.[18] For instance, he submitted the preliminary findings he presented to the AMA for publication in its journal, *JAMA*.[19] He also accepted an invitation to speak at an international symposium on food in September 1973 at the Royal Institution of Great Britain and submitted another article for publication in the *British Medical Journal* (*BMJ*).[20] Feingold also agreed to write a signed editorial for the medical journal *Hospital Practice*, which appeared in October 1973.[21] Finally, towards the end of 1973, Feingold accepted a second invitation to speak at the AMA's 1974 meeting, this time in Chicago.[22]

Nevertheless, the reaction of many influential medical associations to Feingold's theory during this period was ambivalent. On the one hand, the AMA and the California Medical Association (CMA) invited Feingold to present his theory to their annual meetings in 1973, 1974, and 1975. As they had done the previous year, the AMA scheduled another press conference in 1974 to precede Feingold's presentation and, again, media coverage was heavy, resulting in almost daily stories in American print, radio, and television media.[23] But on the other hand, *JAMA* refused to publish Feingold's findings in either 1973 or 1974 and the CMA refused to publish his findings in its journal, then called the *Western Journal of Medicine*, following Feingold's presentation to them in 1975. Feingold's submission to the *BMJ* was similarly rejected.

Feingold had been published in both *California Medicine*, one of the predecessors of the *Western Journal of Medicine*, and *JAMA* in 1949 and 1951, respectively. One possible reason that the CMA was reluctant to publish his findings with regards to hyperactivity involved not only the controversial nature of his research but the fact that he worked for the medical insurance firm Kaiser Permanente. According to Feingold's colleague Alice Friedman, Feingold had been a member of the CMA when he worked in private practice in Los Angeles, but when he joined Kaiser Permanente in 1951, the San Francisco branch of the CMA "blackballed him" and prevented him from joining them. This was because Kaiser Permanente provided private medical insurance, a concept that was viewed by many American physicians as being socialist and a threat to their income during the 1940s and 1950s.[24]

Feingold's history with the CMA notwithstanding, the mixed response to Feingold's theory during this early period is perplexing. Why did the AMA promote Feingold's thesis by inviting him to their meeting and arranging large press conferences, only to reject Feingold's submission for *JAMA*? Given the fact that the first clinical trials that tested the Feingold diet were not performed until 1976, it is clear that the AMA's decision not to publish Feingold's findings was not based upon scientific evidence or the reports of other researchers. Although the reasons for the AMA's reversal are difficult to pinpoint, a number of factors help to explain why Feingold ultimately abandoned his goal of achieving the sanction of the medical community.

The chief reason for the AMA's initial interest in Feingold's theory seems to have been his excellent reputation as a pediatric allergist. According to C. Keith Conners, a pioneer in hyperactivity research and key player in the investigations into the Feingold diet, "The weight of his authority at first caused Feingold's theory to be taken seriously by scientists. He had already made some fundamental discoveries in allergy and had written a well-regarded textbook of pediatric allergy."[25] Morris Lipton, the University of North Carolina psychiatrist who headed the Nutrition Foundation's investigation into Feingold's claims, stated in 1977 that "Dr. Feingold and his work are well known to me, and as a reputable physician I must take him seriously—up to a point."[26] Not only was Feingold a leader within the allergy community in California, with impressive clinical experience and publications, but he sat on the AAA's Committee on Food Allergy and Committee on Insects and Insect Allergy during the 1960s and 1970s.[27] Feingold's antipathy for the clinical ecology movement might have reassured the AMA that they were inviting a conservative allergist to speak to the media, and not a radical such as food allergist and clinical ecologist Theron Randolph.[28] Others have suggested, however, that the AMA invited the allergist back in 1974 because "he was controversial and [they] knew it would raise attendance."[29]

It may be precisely such controversy that ultimately caused the AMA to distance itself from Feingold and his theory.[30] Despite Feingold's reputation as a conservative allergist, his theory about hyperactivity had profound implications for food, chemical, and pharmaceutical companies. As *Business Week* contributor Geraldine Pluenneke described in her review of *Why Your Child Is Hyperactive*:

> . . . a time bomb is ticking beneath the dust wrapper of this book, and it could explode into another widespread controversy over food additives. . . . Count Chocula and Boo Berry cereals. Decongestants and bear-shaped vitamins. Cavity-tracking toothpastes, self-basting turkeys; corn oil margarines, colas . . . a San Francisco allergist is advancing an empirical theory linking the common ingredients in such products— synthetic colors, flavors, and enhancers—with a seemingly epidemic rise in learning problems.[31]

Pluenneke went on to state that some "companies are already keeping a low profile while test-marketing new products to avoid provoking attacks by food naturalists who already question the long-term dangers of food chemicals. Feingold's theory has an immediacy that could have an impact at the checkout counter: the promise of a rapid dietary escape from a problem that is now routinely handled with a battery of stimulant, tranquilizing, and antidepressant drugs."[32]

By the early 1970s, Feingold's previous work on reactions to food additives, as well as similar work conducted by researchers such as Stephen D. Lockey, Frederic Speer, Guy Settipane, and F. H. Chafee on reactions to food dyes such as tartrazine, had caught the attention of food chemical companies.[33] Although links between the AMA and the food industry are difficult to establish, other medical associations such as the AAA had close ties with the food industry. One of the proposed projects of the AAA's Food Allergy Committee in 1984, for example, was the "creation of formal relationships with our Committee, and the American Academy of Allergy and Immunology, to scientists connected with the food industry." The rationale behind such a relationship was not to warn the public about possible food allergies but to reassure them about processed food in restaurants.[34] Since the AMA does not currently allow the vast majority of its records to be viewed by historians, it is difficult to shed light on the AMA's contradictory decisions regarding Feingold's hypothesis. It is only apparent that at some point following Feingold's 1973 and 1974 presentations to the AMA, a decision was made to stop promoting his diet and prevent his ideas from being published in *JAMA*.[35] The decision might not have been influenced by the food chemical industry, but it did parallel initiatives made by the food chemical industry in 1974 and 1975 under the auspices of its research organization, the Nutrition Foundation, to investigate the Feingold diet and downplay its significance.[36]

The steps taken by the Nutrition Foundation to investigate Feingold's hypothesis included a December 1974 report and a January 1975 conference on the subject. Despite the fact that the last paragraph of the Nutrition Foundation's proposal stated that "no publicity will be given to the findings until the Committee has approved the report for release," a week later a preliminary report was published with a number of conclusions about the theory. Among them were the warnings that no "controlled studies have demonstrated that hyperkinesis is related to the ingestion of food additives" and the "nutritional quality of this diet has not been evaluated and it has not been determined if it meets the long-term nutrient needs of children."[37] Although these preliminary conclusions were originally intended to stay out of the press, they were given a great deal of exposure in the American media.[38] The American Academy of Pediatrics (AAP) proceeded to print the Nutrition Foundation's statement verbatim in their newsletter, along with the Nutrition Foundation's New York address.[39] Other medical organizations, including the AAA, also served notice to the public that they were unwilling to endorse Feingold's theory.[40] It is important to note that the responses of all of these medical associations, not to mention the Nutrition Foundation, occurred well before any controlled studies into the diet had been conducted. The AMA might have instigated interest in the Feingold diet by organizing the press conferences that accompanied Feingold's presentations, but they, like other medical associations, were also quick to distance themselves from his theory when it appeared to be too contentious.

The Popularization of the Feingold Diet

Ultimately, the reasons that prompted the AMA to reverse their position on Feingold's hypothesis proved to be less important to the fate of the Feingold diet than the impact of this reversal on how Feingold subsequently chose to promote his ideas. Faced with the rejection of his colleagues while simultaneously inundated by queries from parents and media, and continuing to experience clinical success with the diet, Feingold had to decide how to spread the word about his hypothesis. The allergist would continue to speak to medical audiences such as the AAP in 1977 and publish his ideas in medical journals, but these tended to be less renowned journals such as *Ecology of Disease* and the *Delaware Medical Journal.*[41] Feingold's post-1975 publications in the *Journal of the American Society for Preventive Dentistry*, the *American Journal of Nursing*, the *Journal of Learning Disabilities*, the *International Journal of Dermatology*, *Academic Therapy*, and the *International Journal of Offender Therapy and Comparative Criminology* suggest that Feingold turned his attention away from physicians and towards dentists, nurses, special educators, dermatologists, psychologists, and counselors working in the criminal justice system.[42]

For the most part, however, Feingold's efforts after 1974 focused on parents and the media. Feingold gave dozens of media interviews, presented his views at countless speaking engagements, and addressed the public on the radio and television to the extent that he mentioned to a colleague that he had "actually been in a tailspin with so much to do and so many requests."[43] Despite his eagerness with the media, Feingold's shift towards a popular audience also reflected his belief that he had been slighted by his colleagues. According to his associates, Feingold was surprised and disappointed by the

decisions of *JAMA*, the *Western Journal of Medicine*, and the *BMJ* not to publish his findings on hyperactivity and food additives. One of his colleagues
stated that Feingold "was dismayed. Dejected. I remember how he looked at his
wife as he tried to rationalize it. You could see the tears in her eyes. At times he
would just stare at the San Francisco harbor from his high rise apartment when
looking back at his career and realizing that it had no influence on his peers . . .
He became disillusioned with these journals afterwards. He realized that
politics played a more important role than science. He said, 'If I had a drug for
these kids, I would have no problem having these same journals accept my
papers.'"[44] Others have also stressed that he was "shocked by the rejection and
criticism," responses that "left him bewildered" and "pained."[45]

Despite his disappointment, Feingold was not reluctant to recount his
humiliating experience to various audiences and, when doing so, expressed
a degree of bitterness with regards to the episode. In response to criticism
from Robert L. Sieben, a Connecticut-area pediatric neurologist who accused
Feingold of publicizing his theory before adequately testing it, Feingold first
defended his reputation by stating that "as a practitioner of international reputation for over fifty years, I am well acquainted with the proprieties of medical
practice, so that moralistic and ethical innuendos are completely unjusti-
fied."[46] He outlined why he chose to write for the broader public, stating that
"it may be of special interest to Dr. Sieben to learn that in each instance, 1973,
1974, and 1975, organized medicine rejected my manuscripts for publication"
and that *Why Your Child Is Hyperactive* "was written for a general public
following the rejection of my manuscripts."[47]

Feingold expressed a similar degree of resentment in response to a March
1975 syndicated newspaper column by Frederick Stare (1910–2002), who was
the founder of the Department of Nutrition at Harvard University and a keen
supporter of the food industry:

Dr. Stare resorts to additional innuendos which have been copied
repeatedly by the lay press and at times even scientific publications.
Dr. Stare states: "Interestingly, to our own knowledge Dr. Feingold
has not published a single paper in the medical literature so physicians
and scientists can evaluate his results." The word "interestingly" seems
meant in this context to imply I have purposely withheld publication,
an implication that is strengthened by his next statement, "He apparently
prefers talk shows." Dr. Stare fails to report that my initial presentation
was by invitation from organized medicine—the AMA and the
California Medical Association—that both the AMA and the California

Medical Association rejected for publication the manuscripts of my presentations in 1973, 1974 and 1975. It was following the rejection in 1974 that I accepted an invitation from the publisher [Random House] to author a book *Why Your Child Is Hyperactive* for the general public. Dr. Stare and the other critics fail to mention that since 1973 I have authored twelve publications on the subject of food additives in various scientific periodicals. As for my appearances on talk shows, I must point out to Dr. Stare and his cohorts that practically all the publicity which has led to worldwide awareness of this new modality for hyperkinesis was initially generated by the press conferences scheduled by the AMA and California Medical Association. Furthermore, I continue to feel privileged whenever the media extends an invitation to me to explain my research directly to the public.[48]

Feingold's sharp responses to Sieben and Stare highlight how he resented being seen as a publicity seeker and not an experienced, honest, and responsible physician. By indicating the AMA's role in publicizing his theory, as well as the fact that he accepted Random House's invitation to publish his hypothesis only after he had been thrice rejected for publication in leading medical journals, Feingold emphasized that it was not his decision to take his ideas directly to the public without first gaining the approval of the medical community. The scientific content in *Why Your Child Is Hyperactive*, Feingold's unwillingness to link his research with that of food allergists and clinical ecologists, as well as his ongoing efforts to respond to his medical critics and publish his ideas in less renowned journals, all indicates that, while he was discouraged by the response of the medical community, he still wanted to be considered as a respected scientist. Although Feingold increasingly shifted his efforts to convincing the public, he nevertheless hoped and even anticipated that his theory would eventually be accepted by his medical peers. As he wrote in a letter to a colleague in late 1979, "We are making progress, but slower than I would like. The professional climate is gradually changing, and they are beginning to grasp my basic hypothesis."[49]

Despite Feingold's desire to be taken seriously by his colleagues, there were other, more pragmatic, reasons for him to disseminate his theory through the popular media. Both scientists who were supportive and who were critical of Feingold demanded that he prove the efficacy of his hypothesis through double-blind clinical trials.[50] Such trials, for example, the ones conducted by Leon Eisenberg and C. Keith Conners during the 1960s to test the effect of Ritalin on hyperactive children, were intended to determine both the efficacy

and the safety of proposed treatments.[51] Feingold, however, had not conducted
such trials. In criticizing Feingold's decision to report his theory before conducting trials, prominent New Zealand pediatrician John Werry pointedly
stated,

> I personally feel there is no greater breach of medical ethics than that of
> foisting a potentially worthless or dangerous treatment on to a credulous
> public. Theirs may be the right to believe in magic and panaceas but
> ours as a profession is to act responsibly, cautiously and scientifically,
> though not prejudicially. Why should all of my U.S. colleagues in pae-
> diatric psychopharmacology research, no more than a handful, have to
> drop their work to show a clamouring public that Feingold's hypothesis
> is or is not correct and is or is not safe. Surely the obligation is his before
> he announces it to the public?[52]

Although Feingold had expressed some interest in subjecting his theory to
controlled clinical trials when he initially reported it in 1973, his interest and
faith in this process waned soon after. His decision to write *Why Your Child Is
Hyperactive* before the publication of any such trials, conducted by himself or
others, is indicative of this. One of the reasons for this was Feingold's impatience to get his ideas out to the public, impatience due partly to his advanced
age and health concerns. Not only was Feingold in his mid-seventies, he had
already undergone two surgeries for cancer and experienced ongoing heart
problems that would see him have a pacemaker operation in 1979.[53] He also
commented to a journalist that it would take as many as thirty to fifty years
to prove unequivocally through trials that his hypothesis was correct.[54]
Feingold's colleagues nevertheless urged him to conduct clinical trials, but
Feingold demurred, citing his age.[55] According to Conners, "Dr. Feingold at 75 is
a man in a hurry. He once told me while we were on a radio program together,
'I don't have time for sacred cows of science, the double-blind placebo controlled trials' . . . Rather than support these assertions with laborious and time-
consuming studies, he preferred to take his message directly to the consumer."[56]
    Given the fact that Feingold attempted to present his ideas to his medical
colleagues, Conners's assertion that Feingold "preferred to take his message
directly to the consumer" is not altogether accurate. Regardless, there was
another, more epistemological reason that Feingold questioned the desirability
of conducting controlled clinical trials. Feingold's experience trying to develop
an allergen to desensitize people allergic to flea bites during the 1960s had
demonstrated to him many of the pitfalls and frustrations of trying to derive
knowledge through scientific experimentation. In one article, for example,

Feingold elaborated on the difficulty of even determining if in fact his flea bite allergy patients were suffering from flea bites:

> One unfortunate factor in most of this work has been the dependence of workers on subjective reports from patients regarding the insect causing clinical symptoms. In our experience many patients never see the insect biting them except in the case of mosquitos and biting flies. Inconspicuous insects, such as fleas and bedbugs, may possibly bite these people for years without being noticed, and even when seen may be misidentified. During our work individuals have brought "fleas" to the clinic which have proven to be anything from sawtooth grain beetles to small weed seeds. Needless to say, under these conditions it is difficult to ascertain whether clinical lesions are due to actual flea bites, and, if hyposensitization is attempted, whether any reported relief is due to treatment or to the cessation of flea activity.[57]

Feingold proceeded to explain that no fleas were to be found in many of the houses of patients who complained of flea bite allergies. Moreover, Feingold's research, while important to the development of allergy theory, failed to develop techniques for desensitizing people to flea bite allergies.[58] Not only was it difficult to design such experiments and eliminate potentials for error, but it was also clear to Feingold that such experiments did not always yield the results that were intended.

As an allergist, Feingold was also aware of the potential for individual differences in patients, differences that could affect the outcome of even carefully designed and controlled trials. His research during the 1960s on psychosomatic allergy, for example, suggested to him that "psychological factors are of importance in understanding allergic illnesses," but it was "unlikely that any typical allergic pattern will emerge" and the allergy population was "quite heterogeneous."[59] In other words, not only was it complicated to determine the degree to which allergic symptoms were dependent on psychological factors, but it was also difficult to develop a reference point from which to assess such influences. Environmental differences could also play a role, as described by Alice Friedman:

> It's extremely difficult in allergy and allergy treatments to have a firm scientific basis because what individuals do has such an important bearing. You know, if you smoke and irritate all your membranes very obviously your symptoms are going to be there no matter what else you do. If you have five dogs and three cats and you're sensitive to dander, you're going to have problems no matter how you're treated for your hayfever.

Allergy, more than almost anything else, gets into what you do in your everyday life. To document all these things is very difficult. If you live in a moldy house, which can certainly happen in San Francisco, you may have terrible problems that nobody can solve until you get out of that house. So there are so many factors that are parts of everyday living that can affect the outcome of your scientific endeavors. But it's extremely difficult to document these things.[60]

Given such experiences, it is somewhat understandable that Feingold considered controlled clinical trials a daunting, laborious, and unpromising undertaking at his late stage in life. In addition, however, Feingold had one other reason for refusing to conduct clinical trials by the time he decided to publish *Why Your Child Is Hyperactive*. This was his strong belief, reinforced by an increasing number of clinical encounters, that his diet worked. Although Feingold's naturally conservative tendencies were reflected in his initial hesitance to promote his idea before he was certain of its validity, such caution was eventually overcome by his high degree of self-assurance. Feingold's confident nature may have made him "despotic" and "exceedingly autocratic," to some of his colleagues, but also made him a "very positive" individual who had great faith in his own ideas and the ability to convey this faith to others.[61] In other words, once Feingold believed that his theory was correct, he steadfastly defended it, was willing and able to disseminate it, and was not likely to change his opinions in the face of results from poorly designed trials.

Conclusion

After initial encouragement, the AMA and other medical associations were ultimately unwilling to provide Feingold with a venue to disseminate his theory to fellow physicians. Disillusioned and frustrated by this about-face, and doubtful that much would be gained by conducting the trials demanded by physicians such as Werry and Sieben, Feingold became more willing to take his theory directly to the public, often using the media to do so. After half a century of being an orthodox and respected leader in the pediatric allergy community, Feingold chose to become a radical figure, a pariah who eschewed the "sacred cows of science, the double-blind placebo controlled trials" and took his message directly to parents. Although he would continue to couch his theory in scientific language and associate it with those of others studying neurology and toxicology, Feingold realized that, if his theory was ever to achieve medical respectability, it would be because of bottom-up pressure from parents, journalists, activists, and unorthodox physicians rather than top-down recommendations from bodies such as the AMA.

According to historians Roger Cooter and Stephen Pumfrey, the popularization of scientific theories can transform how such ideas are understood not only by the public but also by the scientific community. Scientists often enroll a "network of alliances" in order to communicate their theories to popular audiences and, during this process of translation, the meaning and application of their ideas may change.[62] As Cooter and Pumfrey explain, "There is no reason to suppose that popular science takes the form intended by its popularizers," largely "because it is developed by its recipients for different purposes."[63] Depending on what these purposes might be, and according "to its position and influence in the 'network,' the public alters the kind of science pursued in future."[64]

In the strangely similar case of Hans Selye's theories about the physiological impact of stress, popularization had a considerable effect on how stress would be conceived by both the public and scientists. Russell Viner has explained how Han Selye attempted to promote his ideas about stress and the general adaptation syndrome, "a universal truth regarding the relationships of organisms with their environment, a truth he would sell to whoever would listen."[65] Selye found that, despite initial interest during the 1930s and 1940s, his colleagues in laboratory research felt that his theory was "too vague and teleological to be scientifically credible," and questioned his research methods and personality.[66] Selye then enrolled allies in other domains, first in the field of military medicine and later among American conservatives, who were enticed by his notion that societal strife could manifest itself in disease.[67] Although the general idea that stress played a key role in affecting physiology would become accepted by numerous scientific disciplines during the 1970s, many specifics underlying Selye's theory were undermined, and stress became a more elastic concept than Selye had originally envisioned.[68]

In the case of the Feingold diet, popularization had more of an impact on the reception of Feingold's hypothesis than on its substance. This is partly because, as a clinician, the interests Feingold had in disseminating his hypothesis were roughly parallel to those of the parents who employed his diet; both were dissatisfied with contemporary treatments of hyperactivity and desired an alternative. Feingold and parents equally desired a dietary regimen that was comprehensive but not unnecessarily restrictive. Feingold's hypothesis was also based more on the accumulation of clinical experience, which was itself dependent upon the ability of patients to observe and recall how and when their symptoms arose, than on an underlying theoretical model. As such, Feingold was happy to work with parents and with Feingold Associations to refine the diet, for example, eliminating synthetic preservatives from the diet after *Why Your Child Is Hyperactive* was published, but resisting calls to include refined sugar to the list of banned substances. After Feingold's death, FAUS continued to adjust the list of approved substances, often in response to parent suggestions. Nonetheless, FAUS adhered closely to Feingold's general principle that the diet had to be kept as liberal as possible, and the organization stubbornly rejected suggestions to ban foods such as refined sugar criticized by other theorists. Although Feingold's theory was shaped by parents, his most important allies, it is probable that this also would have been true had he not decided to write a popular book.

The popularization of the Feingold diet, however, did expose the belief of many physicians during the 1970s, such as Seiben, Stare, and Werry, that untested medical ideas posed a danger to the public. Such thinking could be seen as protecting patients from quackery and snake oil salesmen, not to mention unscrupulous drug companies. But it also implied that patients and their families should not be involved in the assessment or formulation of novel medical ideas and that members of the public were not capable of informing medical opinion about the provision of treatment. Not only was such thinking naïve, in that it underestimated the agency patients and their families exhibited in selecting or refining medical advice, but it also failed to recognize that when patients were dissatisfied with a particular medical approach they would simply look elsewhere. In the case of the Feingold diet, dissatisfaction with conventional explanations for and treatments of hyperactivity led patients and their families to consider alternative approaches.

Chapter 4

The Problem with Hyperactivity

Without the support of the AMA, it was difficult for Feingold to gain the credibility he desired for his diet, and this problem was compounded by the difficulty of communicating his idea to parents via their physicians. Fortunately for Feingold, Random House's offer to publish his book in 1974 provided him with an ideal opportunity to present his idea directly to parents and foment a debate about the etiology and treatment of hyperactivity. Random House's interest also affirmed that while the medical establishment was unwilling to endorse Feingold's hypothesis, the public was intrigued by the notion that food additives could cause hyperactivity. The following two chapters explore how the public's interest in Feingold's theory reflected not only concern about increasing rates of hyperactivity, and the controversial ways in which the disorder was treated, but also growing alarm about chemicals in the food supply.

Although these issues were separate on the surface, they both indicated a growing distrust of corporate America—in this case the pharmaceutical and food manufacturing industries—as well as the professional associations and government departments, such as the AMA and the FDA, that were supposed to safeguard the public against corporate irresponsibility. As Canadian psychiatrists Ivan Williams and Douglas Cram suggested, the Feingold diet became popular because (1) it was an alternative to drugs, (2) it shifted guilt from parents to the food industry, (3) it removed blame from schools, (4) it fitted the growing consciousness about ecology and pure foods, and (5) it enabled parents to be the primary therapeutic agents, since they were in control of the diet.[1] Feingold's hypothesis fitted into other "radical critiques" of hyperactivity, which echoed "the spirit of the times when American society came under systematic questioning and attack."[2] The Feingold diet provided a particular treatment for a specific childhood disorder, but it simultaneously represented a critique of American psychiatry and of corporate practices relating to the environment and the food supply. Interest in the Feingold diet was a grassroots response to a medical problem at a time when Americans were increasingly disillusioned with their political leadership in the light of crises such as the Vietnam War, the Watergate scandal, and energy shortages.

Hyperactivity emerged during an era of considerable cultural, educational, demographic, and political turbulence within American society. It was also an era in which the American psychiatric community was undergoing upheaval and was fraught with interdisciplinary strife. The psychiatric community of the 1960s and 1970s could be divided into three primary disciplines: psychoanalysis, social psychiatry, and biological psychiatry. The theoretical underpinnings and modes of treatment could overlap in practice: for example, psychoanalyst George A. Rogers found that Ritalin facilitated psychotherapy in his neurotic patients.[3] However, each approach essentially represented a significantly different way of understanding mental illness, and psychiatrists typically favored one methodology over the others. The profound differences in each discipline's approach to mental illness were reflected in their explanations of what caused hyperactivity. Although some psychiatrists spoke of hyperactivity as being multicausal, and suggested that a variety of treatments to help hyperactive children, most research papers stressed the validity of one approach as opposed to others and, in clinical practice, psychiatrists tended to privilege one treatment modality over another.

By the early 1970s, most psychiatrists believed that hyperactivity was a neurological dysfunction passed on genetically or caused by brain damage, but they were unable to provide specifics on the mechanisms of the dysfunction, and psychoanalytic and social explanations remained common.[4] Whereas psychoanalysts blamed strained family relationships for hyperactivity, social psychiatrists looked to social conditions such as poverty, overcrowding, and crime-infested neighborhoods.[5] Feingold's hypothesis differed considerably from these theories, but what it had in common with them was the notion that some aspect of American society, whether it be rooted in family structure, socioeconomic conditions, or exposure to chemicals, was pathological to children.

Psychiatric debates about hyperactivity might not have mattered a great deal to the parents of hyperactive children. Nevertheless, these disputes, as well as the wide range of opinion represented, highlighted the controversial nature of hyperactivity and suggested that its diagnosis was not straightforward. Parents were also concerned that the methods psychiatrists used to treat hyperactivity were ineffective, inappropriate, or dangerous. By the 1970s, the most common method for treating hyperactivity was with stimulant drugs, such as Ritalin, Cylert, and Dexedrine, although psychotherapy, family counseling, and behavioral therapy were alternatives. Despite the variety of explanations and treatments for hyperactivity, many parents were hesitant to accept conventional explanations or solutions for their child's behavioral problems. Dissatisfaction with the primary methods of treating hyperactivity led parents to consider alternative approaches and, during the 1970s, the Feingold diet was by far the most successful of these alternatives.[6]

Psychoanalysis: The "Most Productive and Cohesive Theory Available"

Following World War II, psychoanalysis was the dominant discipline within American psychiatry, influencing not only clinical practice and research but how the public perceived psychiatry.[7] For example, the editorial board of *JAACP*, founded in 1962 to reflect the increasing interest in child psychiatry, consisted primarily of psychoanalysts, and most of the articles published by the journal during the 1960s were oriented towards psychoanalysis. In a special series on childhood behavioral problems in 1963, all articles were based in psychoanalytic theory, including those by Eveoleen N. Rexford (1911–1992), the series' editor.[8] The journal continued to be dominated by psychoanalysis unto 1976, when Melvin Lewis (1926–2007) replaced Rexford as editor and its focus shifted to biological psychiatry. The first article of the new era was Dennis P. Cantwell's "Genetic Factors in the Hyperkinetic Syndrome."[9] But during the 1960s, psychoanalytic explanations for childhood disorders remained prevalent. This was reflected in the *Diagnostic and Statistical Manual of Mental Disorders-II* (1968), which included a psychoanalytically oriented description of hyperkinetic reaction of childhood.[10] Psychoanalysts also regularly took up the presidency of the American Psychiatric Association (APA) during the postwar period.[11]

Psychoanalysts tended to guard jealously their hegemony over American psychiatry, especially as rival theories became popular during the 1950s and 1960s. A letter written by Iowa child psychiatrist Mark Stewart to the editor of the *AJP* in 1960 demonstrated the psychoanalytic dominance of American psychiatry but also implied that not all psychiatrists were happy with the situation. Stewart argued that jobs advertised in the APA's "Mail Pouch" nearly always stressed the importance of a psychoanalytic orientation, and he complained that "this phenomenon, which unhappily is symptomatic of the general situation of psychiatry today, can make our profession seem ridiculous to other physicians and to scientists in general."[12] Although Stewart's criticism foreshadowed the ultimate demise of American psychoanalysis, for many post-war psychiatrists there was no "magical belief in some kind of correspondence between psychical processes and central nervous processes."[13]

Psychoanalysts believed that hyperactivity, like many other psychiatric conditions, was rooted in family dynamics and involved disruption of the superego, which, in turn, resulted in poor impulse control.[14] Although this explanation appeared simple superficially, the key for psychoanalysts was to determine what initially caused such disruption in order to provide effective psychotherapy. As a result, most of the psychoanalytic articles in psychiatric journals during the 1960s about hyperactivity were case studies featuring the clinical observations of a single patient. The patient would be introduced along with a detailed description of his or her behaviors, personality, history, and family situation. The authors would then describe how they were able to unravel the reasons for the patient's hyperactivity and recount the course of treatment. One instance of this is found in a 1960 edition of the *Archives of General Psychiatry*, in which "Jean" was described. Jean was a twelve-year-old girl whose impulsive behavior, her psychiatrist determined, was the result of penis envy stemming from the relationship that she had with her father. Jean's impulsivity ceased only when she was able to come to terms with this explanation.[15] The root causes of hyperactivity in other children could originate in the child's weaning, toilet training, adjustment to a new sibling, or other types of trauma.[16] In other cases, inappropriate, unhealthy, or inadequate relationships with parents were believed to be the problem.[17]

Case studies were an attractive means by which to depict hyperactivity and the course of psychoanalytic treatment. The reader was provided with a mini-narrative that usually resulted in a happy ending; the child who was so disruptive at the beginning of the case study was usually thriving at both school and home by the end of it. Although skeptics could question the reliability of such descriptions, case studies had an emotional impact upon readers that the impersonal accounts of double-blind clinical trials lacked. In keeping with a similar tradition in allergy, Feingold used case studies to great effect in *Why Your Child Is Hyperactive*.

Nevertheless, Feingold, like many parents and other physicians, was less satisfied by how psychoanalysts explained hyperactivity. Although Feingold agreed that the stress and disruption of having a hyperactive child could strain relationships both at home and at school, even compromising the efficacy of his diet, for him the root of such problems were reactions to food additives.[18] For parents of hyperactive children, including many of those who would employ the Feingold diet, psychoanalytic explanations of hyperactivity were often confusing and contradictory, and seemed to imply, if not explicitly state, that parents were to blame for their child's hyperactivity.[19] Mothers in particular were singled out as being responsible for causing behavior problems in their children. According to journalists Barbara Ehrenreich and Deirdre English, "By the mid-twentieth century the experts were grimly acknowledging that despite constant vigilance the American mother was failing at her job."[20] The ubiquity of such notions during the postwar period meant that physicians often pinned a range of health problems on poor mothering.[21] For example, overprotective, smothering mothers were believed to be pathological in the cases of schizophrenia and asthma. While German psychoanalyst Freida Fromm-Reichmann (1889–1957) described the "schizophrenogenic mother" in 1948, the "asthmogenic home" was a concept employed by pioneering English allergist John Freeman (1877–1962) during the same period.[22] Mothers who turned to the Feingold diet also found that physicians blamed them for their children's health problems. As Lesley Freeman described when she tried to find help for her son's tics, "I took him to an ENT [ear, nose, and throat] doctor who examined him and said, 'There's nothing wrong, Mother, he needs more attention.' I took him to an eye doctor . . . and he said, 'There's nothing wrong with his eyes, Mother, he needs more attention.' This kid gets all the attention in the family. How could he possibly need more attention?"[23] Although Feingold's theory could also be interpreted as having an element of mother blame, in that mothers were largely responsible for feeding their children harmful additives, Feingold and FAUS almost always refrained from questioning mothers and, instead, criticized corporations, medical associations, and federal agencies.

Other psychiatric theories, particularly those of biological psychiatry, not only absolved mothers from blame but provided promising new remedies for psychiatric problems. Drugs such as the antipsychotic Thorazine and the antidepressant Miltown were advertised as treatments for patients ranging from the institutionalized schizophrenic to the depressed housewife.[24] As such drugs became more popular during the late 1950s and 1960s, psychoanalysis was increasingly seen as anachronistic and unscientific. This was particularly pertinent to psychiatrists who believed their profession was disrespected by other physicians.[25] As child psychiatrist John Werry described, encouraging his colleagues to employ "pediatric psychopharmacology," "child psychiatry . . . is not simply a humanitarian exercise, but an applied biological science."[26]

Despite the excitement and sales generated by the new medications, however, many psychoanalysts insisted that neurology and psychiatry were incompatible. As Albert J. Solnit (1919–2002), one of the first American child psychiatrists, asserted, "There is considerable doubt that the use of research models derived from the physical sciences can be of more than limited usefulness in child psychiatry research." According to Solnit, psychoanalysis was the "most cohesive and productive theory available."[27] Solnit's assertion, however, was increasingly unpopular among American psychiatrists, and his article generated a heated response from Leon Eisenberg (1922–2009), who had conducted the first large-scale Ritalin trials with C. Keith Conners. Eisenberg stated that psychoanalysis had "a constricting influence" on psychiatry and that psychoanalytic case studies should be replaced with "epidemiological, pharmacological, and psychological studies."[28]

More important, perhaps, was the practicality of treating the vast numbers of hyperactive children with psychotherapy.[29] Psychoanalysis required that each case be treated individually or, as described by an anonymous writer in *AJP*, "Individual psychotherapy is the only treatment that roots out the trouble. You can't apply this on a mass basis." Although practitioners of group therapy would object to such a comment, few practitioners recommended group therapy for hyperactivity.[30] Many psychiatrists recognized, however, that there were "more people struggling in the stream of life than we can rescue with our present tactics" of psychotherapy, and they argued that there were nowhere near enough psychotherapists to treat the "extraordinary numbers of disturbed children in the country."[31] Others criticized the effectiveness of psychotherapy in treating hyperactivity altogether, charging that "unfortunate children with minimal brain dysfunction [a contemporary term for hyperactivity] are still being condemned to months of fruitless and frustrating psychotherapy in various guidance clinics, while guilt and resentment builds upon their bewildered parents"; "misdirected psychotherapy can be every bit as dangerous as misdirected surgery."[32] Although the previous quotation came from an advocate of using stimulants to treat hyperactivity, psychoanalysts themselves admitted that psychotherapy was a time-consuming, expensive, and emotionally demanding intervention.[33]

Even psychoanalysts who were confident about the efficacy of psychotherapy could find that hyperactive patients were not particularly easy to treat. Psychotherapy required that a patient concentrate, be reflective, and follow dutifully the psychotherapist's suggestions. Understandably, this was an arduous requirement for hyperactive children to meet. Although the play therapy advocated by child psychoanalyst Anna Freud (1895–1982) might have been an effective intervention for hyperactive children, it was not commonly employed, and psychoanalysts found their hyperactive patients to be difficult.[34] One psychoanalyst described how her patient's "hyperactivity increased and all in a manner of a few minutes, she sat on my desk, wrote on the blackboard, and picked her nose excessively."[35] She concluded that her inability to help this particular patient was an indication that her hyperactivity was due to neurological, rather than familial, factors. Nevertheless, in a market saturated with potential patients but lacking enough psychoanalysts to meet demand, many psychiatrists accused psychoanalysts of turning away hyperactive children because they were difficult to treat successfully.[36] Psychoanalytic explanations and solutions to hyperactivity might have helped to explain some aspects of the disorder, but as diagnoses of hyperactivity expanded rapidly during the 1970s, and as psychiatrists increasingly looked to neurology to explain mental illness, psychoanalysis failed to remain viable for most families.

Social Psychiatry: "A Preventative Psychiatry"

Social psychiatrists not only recognized the impracticality of providing psychoanalysis to hyperactive children, but also attempted to put forth their own, presumably more pragmatic, solutions. During the late 1950s and early 1960s, psychiatrists concerned with preventing mental illness as well as the psychological effect of both geopolitical tension and domestic civil unrest increasingly looked to society as a source of psychiatric problems. For some social psychiatrists, mental illness could be prevented by alleviating its social causes, particularly poverty, overcrowding, crime, and substance abuse. For others, social psychiatry was more concerned with providing psychiatric services, often in community mental health centers, to the poor, who were believed to be disproportionately affected by mental illness. The corollary to both of these premises was that psychiatrists were expected to be both political and medical actors who had the specific skills and authority to foster social change.

Despite its seemingly radical foundation, the preventative strategies espoused by social psychiatrists reflected the beliefs of many psychiatrists during the 1960s, as well as the official policy of the APA, especially with respect to children and adolescents.[37] Many presidents of the APA during the 1960s supported the tenets of social psychiatry and urged their colleagues to study the pathological effects of social problems.[38] Much as the founding of *JAACP* was a response to growing interest in child psychiatry, the *International Journal of Social Psychiatry (IJSP)* and *Social Psychiatry* were founded in 1956 and 1966 respectively to reflect such concerns. The editorial statement that graced the inaugural edition of *Social Psychiatry* stressed how such journals would "disseminate this growing body of pertinent knowledge." It emphasized that the "world-wide movement toward a social orientation affects psychiatric practice, education and research" and went on to describe the editors' interest in papers that reported "on the social, cultural and familial determinants of psychic disorders, and their implications for social and psychological treatment."[39]

As Sir David Henderson (1884–1965), British psychiatrist and professor of psychiatry at the University of Edinburgh, indicated in his letter supporting the founding of *IJSP*, social psychiatry had its roots in the theories of previous generations of psychiatrists, especially the pioneering work of Adolph Meyer (1866–1950) in New York.[40] Henderson went on to stress that "social psychiatry is first and foremost a preventative psychiatry. It strives to combat all those causes of social and environmental nature which are manageable" and "concerns itself with public welfare in the widest sense."[41] A letter in the subsequent issue put matters more bluntly, stating that "social life is a prolific breeder of mental disease," and that "we would do, both for the patient and for society as a whole, immediately better if we could go to the roots of these troubles."[42]

Taken in the context of the 1960s, in the midst of the civil rights movement, protests against the Vietnam War, and the New Frontier and Great Society initiatives of Presidents Kennedy and Johnson, it was understandable that many psychiatrists were interested in social psychiatry. If President Kennedy's 1963 "Message to the United States Congress on Mental Illness and Mental Retardation" is any indication, social psychiatry was poised to challenge psychoanalysis for dominance during the 1960s. Kennedy's emphasis on eliminating the environmental causes of mental illness mirrored many of the preventative strategies of social psychiatry and was a significant aspect of his New Frontier policy.[43] His stress on the need for psychiatry to rely less on massive, isolated state hospitals, a system he called "social quarantine," and instead shift towards more numerous, smaller, and localized community mental health centers also echoed the calls of social psychiatrists.[44]

By the 1960s, social psychiatric research had indicated that preventative social strategies could help to explain and address hyperactivity in children. Researchers found that children brought up in poverty and exposed to vices such as petty crime, prostitution, and violence were much more likely to be hyperactive, impulsive, and distractible in school and succumb to mental illness later on in life.[45] Influential child psychiatrists Stella Chess (1914–2007), Alexander Thomas (1914–2003), Michael Rutter (b. 1933), and Herbert G. Birch (1918–1973) claimed that environmental factors could cause childhood behavioral disorders.[46] Psychiatrists were discovering that hyperactivity was most commonly diagnosed in poor children, often representing marginalized visible minorities.[47] Even some biologically oriented psychiatrists, such as Leon

Eisenberg, were sympathetic towards social psychiatric principles. Eisenberg not only lamented that psychiatrists "neglected prevention in our preoccupation with treatment," but also believed that "much . . . difficult behavior . . . stems not from the anatomical deficits, but from the social consequences of personality development."[48]

Feingold incorporated some aspects of social psychiatry into his theory of hyperactivity. Social factors might not necessarily cause hyperactivity, but they could undoubtedly exacerbate the disorder and contribute to other behavioral problems. Although "the ghetto can no longer claim sole ownership . . . without question, socioeconomic pressures influence instinctive behavior, and such behavior becomes imprinted on the patterns of the individual. . . . Deprived infanthood and adolescence can add up to a troubled adult."[49] What complicated matters for Feingold, however, was that disorders such as hyperactivity were not restricted to the ghetto but had "spread to the stamping grounds of the middle class and into wealthy suburbia."[50] Socioeconomic inequality might indeed cause much strife, and might even cause mental illness, but it did not entirely explain disorders such as hyperactivity, which were thriving in both lower- and middle-class populations.

Although the socioeconomic solutions put forward by social psychiatrists garnered much support during the 1960s, they required more political fortitude than psychiatrists could muster, especially after federal funding shifted from welfare and education programs to waging the Vietnam War. Indicative of this trend was Henry Brosin's "Presidential Address" to the APA in 1968/1969. In his "Response to the Presidential Address" the previous year, Brosin was optimistic about prospects of reducing poverty and improving mental health.[51] A year later, Brosin's comments were much more cautious. He noted that American involvement in Vietnam was drawing resources away from mental health programs and that difficult choices must be made regarding the direction of American psychiatry's focus.[52] Quoting John W. Gardner, the secretary of health, education, and welfare, Brosin indicated that a "crunch between expectations and resources" was occurring, especially with regards to "early childhood education, work with handicapped children, special education for the disadvantaged."[53]

More important to the parents of hyperactive children, however, was the fact that social psychiatry's focus on prevention did little for children currently experiencing academic and social difficulties due to their behavioral problems. As many parents were also aware, not all hyperactive children came from impoverished backgrounds.[54] Despite Kennedy's endorsement, APA sympathy, and the appeal of its preventative philosophy, social psychiatrists had difficulty addressing the escalating rates of disorders such as hyperactivity. By the 1970s, psychiatrists and parents were looking to more immediate solutions.

Biological Psychiatry: "No Twisted Thought without a Twisted Molecule"

The field of psychiatry that seemed most able to provide the immediate solution to hyperactivity demanded by psychiatrists and parents was biological psychiatry. Drawing on a long tradition of viewing mental illness as a predominantly neurological phenomenon, biological psychiatrists during the 1960s and 1970s were buoyed by recent advancements in pharmacology, particularly the development of psychoactive drugs. By the time the Feingold diet emerged, most, though not all, psychiatrists agreed that there was "no twisted thought without a twisted molecule."[55] Biological psychiatrists looked to the brain for the explanation of hyperactivity, and employed not only stimulant drugs but tranquilizers and antidepressants as treatment.[56] For many psychiatrists, biological psychiatry's emphasis on the neurological causes of mental illness gave the profession renewed respectability within the broader medical community, something that they believed was lacking during the years when psychoanalytic interpretations of mental illness dominated.[57]

Although the shortcomings of psychoanalysis and social psychiatry in treating hyperactivity helped to create a vacuum in which neurological approaches to the disorder could flourish, there were other factors that contributed to biological psychiatry's dominance of hyperactivity. First, biological psychiatrists could point to a long tradition of viewing childhood behavioral problems as neurological phenomena. They could also demonstrate, by highlighting the work of Charles Bradley during the late 1930s, that there was a long history of treating disturbed children with stimulants. For example, the first significant trial of methylphenidate by C. Keith Conners and Leon Eisenberg in 1963 pointed to Bradley's research on amphetamines and scholastic achievement.[58]

Similarly, biological psychiatrists had key allies in pharmaceutical companies such as Ciba, the manufacturers of Ritalin, which were understandably interested in profiting from the epidemic. Not only did Ciba fund research and conferences on hyperactivity, they produced films and pamphlets and raised awareness of the disorder at parent teacher association (PTA) meetings during the late 1960s and early 1970s.[59] Such marketing not only helps to explain the rise in rates of hyperactivity diagnoses, but it also hints at why Ritalin became "the treatment of choice [despite] . . . very little empirical basis for its supposed superiority" to other drugs such as dextroamphetamine.[60] Although the Convention on Psychotropic Substances in 1971 curtailed the practice of marketing directly to parents and teachers, physicians remained a target of drug companies, as pharmaceutical advertising in medical journals increased enormously during the 1960s and 1970s.[61] As historian Nancy Tomes has observed, "Under the American patent system, drug companies had roughly twenty years to profit from a new prescription drug; to build market share in a brutally competitive industry, they had a strong incentive to court physicians aggressively. Doctors were deluged with advertisements through the mail and the pages of their medical journals. . . . Whereas once doctors had been a relatively small side specialty in drug advertising, they now became its main target."[62]

Two final factors were, arguably, the most crucial to the acceptance of biological interpretations of hyperactivity. One of these factors related to how biological psychiatrists accounted for hyperactivity, and the other concerned the treatment of the disorder. First, by treating hyperactivity as a genetic, neurological condition, biological psychiatrists abandoned the implication made by both psychoanalytic and social psychiatric interpretations of the disorder that parents, and especially mothers, were to blame for their children's mental health problems. As sociologist Ilina Singh has noted, "Weary of mother-blame . . . for mothers with problem boys, the news about drug treatment and the emphasis on the organic nature of children's behavior problems appears to have been very welcome."[63] Many of the mothers who turned to the Feingold diet were ones who had been blamed for their child's behavioral problems. Lesley Freeman's interactions with both mental health workers and people in her neighborhood made her believe that, "whatever is wrong with the kid, obviously, it's the mother's fault. She feels like a failure, like a bad parent." When Freeman was told that her son's problem was genetic, due to neurological dysfunction, and had little to do with her parenting skills, she "was happy," stating, "I was off the hook, it wasn't my fault."[64]

. She felt "off the hook" in a different way when she was told by her physician that all her son needed was a pill, specifically Ritalin. Her first impression of Ritalin, like that of many parents, was that it "was amazing . . . a wonder drug."[65] Biological psychiatrists had an enormous advantage over their disciplinary rivals in that their method for treating hyperactivity could evoke immediate, and often dramatic, improvements in behavior. As Maurice Laufer stated in an interview for the *New York Times*, stimulant drugs provided psychiatrists with "one of the few situations in which you can do something quickly for people."[66] Laufer's colleague Eric Denhoff was so impressed by the efficacy of stimulant drugs that he considered "it as 'sort of criminal' to withhold treatment from those who can use it."[67]

Although some biological psychiatrists were puzzled by the fact that stimulants seemed paradoxically to calm hyperactive children, the belief in their effectiveness was such that stimulants were, in some cases, used as a diagnostic tool: if they calmed down an overactive, impulsive child, then the child likely had hyperactivity.[68] More importantly for parents, however, was the fact that ensuring that their hyperactive children had their medicine was a quicker, easier, and less expensive treatment modality than arranging for psychotherapy or analyzing and attempting to change the social factors that might be contributing to such behavior. Unlike other psychiatric approaches to hyperactivity, biological psychiatrists appeared to be able to establish the efficacy of Ritalin, and for many parents of hyperactive children, the drug seemed to be a veritable magic bullet.

Despite this apparent success, however, there were enough gaps in biological explanations of hyperactivity and concerns about drug treatment for Feingold's idea to gain considerable attention. Ironically, the chief argument against the biological method of treating hyperactivity involved precisely what had made their approach so popular, namely, the use of stimulants to treat hyperactive children. According to *New York Times* columnist Jane E. Brody, "Many parents dislike the idea of giving their children a potent drug day after day and are readily attracted to seemingly safer therapies, such as the diet Dr. Feingold has devised."[69] Interviews with parents who used the Feingold diet to treat their hyperactive children demonstrated that fears about the side effects of Ritalin, as well as uneasiness about drugging children, were among the most important factors leading to their employment of the Feingold diet.[70]

As Trevor Davidson explained, "I know medication works for a lot of people, but it didn't seem like the thing to do to take a 6-year-old kid and give him Ritalin or something of that nature, you know, and drug him up to behave the way you want him to behave."[71] Davidson's wife Gayle added that she was also concerned that Ritalin might affect her son's growth, and that he would use it as "a crutch," avoiding responsibility for his behavior.[72] Rosemarie Kushner worried not only that Ritalin could suppress her son's appetite but recalled news stories about amphetamine abuse that described "Ritalin being like an upper for regular folk." The combination of these factors made her "dead set against Ritalin."[73] Theresa McKay concurred, stating that hyperactivity "is probably what he'll always have and he needs to learn to deal with it. He needs to learn to recognize it. He needs to learn to control himself. . . . A pill doesn't teach you that." McKay added, however, that medication had value as a last resort.[74] In contrast, Maggie Jeffries's experience working in mental health care meant that she "certainly wasn't going to put my child on Ritalin."[75]

Some parents had been inclined to try drugs, but abandoned them due to side effects or ineffectiveness.[76] Sylvia Terry found that Ritalin made her five-year-old son "even more aggressive and . . . exasperated. . . . He started cursing quite a lot, . . . and I wasn't like that. I don't know where all that came from."[77] In order to deal with his hyperactivity, depression, and other psychological problems, Terry's physician had him taking up to three different medications, totaling nine pills per day. Not wanting him on so many medications, Terry sought the opinions of other physicians, but they all tried "to convince her that finding that right combination of drugs or getting the dosage adjusted would be the key."[78]

Lesley Freeman was initially impressed with some of the drugs prescribed to her son, but she soon found that

> after a little while they couldn't get it right. He was either a zombie or as it wore off he was crazy and throwing furniture. And I remember thinking, I'm so glad he's small for his age. And he was small, he wasn't growing on Ritalin, either. . . . And the neurologist said . . . "Oh it's okay that he's not growing, I'll give him growth hormones." . . . They changed his medication to Cylert and that was another wonder drug. It really kept the lid on. He was not the same child anymore. He was quiet . . . [but] he was hallucinating. It's hard to know if you're child's hallucinating when they're very young and they're not communicating very well. . . . Well, he was hallucinating and eventually I understood it because he told me, "You know today my teacher's tongue was long and green and furry."

Eventually he told his mother that he did not "want anybody to mess with my brain anymore" and she took him off all medication.[79]

Although one of the reasons Ritalin became preferred over stronger amphetamines and tranquilizers was that it was less dangerous, the drug nevertheless boasted its share of worrying side effects. Parents were warned about inhibited growth, insomnia, anorexia, irritability, heart rate changes, hallucinations, and unknown long-term effects. One clinical trial found that hallucinations associated with Ritalin use were so "severe, dramatic, and very frightening to the families it was not considered ethical to attempt replication."[80] Concern about side effects was so acute that a number of medical articles were published during the mid-1970s that advocated prescribing hyperactive children caffeine instead of Ritalin. The chief proponent of this alternative, psychiatrist Robert Schnackenberg, observed that many of his hyperactive patients self-medicated with coffee, which, he noted, was cheaper and less controversial than Ritalin. Although some researchers replicated

Schnackenberg's findings, most found that caffeine was not as effective as Ritalin.[81]

While physicians could read about the side effects of Ritalin in medical journals, parents were more likely to learn about such drugs from the media. American newspapers began reporting on the increasing numbers of prescriptions for hyperactivity drugs as early as the mid-1960s. Although stories differed with regards to whether stimulant drugs were good or bad for children, nearly all stressed that such drugs were contentious.[82] As *New York Times* science columnist Robert Reinhold (1941–1996) described, "The increasing use of drugs to help children with learning disabilities is generating a sharp controversy among medical men."[83] Reinhold quoted physicians who debated whether the long-term effects of hyperactivity drugs should be considered or not. While pediatrician Sidney J. Adler from California admitted, "I don't know what the drug will do in twenty years . . . but I have to try to do what we can do now to keep the kid from winding up in juvenile hall," Richard D. Young, a psychology professor at Indiana University, stated that "I shudder when I hear my colleagues suggest you can go ahead and give drugs to children . . . We really don't know what are the effects of a lot of these drugs on a lot of processes over the long run."[84] The headline of the story Reinhold wrote two years later, "Drugs Seem to Help Hyperactive Children," suggested a conclusion to the debate, but Reinhold continued to emphasize that the issue was divisive. He warned that "the treatment often involves keeping the children on amphetamines, which are widely abused, for many years. This has led to fears of long-term damage and charges that youngsters were being drugged into submission."[85] In another article, Reinhold reported "children swapping their pills in the school yard with unfortunate effects."[86]

Reinhold's comment that amphetamines had been "widely abused" highlighted one of the other reasons why many parents were wary about hyperactivity drugs. Ritalin, which had largely replaced more powerful amphetamines such as Dexadrine by the late 1960s, was nevertheless related chemically to a wide range of illegal amphetamines known generally as "speed," but also by the street names "'splash,' 'crank,' 'rhythm,' 'meth,' or 'crystal.'"[87] According to a *New York Times* story titled "The Speed that Kills," the "cannibalism of speed" had transformed "quiet flower children [into] ravaged scarecrows" or "speed freaks," whose high-risk behavior led to violence, suicide, and health problems such as "colds, infections, muscle tremors, cardiac problems, nausea, cramps, respiratory problems and hepatitis."[88] Such concerns in Sweden led to a complete ban on amphetamines, including Ritalin, during the late 1960s.[89]

The gateway to abusing such drugs was often attempts to improve academic performance. The opening paragraphs of "The Speed that Kills," for example, focused on a college student who, facing a deadline, accepted his girlfriend's offer of some mild amphetamines:

> With the first pill, Norman's mind clicked into gear and his fingers pattered over the keyboard as intricate insights streamed out of his head. After 10 hours he took a break and cleaned out all the drawers of his desk, arranged the pens and pencils in precise parallels, and stacked all his books so that the bottom corners were exactly even. Then he slid the pile so it coincided perfectly with the right angle at the corner of his desk. He stared at the pile for 20 minutes. Then he popped another pill, whistled through 10 more hours of typing and polished up the conclusion of his thesis with some more rather arcane insights. Norman drank half a quart of orange juice, emptied the icebox, and cleaned out all the shelves. Then he retyped some earlier pages which a dirty eraser had smudged, called up his girl and chattered gaily for 40 minutes. Then Norman passed out for 10 hours with dreams of an A in his head. He got a B-plus. Norman was speeding, but well under the limit.[90]

Although Norman's flirtation with speed might have been innocent enough, the euphoria associated with amphetamines, reported to be "potentially as addictive and debilitating as heroin," meant that such experiments could lead to abuse.[91] More subtly, however, the scenario of a college student taking speed to finish an assignment was not so different than parents taking a physician or teacher's advice to put their child on Ritalin. In both cases, academic difficulties could be allayed with the help of stimulants. While some parents and students found the potential benefits tempting, others were alarmed that it could lead to overdependence on medication and experimentation with other drugs. As child psychiatrist Mark Stewart described, "By the time a child on drugs reaches puberty, he does not know what his undrugged personality is and, even worse, his family does not know how to accept it."[92]

Illicit use of Ritalin also proved to be problematic. A Seattle health worker warned that Ritalin was "the No. 1 drug-abuse problem in that city," and was responsible for "severe medical problems including multiple abscesses, and damage to heart valves" when it was dissolved and injected.[93] Ritalin's legitimate use also courted controversy. Of particular concern was the notion that school officials were too eager to convince parents that medical intervention was required to improve their child's school performance or behavior. A Rhode

Island mother, for instance, felt "forced by school officials into drugging her child. . . . She said she had been constantly harassed by the school about her child's behavior and got a note from the school nurse which stated simply: 'Your child is hyperactive. He doesn't sit still in school. Please see a physician.'"[94] Another article reported a six-year-old girl in Michigan whose teacher convinced her father to consider Ritalin. The father reported that "the drug made her so withdrawn that sometimes she would sit for hours doing nothing." After getting "panicky" about her behavior, he brought her to a psychologist who determined that she "was perfectly healthy . . . [and needed] drill in basic reading, not drugs."[95] Sylvia Terry was told by her son's private Christian school that, unless her son was put on medicine, he could not come to school. This was ironic, since Terry had taken her son out of a previous school because they insisted that she employ corporal punishment. As she described, "They would not let him stay unless I paddled him . . . so he was being spanked a lot and I really think that when you add the low self esteem to whatever other problems he had that does more damage than anything."[96]

The extent of Ritalin use became national news in 1970 when it was reported that between 5 and 10 percent of the school-age population in Omaha, Nebraska, or approximately sixty-two thousand children, was on drugs for behavior and learning problems.[97] The story, reported on the front page of the *Washington Post*, prompted not only national outcry but congressional hearings, led by New Jersey congressman Cornelius E. Gallagher, and a 1971 conference organized by the Office of Child Development.[98] Although the conference would tacitly approve the prescription of stimulants for hyperactivity, provided parents were not coerced into agreeing to such measures and long-term follow-up was conducted, the mixed messages about Ritalin in the media did much to counter the glowing reports of its efficacy found in medical journals.[99] Although some Ritalin advocates, such as Eric Denhoff, were describing the drug in 1970 as "the penicillin of children with learning disabilities," to parents it might have seemed less like a magic bullet and more like "black magic," a drug whose benefits might not outweigh its costs.[100]

Conclusion

Feingold's explanation for hyperactivity was one of many that contended for legitimacy during the 1960s and 1970s. Although some psychiatrists such as Leon Eisenberg favored a more pluralistic approach, by the time *Why Your Child Is Hyperactive* was published, biological interpretations and pharmaceutical treatments of hyperactivity prevailed, and most of what social psychiatrists and psychoanalysts posited about the disorder had been either rejected or disregarded. The resolution of such debates occurred not because the biological approach was necessarily more valid, but rather because it was more direct, facile, and inexpensive, and because it capitalized on contemporary developments in psychopharmaceutical research. Nevertheless, none of the psychiatric approaches to hyperactivity, especially when viewed singularly, escaped criticism. Given the unwillingness of American psychiatrists to compromise on the cause of hyperactivity, it is interesting that Feingold himself acknowledged that hyperactivity had a social and interpersonal dimension. It is possible that, had American psychiatry agreed that hyperactivity was a multidimensional phenomenon, the Feingold diet would have been less controversial and, instead, viewed as another facet of a complicated and recalcitrant disorder. Feingold's acceptance of certain elements of psychoanalytic, social, and biological psychiatry made his theory appear more acceptable to parents who were less dogmatic about psychiatric theory than American psychiatrists.

The complex manner in which conceptualizations of hyperactivity were developed, debated, and either accepted or rejected highlights not only the contentious nature of psychiatric knowledge but also how explanations of mental illness could be open to interpretation. When it came to the biological approach to hyperactivity, parents who favored the Feingold diet found themselves in a difficult position. While they accepted the premise that hyperactivity had something to do with the nervous system, they rejected the pharmacological treatment of the disorder. Although most parents with hyperactive children during the 1970s ignored the warnings about Ritalin and, instead, concentrated on the positive effect it seemed to have, others were either not willing to do so or found that drugs were not effective or safe. Often desperate for any form of succor, these families turned to the Feingold diet.

Feingold's specific explanation for hyperactivity also capitalized on the etiological shortcomings of biological psychiatry. Unlike biological psychiatrists, whose vague explanations implied that some imprecise genetic defect was at fault, Feingold delineated a clear cause for hyperactivity, one that he claimed to be able to prove by "turning the disorder on and off" with food additives.[101] Although Feingold's theory became an explanation for hyperactivity that thousands of families found plausible, and food additives proved to be a tangible culprit against which they could take action, dissatisfaction with conventional explanations for and treatments of hyperactivity was only one reason why the diet was attractive. Feingold's idea also tapped into contemporary fears about the chemicalization of the food supply and broader concerns about the effects of a wide array of pollutants on human health.

Chapter 5

"Food Just Isn't What It Used to Be"

The role of chemicals in the food supply was an enormous debate during the postwar period, dividing opinion not only about food but technology, modern lifestyles, and the etiology of disease. While some, such as English psychiatrist Richard Mackarness, advocated a return not only to a chemical-free diet but to a "stone-age diet" based on protein rather than carbohydrates, others, such as nutritionist Frederick Stare and epidemiologist Elizabeth Whalen, believed that food additives were of enormous benefit and a sign of progress.[1] By the time of the emergence of the Feingold diet, most Americans would have agreed with journalist Jacquin Sanders that "food just isn't what it used to be," but not all would have agreed that the changes had been detrimental.[2] Such divisions accentuated the controversy surrounding the Feingold diet in both the public press and medical literature.

For parents who already believed that food additives were unhealthy and had either made or considered making their diet more organic, success with the Feingold diet confirmed their suspicions about the food supply. Other parents came to the Feingold diet from the other side of the debate, believing that there was nothing wrong with such chemicals or without any clear sense that such debates were occurring. Once these parents began investigating Feingold's theory, however, they tapped into a vast array of literature, dating primarily to the late 1960s and early 1970s, that claimed that the modern American diet was unhealthy. On the one hand, this legacy of suspicion helped to legitimize the Feingold diet for parents who might otherwise have questioned how food additives could cause behavioral disorders. On the other hand, the divisive nature of debates surrounding food additives meant that, no matter how Feingold distanced himself from such critics and attempted to make his diet appear scientifically valid, it was perhaps inevitable that it would be perceived as being on the radical side of the debate.

Although Feingold linked the rise in hyperactivity to postwar changes in how food was produced, packaged, and preserved, there had been concerns about food adulteration and food safety well before the emergence of TV dinners and microwavable meals. In Britain, as historian Derek Oddy indicates, concern about food chemicals had grown by the 1880s, as "chemical preservatives, such as borax or formalin, were used extensively in foodstuffs to extend shelf life. The opportunities for adulteration and the use of additives and improvers was irresistible, and there were some notable instances when consumers' health was seriously affected as producers cut corners."[3] Processed food products could be found on American store shelves at roughly the same time and, within two decades, spurred on by the publication of *The Jungle* (1906) by Upton Sinclair (1878–1968), American journalists had begun warning their readers about food additives.[4] *The Jungle*, which described the deplorable working and sanitary conditions in Chicago meat-packing plants, contributed to the passage of the Pure Food and Drug Act of 1906, which was intended to prevent "the manufacture, sale, or transportation of adulterated or misbranded or poisonous or deleterious foods, drugs, medicines, and liquors."[5] The path to legislation began when Sinclair sent a copy of *The Jungle* to President Theodore Roosevelt (1858–1919), who ordered two commissioners to investigate the author's claims. Despite the fact that the packers were given two weeks' notice of the commissioners' visit, nearly all of Sinclair's allegations were verified.[6]

There was a key difference, however, between the adulteration targeted by legislation such as the 1906 act and that which attracted attention during the 1960s. The adulteration described in *The Jungle* and other publications tended to focus on producers who added inedible or unsanitary substances to food in order to improve profit margin. For example, an anonymous physician writing in 1885 warned of the "man who willfully adds a non poisonous substance to an article which he sells, for the sake of increasing its bulk or weight, and afterward retails that to his customers as pure," as well as the "man who adds that to his goods which shall injure the health of the partaker." Such practices, according to the writer, "greatly effects the public health, and . . . thousands annually owe their deaths to the tricks of the trade." Even bread could be adulterated with "chalk, pipe clay, plaster of paris, alum, carbonate of ammonia, sulphate of zinc."[7]

Although the introduction of chemicals into the food supply following World War II also had much to do with increasing profits, postwar food additives were there purposefully to enhance flavor, retain color, and preserve, as well as to facilitate the invention of a whole new range of food products and fast food restaurants in which such products were sold.[8] Moreover, as historian Harvey Levenstein discusses, "Most American consumers were impressed by these achievements, and until well into the 1960s they showed little concern for the methods and ingredients which food processors employed to turn out a host of new products. . . . There was little inclination to question the products of the food business, which seemed to make life easier for the housewife with each new chemical breakthrough."[9]

The sales of processed foods such as Betty Crocker instant cake mixes and Swanson's TV dinners were profitable not only because of their novelty but also because they appeared to liberate housewives and working mothers from the drudgery of the kitchen. During the postwar period, most academic nutritionists and government agencies supported the proliferation of food additives.[10] One of the manifestations of the tight relationship between academic nutritionists and the food industry was the creation of the Nutrition Foundation in 1941. Envisioned and funded by food producers, the Nutrition Foundation published an academic journal entitled *Nutrition Reviews*, which included articles by academic nutritionists and was edited by Harvard nutrition scientist Frederick Stare. According to Levenstein, the Nutrition Foundation was often "used to marshal scientific opinions to correct 'superficial and faddish ideas' and to combat those questioning any of the 704 chemicals that by 1958 were commonly used in foods."[11] Although such chemicals were seen by the Nutrition Foundation as improving the food supply, the potential danger posed by ingesting synthetic colors, flavors, preservatives, and pesticides also prompted both considered and visceral reactions from many ecologists, politicians, journalists, and physicians. The debates about food additives reflected a broader climate of suspicion in American society that, in turn, contributed to interest in the Feingold diet. Although most Americans trusted the food industry and the governmental agencies that regulated it, many others had lost faith in American food and turned to theories that blamed it for ill health.

The Delaney Clause, *Silent Spring*, and the Fear of Food Additives

Despite the influence of the Nutrition Foundation and the proliferation of processed food, by the late 1950s and early 1960s trust in the American food supply was beginning to be shaken.[12] Ironically, this concern was partially due to a shift in American government policy regarding nutrition and health. As nutritionist Marion Nestle describes, until the 1960s government policy regarding food consumption was concerned with preventing nutritional deficiencies that could lead to diseases such as rickets, pellagra, and scurvy.[13] As such, government advice was for Americans to eat more calories, rather than fewer, and not to worry about restricting their intake of any particular foods. By the 1960s, however, amid concerns about certain chronic diseases, including heart disease, cancer, and diabetes, government opinion had shifted and now encouraged Americans to eat fewer calories. Americans were instructed to avoid certain foods, particularly those containing high levels of fat, cholesterol, sugar, and salt, as well as alcohol.[14] In the eyes of government nutritionists, food had shifted in many ways from being a protection against disease to being a cause of disease. But if traditional foodstuffs such as beef, butter, and eggs could be vilified by the new approach to nutrition, what did this imply for synthetic food additives?

If rising rates of chronic disease altered how nutritionists perceived food generally, two developments during the postwar period targeted food additives as being specifically harmful to health. These were the passing of the Delaney Clause in 1958, which affected the process by which food additives were approved by the FDA, and the publication of Rachel Carson's *Silent Spring* in 1962. The reception of both the Delaney Clause and *Silent Spring* highlight how the chemicals used in postwar food processing were a matter of intense debate. While consumer groups, environmental activists, and concerned physicians warned that such chemicals were a major threat to human health, food and chemical processing companies, the FDA, and skeptical health professionals argued that additives posed no harm or, in some cases, benefited health.

Although the Chemicals in Food Products hearings occurred during 1950 and 1951, the Food Additive Amendment, nicknamed the Delaney Clause after committee chairman Congressman James Delaney, was not added to the Food, Drugs, and Cosmetics Act of 1938 until 1958. The Delaney Clause specified "that no additive shall be deemed to be safe if it has been found to induce cancer when ingested by man or animal."[15] Two years later such principles were reapplied in the Color Additive Act.[16] The fact that it took so long to pass the amendment suggests that there was little political will during the 1950s to examine, let alone curtail, chemicals entering the food supply. According to the Senate Labor and Public Welfare Committee, whose members wrote the legislative history of the bill, the Delaney Clause was the result of "the most extensive and intensive hearings on legislative proposals in a particular field in which we have knowledge."[17] Indeed, Delaney had difficulty recruiting scientists to testify when he first launched the hearings.[18]

Nevertheless, in 1958 the bill received support from two sources, one conventional and one unexpected. First, the National Cancer Institute, spearheaded by the work of controversial pathologist Wilhelm Hueper, reported that "a number of chemicals long used in food might cause cancer in humans."[19] Unlike previous warnings from individual clinicians, this report from a national organization received a great deal of press. According to Delaney, however, who felt that his efforts to gain support for his bill were akin to "screaming at the wind," more influential were the efforts of Hollywood actress and health food advocate Gloria Swanson (1899–1983), who urged the wives of numerous congressmen to convince their husbands to support the amendment. The congressman had faced considerable opposition, and he claimed that the "the chemical lobby spent $90,000 to defeat" him in the 1956 congressional election. Delaney won by forty-five votes when normally he won by a ratio of two or three to one.[20]

The Delaney Clause was divisive for a number of reasons. First, it threatened the use of food additives in both agricultural production and food processing because the cost of proving that these additives were safe was believed to be onerous.[21] Food industry representatives also disagreed that substances found to be carcinogenic in animals should be automatically thought to be carcinogenic in humans.[22] Related to this was a debate regarding the point at which a substance should be classified as a carcinogen.[23] Some food additives were found to be carcinogenic but only when consumed by humans in extremely large amounts (see the cranberry example below) or in combination with other substances. Moreover, it was not easy to determine if links between supposed carcinogens and disease were examples of correlation or causality. As historian Christopher Sellers explains, the establishment of tobacco as a carcinogen made it difficult to determine if certain workplace chemicals, such as asbestos, were also causing cancer because so many workers smoked.[24] Finally, there was the argument that certain substances, such as the artificial sweetener saccharin, which could be carcinogenic at high levels of consumption, could also be beneficial to health, since it could help individuals lose excess weight.[25]

Given these complaints, according to Thomas H. Jukes (1906–1999), a prominent Anglo-American biologist then working for the American Cyanamid Company, the Delaney Clause represented "a serious concern to all manufacturing groups concerned with chemicals which come into contact with food."[26] Confirming such fears, the clause was invoked soon after its passage in the case of the chemical amintriazole, an herbicide used in cranberry bogs.[27] Although the FDA had banned the use of the herbicide in May 1959 because it had been shown to be carcinogenic, it was discovered nevertheless to have been used in a proportion of that year's crop. The contaminated cranberries were taken off the market with the assurance that even if some of the berries made it into Thanksgiving dinner, people would have to consume 15,000 pounds of them to suffer any harm.[28] Nevertheless, Americans refused to buy cranberries that November, and the government eventually reimbursed producers the $8.5 million lost due to the scare.[29]

The fear of carcinogens also contributed to the impact of Rachel Carson's *Silent Spring*. This was partly due to the book's content, particularly its chapter "One in Every Four," which linked environmental pollutants to cancer, but also to the fact that Carson spent many of her later years battling the disease, succumbing to a cancer-related heart attack in 1964.[30] But despite the unquestionable influence of *Silent Spring* in sparking environmental awareness and activism in the United States, Carson's book, like Delaney's amendment, was contentious. *Silent Spring* was, on the surface, about the broad environmental dangers and health problems caused by the overuse of pesticides. Underlying the sordid story of pesticide use, however, was a message about ecology, and how plants, animals, and humans were bound symbiotically to each other and the state of the environment. The songbirds rendered silent by pesticide use were a tragedy unto themselves but also a warning about what was in store for humans if the wanton use of DDT and other chemicals went unchecked.

While Carson's ability to describe chemical and ecological phenomena in a lyrical, poignant, yet scientifically rigorous manner captivated countless readers, it also threatened the chemical industry and the scientists and politicians allied with it. The ensuing debate was played out not only in industry journals but in the media, as both scientists and members of the media argued about Carson's claims. At the heart of the dispute was where to strike the balance between agricultural development, and the resulting availability of inexpensive food, and environmental stewardship. U.S. Department of Agriculture (USDA) spokesman Ernest G. Moore, interviewed in the *Washington Daily News*, suggested that Americans were unwilling to return to life without pesticides: "the balance of nature is a wonderful thing for people who sit back and write books or want to go out to Walden Pond and live as Thoreau did. But I don't know of a housewife today who will buy the type of wormy apples we had before pesticides."[31]

Although the issue of how to mediate between agricultural development and environmental sustainability was perceived to be a crucial debate that had global implications, much of the criticism centered not on Carson's scientific arguments but upon her manner of presenting it and whether she had the expertise to discuss the topic at all. According to her biographer, Linda Lear,

Carson "deliberately employed the rhetoric of the Cold War and the tone of moral crisis to persuade her readers of the urgency of her message."[32] Such tactics helped to propel the book to the top of the *New York Times* best-seller list during late 1962 but resulted in a virulent response mounted in "equally ideological terms."[33] As Lear suggests, these criticisms tended to focus on three factors, unrelated to her ecological argument. These included the fact that she had written for a public, rather than a scientific, audience, her relative lack of scientific training—although she had a master's degree in zoology, she had never published in peer-reviewed journals or held an academic post—and her status as an unmarried woman. Carson was branded as an overly emotional, manipulative spinster whose "reason had been sacrificed to sentiment."[34]

In many ways, these criticisms foreshadowed those directed at Feingold a decade later. Feingold, too, was criticized for writing for a popular audience. Although he was a qualified physician, he was perceived as a clinician, rather than a medical researcher, and was criticized for reporting his clinical observations rather than submitting his hypothesis to large double-blind clinical trials. Although Feingold's gender was not questioned, his age was raised as a complicating factor, as Feingold's detractors claimed that his grandfatherly charm could unduly influence parents' assessments of the Feingold diet.[35]

Perhaps the most striking synthesis of the criticisms leveled against Carson was agricultural company Monsanto's sarcastic parody of *Silent Spring*'s opening lines, which they sent to newspapers across the United States: "Quietly, then, the desolate year began. Not many people seemed aware of the danger. . . . How could the good life depend on something so seemingly trivial as bug spray? Where were the bugs anyway? The bugs were everywhere. Unseen. Unheard. Unbelievably universal. Beneath the ground, beneath the waters, on and in limbs and twigs and stalks, under rocks, inside trees and animals and other insects—and, yes, inside man."[36] *Time*'s anonymous reviewer of *Silent Spring*, while less creative, also focused on these themes, stating that "Miss Carson's . . . emotional and inaccurate outburst in *Silent Spring* may do harm by alarming the non-technical public, while doing no good for the things that she loves."[37] Emphasis on "Miss" Carson's gender, emotionality, scientific qualifications, and prose style was also a hallmark of attacks launched on her by the Nutrition Foundation, which would later target Feingold, and other industry groups such as the National Agricultural Chemicals Association, the Manufacturing Chemists Association, and the National Pest Control Association.[38]

Despite such attacks, the American public was willing to consider Carson's claims, and millions tuned in to a special edition of *CBS Reports* that addressed the controversy.[39] Carson's calm, thoughtful, and dignified demeanor on tele-vision belied the industry's depiction of her and, although the program was intended to be an unbiased account of the debate, the reaction from viewers indicated that the majority had been convinced by her arguments. This was despite the fact that some of Carson's colleagues, including nutrition writer Beatrice Trum Hunter, "found the program to be unbalanced in many ways. Although purportedly the program was an attempt to give equal opportunity to an expression of opposing viewpoints, it was weighted heavily, even if incon-sistently, in favor of the chemical approach."[40] Two weeks later, the public response resulted in political interest, as Carson was invited to testify to a U.S. Senate subcommittee on pesticides in 1963. Following Carson's testimony at the Senate hearings, a number of senators commented that her book would "change the course of history."[41]

It is difficult to say, however, if the senators' prediction came true. While *Silent Spring* is largely acknowledged to have marked the emergence of the modern environmental movement, in some ways its legacy has been more of polarizing opinion on environmental stewardship and the safety of the food supply rather than unifying sentiment around such issues.[42] The controversy surrounding the Delaney Clause and *Silent Spring*, along with governmental reluctance to toughen or even enforce existing food additive legislation, sug-gested to certain Americans that corporations and the government were simply not to be trusted when it came to the question of food safety. While other con-temporary regulatory crises, most notably the thalidomide scare, contributed to such beliefs, the rebellious, antiauthoritarian climate of the 1960s and early 1970s, fostered by the civil rights movement, student unrest, drug culture, Vietnam War protests, and the Watergate scandal, also engendered a general spirit of distrust among a growing number of Americans.[43] One of the many ways Americans expressed such dissent was by changing their diet to an organic or natural regime, free of additives and untainted by industry. As defenders of the food industry Elizabeth Whelan and Frederick Stare remarked in *Panic in the Pantry*, "The 'us versus them' attitude expressed . . . is an example of a broad feeling of suspicion the 'consumer-environmentalists' have for the 'greedy industrialists.' It all started with the publication of Rachel Carson's *Silent Spring*."[44]

Organic Food: "It's No Longer a Fad, It's a Movement"

Although Whelan and Stare proceeded to lambast the "food faddists" who trumpeted the necessity of a natural diet during the 1960s and 1970s, journal-ists such as Sandra Blakeslee observed that "more and more shoppers are beginning to eye the labels on products with suspicion, trying to find out whether the foods they shake, brown, heat and whip are really safe to eat."[45] In turn, the proliferation of natural food cookbooks, health food stores, and organic restaurants during these years suggested that a significant segment of the American population were searching for natural, additive-free foods. For example, in 1972 Alice Waters opened the groundbreaking restaurant Chez Panisse, which emphasized its use of local, seasonal, and unprocessed ingredients. The Berkeley, California, bistro became a model for other similar ventures in the United States. While counterculture publications such as *Rat* and *Good Times* published numerous articles on the political and health benefits of an organic diet, natural food was also discussed in the major newspapers and on television in nationally broadcasted programs such as the ABC and CBS evening news.[46] In a general sense, as journalist Jacquin Sanders described in a 1970 newspaper article,

> There is a growing repugnance to the things people do to the things people eat. As a result, more and more people are turning to organic food—produce that contains no trace of the chemicals, hormones, antibiotics, preservatives and dyes which have changed the appearance and taste of practically everything that goes into the human stomach. . . . It's no longer a fad, it's a movement. . . . Says Louis Martucci, owner of an organic food store in San Francisco: "When we started 12 years ago, our customers were elderly people. High school kids used to open the door and laugh at us. Now the same type of kid is our main customer."[47]

Martucci's comment that his previous customers tended to be older reflected a previous trend in whole food diets, in which vitamin supplements often played a key role in a healthy diet. As historian Catherine Carstairs has suggested, the whole food advocates of the previous generation, particularly Gayelord Hauser (1895–1984) and J. I. Rodale (1898–1971) but also Adelle Davis (1904–1974), focused on sales to middle-aged or elderly Americans and emphasized that their dietary regimes promoted longevity. Hauser's best-selling book *Look Younger, Live Longer* (1950) and Rodale's *Prevention* magazine, founded in the same year, were indicative of this trend.[48] Although Hauser lived to the age of eighty-nine, Rodale died rather infamously of a heart attack while he was a guest on the *Dick Cavett Show*. Minutes before he had bragged that he had "decided to live to a hundred" and that he "had never felt better."[49] The desire for longevity and disease prevention continued to attract older Americans to an organic diet during the 1960s and 1970s, but as Martucci suggested, young people were increasingly interested as well. Health food advocates such as Maryland store owner Oliver Popenoe recognized the division between newer organic food stores that emphasized "the idea of living in harmony with nature, rather than trying to conquer nature" and the previous type of "'pill stores' which tend to be for the old folks with a kind of faintly medicinal atmosphere."[50] Or, as Rodale stated, "Only a few years ago the organic health movement was an old people's crusade. Visitors to our farm were almost always white-haired men and women . . . close to the day of reckoning who wanted to stretch life a few more years."[51]

The dichotomy of old and new health food stores notwithstanding, people chose organic diets for a variety of reasons. Organic food, for example, was a political issue for many advocates. Sharon Grant, the spokeswoman for Mother Nature on the Run Caterers, a cooperative catering company, explained in 1972 that her choice for employment was the culmination of a political transformation that spanned numerous social issues: "I started getting into movements. I got involved with the political campaign of a black guy in New Haven—that's where I got radicalized—then with a businessmen's peace group here in Washington . . . I took off with a friend and went camping in Canada and Vermont. That really affected me. It was the first time I hadn't worked and it opened my eyes, showed me what was good for me. Right then I knew that I wanted my pace of life to slow down."[52] Natural food was also associated with consumer advocates, globally minded socialists, counterculture radicals, and whistleblowers, as books such as Beatrice Trum Hunter's *Consumer Beware! Your Food and What's Been Done to It* (1970), Frances Moore Lappé's *Diet for a Small Planet* (1971), Ita Jones's *The Grubbag: An Underground Cookbook* (1971), and former FDA scientist Jacqueline Verrett's *Eating May Be Hazardous to Your Health* (1974) suggested.[53]

It is important to stress, however, that many different political views and approaches were reflected in the organic food movement. Consumer advocate and Harvard-trained lawyer Ralph Nader (b. 1934) was willing to work within the political system and lobby Congress to force the manufacturers of hot dogs and baby food, for example, to reduce the amount of additives included in their production.[54] "Marcia," the columnist for *Good Earth*, believed that dietary change was "part of our total revolution." Writers for *Good Times* and *Rat* warned that not only was processed food adulterated in order to ensure "a drugged, poisoned, sick, mentally deranged populace" but the "vested interests of the U.S. are far too strong for them to revalue their approach."[55]

Other critics of processed food adopted different perspectives, however. For Beatrice Trum Hunter (b. 1918), whose first foray into writing natural food books was *The Natural Foods Cookbook* (1961), natural food was certainly about health, but it was also a matter of environmental responsibility and consumer activism.[56] Hunter was strongly influenced by Arthur Kallet and F. J. Schlink's *100,000,000 Guinea Pigs* (1933), a best-selling indictment of the American food, drug, and cosmetics industry and the government agencies and legislation expected to protect American consumers. Kallet and Schlink urged consumers not only to be vigilant regarding the products they purchased from the supermarket and pharmacy but to lobby government agencies, legislators, and newspapers about "the uncontrolled adulteration and misrepresentation of foods, drugs, and cosmetics."[57] Similarly, Hunter criticized the FDA for its inability to protect the safety of the food supply, particularly with respect to food additives. She believed that "the FDA has relinquished its mandated control of food additive safety testing to the very industries it was supposed to regulate. The effects are significant insofar as such policies may affect the well-being and very lives of the entire population."[58] Such criticisms of both industry and government with regard to food safety were similar to those made by other contemporary consumer activists, such as Ralph Nader, who also pushed for tougher regulations in the auto and nuclear power industries. Although Hunter was influenced by the philosophy of the clinical ecology movement and Theron Randolph in particular, the tone of her books, as well as her role as food editor of *Consumer Research Magazine*, indicate how improving consumer protection through better regulation was a central aspect of her thinking with regards to food. While they were waiting for government regulations to improve, Hunter advocated that consumers educate themselves about food additives and shop selectively. Only half jokingly, she suggested in a *New York Times* interview that, in order to avoid food additives, people should "shop around the walls of the supermarkets, where you find real food. All the fake food is in the middle aisles."[59] Although Hunter gave this advice "with a laugh," most North American supermarkets were designed with fresh fruit and vegetables, meat, and fish, dairy products, and bread around the edge of the store while packaged and frozen foods were in rows in the middle.[60]

In the case of Frances Moore Lappé (b. 1944), dietary choice was more than a matter of individual health and consumer rights; it was a global political statement. In her chapter "Recipe for a Personal Revolution," Lappé insisted that "what we eat is within our control, yet the act ties us to the economic, political, and ecological order of our whole planet. Even an apparently small change—consciously choosing a diet that is good for both our bodies and the earth—can lead to a series of choices that transform our whole lives."[61] Indeed, Lappé recalled feeling appalled when, following what she believed to be a "rousing political speech" in 1972, she was asked a question about "the difference between long grain and short grain brown rice." Shocked by such a banal question, she "wilted. I had wanted to convey the felt-sense of how our diet relates each of us to the broadest questions of our food supply for all of humanity. I had wanted to convey the way in which economic factors rather than natural agricultural ones have determined land and food use. Was I doing just the opposite? Was I helping people to close in on themselves, on their own bodies' needs, instead of using the information to help them relate to global needs?"[62]

Despite Lappé's concerns, many people continued to choose an organic diet for personal rather than political reasons. According to journalist Jeannette Smyth, there were those who believed that a natural diet could be spiritually as well as physically beneficial, and fit into a lifestyle that might also include yoga and transcendental meditation.[63] For others, diet was the hub around which their desire to return to a more natural, communal form of life was centered. As historian Warren Belasco has described, those Americans who were interested in returning to an era where particularly vilified additives, such as those derived from petrochemicals, were absent observed two maxims: "don't eat anything you can't pronounce . . . and if worms, yeast and bacteria grew on it, then it must be natural, for no self-respecting bug would eat plastic."[64]

Others groups that turned to organic foods included the increasing numbers of people who were sensitive to the additives found in food, people treated by physicians such as Theron Randolph. Mysterious conditions such as "Chinese restaurant syndrome," attributed by Chinese American physician Ho Man Kwok to monosodium glutamate (MSG) in a 1968 letter to the *New England Journal of Medicine*, reinforced the idea put forth by Randolph that food additives could cause chronic health conditions and that certain people were particularly sensitive. Kwok described the most prominent symptoms: "numbness at the back of the neck, gradually radiating to both arms and the back, general weakness and palpitations."[65] Finally, there were those such as English instructor Sylvia Feldman who believed simply that organic food "tastes better. . . . That's why I started buying organic."[66]

The profitability of organic food during the late 1960s and early 1970s meant that many of those who owned health food stores were not primarily spurred by politics. For many shop owners and grocery store chains, organic food was simply a prosperous enterprise, one that was attracting the attention of Wall Street investors.[67] As journalist Jean Hewitt noted in 1971,

> Whether fad or trend, health food stores are multiplying in both city
> and suburb. Some of the shops are individually owned and operated,
> but more and more they are members of chains that must see financial

growth through the increase in ecology-minded consumers who have turned to natural and organic foods. The little dusty health food store with a limited line of products is becoming extinct; the new stores, well-stocked and in busy locations, obviously aren't depending simply on trade from hippie-types who led the crusade for organic foods.[68]

Organic grocer and nonorganic restaurateur Lester Grossman concurred, admitting in 1971 that "I suppose the reason I am this involved is that it's a very good industry to be in. . . . Organic food is on the upswing . . . where most other industries in the country are on the downswing."[69] Another health food store owner added, "Look . . . I'm a merchant, not a missionary. We have no other causes—no political causes, no nothing. I just supply nice, good food."[70] Some store owners even felt guilty for taking advantage of people who appeared to be jumping on the bandwagon of organic food. Although James Kennedy started Kennedy's Natural Foods because he and others "super-sensitive" to additives were tired of "foraging the countryside for food," he recognized how stories in the media about the dangers in a particular processed food resulted in much higher sales for its natural alternative.[71]

Concern about food additives and interest in organic foods also entered the political arena during the early 1970s as a series of governmental hearings weighed in on the issue. Connecticut senator Abraham Ribicoff (1910–1998), for example, expressed his concerns about food additives in his opening address as chair of the "Chemicals and the Future of Man" hearings (1971):

It is a common saying that we are what we eat. If this is true, then Americans are becoming a nation of processed, packaged, and preserved people. Last year, Americans bought more processed than fresh foods for the first time in our history. We spent more than $60 billion for these convenience foods including such items as TV dinners, snack foods of all kinds, and frozen foods. With these foods we each consume every year more than four pounds of chemical preservatives, stabilizers, colorings, flavorings, and other additives. . . . Today more than 3,000 chemicals are deliberately added to our foods. These developments raise three basic questions: (1) How much do we know about the hazards to human health from these chemicals? (2) How much assurance of chemical safety should we require? (3) What must the federal government do to assure that the chemicals we absorb are safe?[72]

Another senator, Gaylord Nelson of Wisconsin (1916–2005), introduced legislation to ban untested additives by stating,

People are finally waking up to the fact that the average American daily diet is substantially adulterated with unnecessary and poisonous chemicals and frequently filled with neutral, nonnutritious substances. We are being chemically medicated against our will and cheated of food value by low nutrition foods. It is time to take a careful look at the prolific use of additives permeating our foods. . . . The profits of the food industry are being placed above the public health as regards the safety, nutrition, and necessity of food additives. Synthetic and convenience foods mean high profits and greater market control of the food industry.[73]

Other senate and congressional hearings were held during the early 1970s, including those on particular food additives such as the cyclamates used as artificial sweeteners, the synthetic hormone diethylstilbestrol (DES), and nitrates.[74] There were other contemporary hearings on more general aspects of food additives and nutrition, often chaired by prominent politicians such as Senator Edward Kennedy (1932–2009) and Democratic presidential nominee George McGovern (b. 1922).

Kennedy and McGovern would also become involved in the debate about the Feingold diet. Kennedy was unimpressed by the FDA's inability to take firm action with regards to Feingold's theory. His frustration with the FDA was expressed at a meeting of the Senate Labor and Public Welfare Committee's Subcommittee on Health. According to the *Los Angeles Times*, Kennedy was

anxious for a study to begin. "We want to run this thing out and test it," he said. "If you're not doing it, we want to know why. If it's because of a lack of funds, we want to fulfill our legislative responsibility." Dr. Albert Kolbye, associate director for science of the FDA's bureau of foods, said, "We're getting ourselves together, Senator." "You'll have to do better than that," Kennedy said. "We will not tolerate a mish-mash of government agencies which all want a piece of the action," Kennedy said, "The commissioner of the FDA must indicate that this is a priority action."[75]

Although Kennedy would be disappointed by the FDA's response to Feingold's hypothesis, the FDA did ban some substances, most notably cyclamates and DES.[76] Ironically, by banning cyclamates, the FDA was accused of bowing to the pressure of the sugar industry lobby.[77] Nevertheless, critics such as Beatrice Trum Hunter continued to charge that the FDA and the USDA were too lenient in allowing harmful additives into the marketplace.[78] Others bemoaned the fact that the FDA investigated individual chemicals only on a case-by-case basis—and only after a great deal of public outcry—rather than considering the safety of broad categories of additives such as those derived from petrochemicals.

In contrast, many nutrition scientists, most notably Harvard's Frederick Stare, argued that the regulators had gone too far and that this was "making eating a less enjoyable experience."[79] With regards to what he and coauthor Elizabeth Whalen called "cyclamania," Stare argued that, because of the Delaney Clause, "a cancerphobic American public was willing to ban a substance upon hearing the merest shred of evidence."[80] The authors proceeded to state that "if the Delaney clause had not been exerting its force, it is unlikely that the general public anxiety about food additives would be as intense as it is now. Healthfoodland would be a remote hideaway for eccentric people, instead of the billion-dollar business it is today."[81] Similarly, an anonymous editorial in the *Lancet* argued that the evidence used to demonstrate that cyclamate was a carcinogen was insufficient. In the study analyzed, only four of the fifty rats tested developed bladder cancer and, since the researchers had fed the rats a mixture of saccharin and cyclamate, it was difficult to determine what caused the carcinoma. The author asked, "Was the fate of the world's sweet tooth decided just on the response of . . . 4 rats?"[82] Ultimately, the editorial blamed the Delaney Clause for oversimplifying how scientists determined the carcinogenicity of food additives. In the case of food additives and cancer, as with food additives and hyperactivity a few years later, many physicians were unwilling to denounce substances before "a detailed understanding of the mechanisms involved" was determined.

Stare's implication that health food advocates were more concerned with profit than health was disingenuous given his own connections to the food industry and the reliance of the Harvard department of nutrition, which he founded in 1942 and continued to chair until 1976, on corporate funders.[83] Other prominent supporters of the food industry had connections to the food, drug, and chemical industries; Stare's Harvard colleague Jean Mayer (1920–1993) served on the boards of directors of Monsanto and Miles Laboratories. Mayer was less comfortable with the connections between nutrition science and the food industry, however, and it is possible that this was one reason why he left Harvard to become president of Tufts University in 1976. With regards to pesticides, Mayer recommended a balanced approach, stating that the "big problem has been the indiscriminate use of pesticides in the past" but there "is no sense in going from one extreme to the other and going back to the Cave Age."[84] Nevertheless, Stare was correct in observing that health food had become big business by the 1970s, as the comments of organic food store owners attested. Another example of the industry's profitability was J. I. Rodale's health-food press, which made over $9 million in 1970.[85] Even as the organic food movement faded during the late 1970s and 1980s, food companies were still able to develop products which capitalized on the desire of "yuppies" for "health" food.[86] The role of economics as well as politics on both sides of the debate over food additives made it difficult for consumers to delineate if there was a boundary between ideology and nutrition science.

For parents, especially those whose politics, environmental concerns, and health had not conditioned them to favor one side of the debate, it was difficult to weigh the opinions of various scientific authorities regarding the dangers of food additives and the benefits of organic food. Both sides of the debate over food additives were represented in the media, providing no easy answers. Even the safety of the humble maraschino cherry was difficult to determine. While the World Health Organization deemed the red dye used in the cherries to be carcinogenic, the FDA believed that the amount of dye used was too minimal to warrant a ban.[87] The familiarity of contested products such as maraschino cherries made it difficult for some families to believe that these foods were dangerous. As journalist Elaine Jarvik described in an article featuring two Utah families on the Feingold diet, "even at a time when Americans had begun to wonder if perhaps they were, indeed, what they ate, Dr. Feingold's diet was not so easy to swallow. Here was a man warning of evils lurking in something as innocuous as frozen french fries, as healthy as toothpaste, as all-American as hot dogs. It sounded, to some, a little paranoid, and about as plausible as grapes and copper bracelets for cancer and arthritis."[88]

Multiple messages also emerged from the medical community. For example, the AMA stated in 1969 that "there is no reason to believe that the present use of chemicals in foods is endangering the health of the people."[89] George Christakis of the Mount Sinai Medical Center in New York described organic foods as a "public health threat" due to the false health claims made about them.[90] In contrast, an editorial in the Lancet warned that "the question of the ultimate effects of food additives on man is unanswered. Human experiments are possible only on a very small scale, and, in any case, they do not mimic the life-long, very low doses to which man is exposed."[91] Geneticist and Nobel laureate Joshua Lederberg (1925–2008) agreed with the Lancet editorial, stating that "it would be held a catastrophe if only a hundred U.S. consumers a year were carcinogized by a food additive they could happily live without."[92]

Parents who would employ the Feingold diet, as with other Americans, came to the notion that food additives could be harmful from a number of different perspectives. While some were already convinced of the benefits of an organic, natural diet, others were skeptical that food additives could be the cause of their child's hyperactivity. Maggie Jeffries, for example, described herself as a "health food freak" who had been influenced in her late teens by Adelle Davis's books on nutrition. Believing that many of her allergies were due to reactions to food dyes, Jeffries avoided them to the point that the only food in her house that was "artificially colored or flavored was margarine, pancake syrup, and occasionally maybe some ice creams that were colored." Although the dyes in these products caused problems for her son, she found out that most of the additives he was consuming were provided in foods he ate at school.[93] Sharon Aubrey "had always been interested in nutrition" and baked her own bread. Her son rarely came into contact with food additives, but nevertheless reacted strongly to many naturally occurring salicylates, particularly in grapes and tomatoes.[94]

In contrast, other parents had little apprehension about food additives before hearing about the Feingold diet. Lesley Freeman had lived in Africa for a year with her children and, since all she could get was powdered milk, she "used to put red food coloring in the milk and sugar because it didn't taste so great."[95] Other parents cooked most meals from scratch but had not been in the habit of reading labels, and thought nothing of giving their children drinks, desserts, and chewing gum containing artificial colors and flavors.[96] Although Rosemarie Kushner refused to give her son Ritalin, she recalled being ambivalent about food additives. When Kushner used her skills as a librarian to research the Feingold diet, however, she discovered literature that warned about food additives and decided to try it.[97] The experiences of parents, the opinions of physicians and regulatory agencies, and the stories found in the press all indicate how much American attitudes about processed food could vary by the time Feingold wrote *Why Your Child Is Hyperactive*.

Conclusion

During the postwar period, the amount of food additives found in the American diet increased markedly. Almost immediately, as the 1950–1951 Delaney hearings indicated, they became a source of controversy, although it took until the late 1960s for the furor over food additives to become front page news. Such developments occurred partly because of the Delaney Clause and Rachel Carson's *Silent Spring* but also because of an emerging culture of mistrust within the United States. By the early 1970s, the debate over food additives also highlighted political schisms within the nation and differentiated between those who had faith in the food industry and federal regulatory agencies and those who did not. Trusting the government over whether food additives were safe was not so different than believing its claims about the war in Vietnam, about the threat posed by drugs such as marijuana and LSD, or about the fidelity of the American president. It was into this divisive context that the Feingold diet emerged. Given the cultural climate of suspicion during the early 1970s, it is not surprising that the media found Feingold's claims so captivating and that the food industry found them so alarming.

Food additives, however, were not simply a matter of politics. Although critics such as Whalen and Stare tended to lump all of those who warned about food additives, including Feingold, into a homogeneous mass, those concerned about food additives came to the issue from many different perspectives.[98] As highlighted by journalist Wade Greene in 1971, the organic food movement included

> a wide variety of food cultists, from old-line vegetarians to youthful Orient-oriented "macrobiotic" dieters . . . plus reactionaries yearning to turn back all clocks, urban dropouts in search of simpler, more natural lifestyles, ecologists who are worried about the long-range environmental effects of some chemicals, Dr. Strangelove paranoids who read poison plots on the ingredient labels of pancake mixes and, increasingly, rather ordinary folk to whom pronouncements about the perils of cyclamates, DDT, mercury, monosodium glutamate, phosphates, etc., have stirred a wariness about all man-made chemicals, particularly those that get in their food.[99]

Food additives may have been despised equally by the counterculture anarchist, the environmental toxicologist, and the food allergy sufferer but for quite different reasons. What the anarchist may have interpreted as a plot machinated by a corrupt government and greedy industrialists, the toxicologist may have seen as another indication of western society's perilous, but perhaps unwitting, descent into an increasingly polluted environment. Food allergy sufferers might have perceived food additives on a much more intimate level, viewing them as simply another barrier they faced to a life free of chronic illness.

In other words, the decisions Americans made about food additives were not usually based solely upon the reading of a newspaper article or the watching of a television program, but were a reflection of political beliefs, cultural background, spirituality, and, most importantly, personal and familial health experiences. This highlights one of the challenges inherent in any sort of preventative health policy: people are resistant to break habits for the benefit of their health unless personal experiences dictate that they do so. As numerous historians of nutrition and food have outlined, it has been difficult for physicians and policy makers to convince people to change their diet, even if such changes were salubrious or economical, chiefly because "everyone thinks that they are an expert on their own diet."[100] But when the development of an ideology or an experience of ill health provides the necessary evidence for an individual that breaking a habit is warranted, then such beliefs and experiences can belie the sanctions of even the highest medical authority.

Chapter 6

The Feingold Diet in the Media

Anxiety about food additives persisted into the mid-1970s, in the face of a recession that threatened to undermine consumers' willingness to pay for expensive organic foods. As journalist Anna Colamosca reported in 1974, "Despite soaring prices, the $600 million health food industry seems to be holding up well." Although Colamosca stated that "hundreds of health food stores across the country have gone out of business because they were over-charging in an effort to make a fast buck," she also believed continuing news-paper stories "related to the food industry have kept many people doggedly returning to their favorite health food stores over the last six months."[1] One story she cited was Feingold's recent linkage of food additives and hyperactivity. Just as interest in the Feingold diet was fueled by concern about food additives as well as dissatisfaction with treatments for hyperactivity, Feingold's theory also kept food additives in the headlines while interest in organic foods began to wane and health food sales began to slump.[2]

It is worth repeating that Feingold did not initially court such attention himself. It was the AMA who invited him to its 1973 and 1974 conferences and organized Feingold's press conferences. Nevertheless, once Feingold decided to reach out to the public with his theory, he did so with an eagerness and energy that belied his age. Ironically, the refusal of the top medical journals to provide Feingold with a forum in which to circulate his ideas among his fellow physicians resulted in his idea receiving much greater exposure in the main-stream media; and just as parents were able to read about the diet in their local newspaper, so too were clinicians more likely to read *New York Times* than *JAMA*.

Feingold's ability to disseminate his ideas through the media was facilitated by increased media interest in health reporting during the postwar period.[3] Given the intertwining relationships between the media, policy makers, physicians, patients, advertisers, and readers, the media's role with regards to health was a complex one. The reliance of mass media on advertising revenue helps to explain some of these ambiguities. Historians Virginia Berridge and Kelly Loughlin have described how "the mass media has been enlisted as a public health tool through the development of mass advertising campaigns, and it has been the focus of opposition and control due to the use of mass advertising by commercial interests such as tobacco and alcohol."[4] The role of the advertiser, however, was passive compared to the media's role as a purveyor and interpreter of news and a teller of tales. Both health scares and miracle cures made for compelling stories, ones that generated interest and could have a profound impact on both public policy and the actions of the general public.

Sociologist Clive Seale has emphasized how reports about food scares were particularly apt to attract media interest, stating that "the depiction of ordinary objects whose ingestion is essential for life, yet nevertheless reveal themselves as threats to life, presents a highly entertaining juxtaposition of opposites for the media health producer."[5] Other researchers have echoed Seale's observations about the popularity of food-scare stories.[6] The divisive nature of many of the nutrition-related health scares during the postwar period probably added to their appeal. Unlike the thalidomide scandal, however, which was presented as a clear-cut case of corporate greed and incompetence, there were almost always two justifiable perspectives represented in stories involving pesticides, food colors, artificial sweeteners, and even the recommended daily allowances of fat, cholesterol, and alcohol. The banning of cyclamate sweeteners, for instance, might have been a victory for organic food advocates and the sugar industry, but it dismayed diabetics, nutritionists, and physicians concerned about obesity.[7]

Seale's tendency to portray journalists as scaremongers who exaggerated the seriousness of such food crises also overlooks the fact that journalists did not act alone in constructing these stories. In the British case of the Aberdeen typhoid outbreak of 1964, for instance, a symbiotic relationship existed between the media and the medical officer of health, Ian MacQueen, with regards to reporting the story of contaminated corned beef. While MacQueen, who had originally studied journalism, was able to use the press to help contain the outbreak and to further his desire to promote health education, the media found the outbreak to be "a good story," one that was "intensely reported," and "began to take on a life of its own."[8] Although the Milne Report, an inquiry into the outbreak, criticized the relationship between MacQueen and the media, stating that "the outbreak and the possible dangers of its spread were exaggerated to such an extent that the incident received publicity out of all proportion of its significance," many Aberdeen physicians supported MacQueen's efforts, and the investigative journalism employed during the outbreak served as a model for later food crises.[9]

With the Aberdeen typhoid outbreak and the bovine spongiform encephalopathy (BSE) crisis of the 1990s, the danger posed by tainted beef was unquestionably real. What was questioned in both cases was the media's role in exaggerating the degree of risk and contributing to consumer panic and financial loss in the agricultural and tourism sectors. In the case of more radical or unsubstantiated health claims, the impact of the media can be even greater, especially when public health authorities are unwilling to support such claims. In his discussion of the media's role in providing alternative nutrition advice to American consumers, Warren Belasco has argued that "as health and nutrition counselors, the media ranked second only to physicians. And since most medical information dealt with weight or acute health problems (like diabetes), the mass media were the principal source of advice and information."[10] Belasco believes that, with regards to counter-cuisine and the organic food movement, the American media "sought the high middle ground of conservative reform," rejecting the extreme views of both sides of the debate.[11] This was not, however, the case with the Feingold diet. Newspapers presented strong opinions on both sides of the debate, often angering both proponents and critics.

From the time of his first television appearance on San Francisco television in 1972 and until his death a decade later, Feingold publicized his theory via hundreds of newspaper editorials, magazine articles, radio debates, and television programs. According to Feingold, by 1976 the number of newspaper articles had reached approximately twenty-seven per month, making it, according to a *Los Angeles Times* reporter, "one of the most widely discussed and controversial topics in American medicine."[12] While the Feingold diet often made the front page, for example in Morton Mintz's story for the *Washington Post* in late October 1973, it was also discussed in sections devoted to food, health, women's issues, parenting, and lifestyle.[13] Feingold's hypothesis even found its way into newspaper quizzes that focused on current events.[14] The Feingold diet was covered by newspapers read by millions, such as the *New York Times*, and low-circulation magazines such as *Utah Holiday*. Feingold was willing to be interviewed not only on nationally syndicated television programs such as the *Phil Donahue Show* and NBC's *Today* hosted by Barbara Walters (b. 1929) but also local programs. During a visit to Texas in 1978, for example, the

Dallas–Fort Worth Feingold Association arranged for Feingold to be interviewed on the local ABC and NBC stations. The NBC interview was conducted
by emerging talent Charlie Rose (b. 1942).[15]

Although most media reports of the Feingold diet, especially during the
1970s, tended to be positive, some were negative and others were fairly neutral,
or emphasized the controversial nature of the issue. Both positive and negative
coverage used arguments about the Feingold diet as a means to achieve political ends that had little to do with helping hyperactive children. As such, discussion of the Feingold diet in the media could become a dispute about the role
of government and regulation in a free market system as much as it was a debate
about how to explain and treat hyperactivity. As the political climate changed
during the 1980s, so too did the tenor of stories about the Feingold diet and
the public's willingness to question clinical approaches to hyperactivity. The
Feingold diet existed in the media not only as a captivating story about a
charismatic physician and his startling discovery, but also as a barometer for
the public's attitude towards the medical community, American corporations,
and the government's ability to monitor and regulate these entities.

"A Precious Commodity to Hyperactive Children?"

The first newspaper articles about the Feingold diet appeared after the allergist
presented his findings to the AMA conference in June 1973, and for the next
decade, stories about the diet appeared regularly in American newspapers.
Reflecting concerns about food additives and hyperactivity, newspapers were
quick to report on Feingold's ideas and the controversy that surrounded it.[16]
Media coverage of the Feingold diet tended to fall into three categories: stories
that supported Feingold's hypothesis, stories that were skeptical or reported on
studies that yielded negative results, and relatively neutral stories that represented both sides of the debate. Newspaper and magazine stories could take the
form of anonymous reports of trial results, regular columns contributed by a
health professionals, science or food writers' reports, editorials written by food
industry representatives or advocates of the Feingold diet, multipage feature
articles, debates between experts, or letters to the editor.

Provocative headlines often made clear the perspectives represented in
the stories. For instance, the titles of a pair of stories favorable towards the
Feingold diet and published in the *Washington Post* in 1975 were "Color It
Dangerous" and "Coloring Food—Who Suffers?"[17] Negative stories included
those written in 1977 and 1978 by health columnist G. Timothy Johnson, titled
"Food Additive Link to Hyperactivity Unproven" and "Diet-Hyperactivity Link
Still Unproved."[18] Similarly, the headlines of neutral stories often focused on

the controversial nature of the Feingold diet or posed a question about his theory, such as "Can Dye-Hyped Foods Cause Hyperactivity?"[19] Depending on which story was read, the Feingold diet could be perceived as either "A Precious Commodity for Hyperactive Children" or "Another 'Miracle' Diet Cure that Failed."[20]

Despite the fact that it is possible to categorize stories about the Feingold diet as positive, negative, and neutral, these categories existed on a continuum stretching from the extremely positive to the utterly dismissive. While a number of relatively positive stories were simply reports of a successful trial or coverage of a family that had benefited from the Feingold diet, some of the most positive stories were written by ideologically motivated columnists who used Feingold's theory to berate the government or the food industry. For example, Colman McCarthy's (b. 1938) glowing review of *Why Your Child Is Hyperactive* was representative of his tendency to criticize the American government and capitalism. As a 1986 article about McCarthy's dismissal from the faculty of American University described, "Mr. McCarthy's espousals of leftist ideas—on everything from civil disobedience to vegetarianism—rarely fail to ignite a reaction."[21] Characteristically McCarthy's endorsement of Feingold's book was inflammatory:

> Feingold's book has the ring of alarm to it, as well it should. Such a message is likely to be dismissed as heresy among the true believers who trust the fake food companies and the Food and Drug Administration. Feingold can be quickly put down by those in power: his studies were "unscientific," they were of limited range, and besides who is he—just a tinkering allergist—to say he has the answers. Doesn't Feingold know that we must see the bodies falling dead in the street before there is "absolute proof" and action can be taken? . . . Too many citizens suspect that they cannot trust the food companies, and they know that the FDA is uncaring or underfunded, or else it would be leading the way to find answers, not telling Feingold to go away merely because he wants the consumer to see clearly that the food he is buying is fake. . . . If parents want to act to protect their child, they will likely have to do it on their own. The best help they may get is not from the medical community, the FDA nor the food companies, but from this book.[22]

Not surprisingly, the last two sentences from the review were used in Random House's print advertising campaign for *Why Your Child Is Hyperactive*.

An anonymous 1975 editorial published in McCarthy's paper, the *Washington Post*, also criticized the manner in which the FDA was handling

Feingold's hypothesis. Reporting on the hearings of a senate health subcommittee, the author urged the FDA to act on the "unsettling" findings of a study
into the Feingold diet, one led by C. Keith Conners of the University of
Pittsburgh, that were made known at the hearing:

> The Food and Drug Administration has promised to make recommenda-
> tions shortly on where to go from here. That is the least the agency can
> do. It is regrettable that the FDA has not taken a position of leadership in
> this crucial health issue, rather than lagging behind until all but forced
> to action because of public opinion. As for the manufacturers of artificial
> foods, little can be expected of them except business as usual. The bur-
> den of proof in these matters seems to rest upon those who believe
> a substance is dangerous rather than those, such as the manufacturer,
> who claim that it is safe. The effect of this attitude, in the case of fake
> flavors and colors consumed by children, is to make guinea pigs of our
> children and laboratories of our homes.[23]

By reacting to Conners's study, which had not yet been peer-reviewed let alone
published, by the time the story was published, the author demonstrated how
both Feingold's supporters and his detractors were guilty of exaggerating or
extending the findings of the clinical trials of the Feingold diet in ways that
supported their own views. Despite the fact that Senator Edward Kennedy
stated during the hearings that Conners's result "probably isn't conclusive," the
editorial insisted that the psychologist's findings indicated that "the need is
now for immediate and expanded testing that will show either that a problem
exists or it does not."[24] In this way, the approach taken by the author of this
positive editorial was not so different from that of the Nutrition Foundation,
which reported negatively on the diet prior to the publication of any controlled
trials and believed that there was little need for such "expanded testing."[25]

Other writers were quick to place credibility in Feingold's claims, even
though clinical trials into his hypothesis had not been completed. Nicholas von
Hoffman (b. 1929), for example, used Feingold's hypothesis to criticize Attorney
General William Saxbe's (b. 1916) argument that increase in crime was due to
"parents, permissiveness and pornography."[26] Stating that "neither the conservative attribution of crime to pornography nor the liberal's blaming it on bad
housing show a convincing chain of causality," von Hoffman wondered if the
increase in crime "may be traceable to the involuntary ingestion of drugs in our
food supply."[27] Von Hoffman posited that Feingold's "hypothesis would also
explain the correlation between crime and family income. It's lower income
people who can't afford fresh, unadulterated food and whose social surroundings

don't frown on the consumption of cellophane-wrapped Blinky-Tinkies and all the other chemically manufactured junk foods."[28] Although von Hoffman's political leanings were less obvious than those of Colman McCarthy, his article, written months before *Why Your Child Is Hyperactive* was published in late 1974, indicated how Feingold's hypothesis could be used to critique many aspects of American society and government.

For Robert Rodale (1930–1990), the son of health food publishing magnate J. I. Rodale and his successor as the head of Rodale, Inc., Feingold's theory had both political and financial relevance. Given that his publishing business depended partly on dissatisfaction with the food supply, Rodale had a clear financial incentive to support Feingold's claims. In his syndicated column "Organic Living," which appeared in numerous American newspapers, Rodale described the food industry's use of additives as "possibly the most heinous 'crime' perpetuated by the food processors on an unknowing public," a crime that affected children the most.[29] Continuing on this theme, Rodale speculated, "Let's imagine, and it doesn't take too much, that Dr. Feingold's theories are proven correct. Does this mean that food processors can be tried for the 'crime of negligence' or can food processors who cause cancer be tried also? Maybe they should, if only in the court of public opinion."[30]

Another article by Rodale that mentioned the Feingold diet emphasized how scientists were unable to predict or explain the potentially hazardous effects of the "2,500 substances currently being added to our food supply" and that the only way to be safe was to avoid additives altogether.[31] Rodale began by discussing how "a strange thing happened recently in a University of West Virginia laboratory when adult house flies were fed a diet containing common food coloring additives. As soon as the flies were exposed to light, they died." A picture of a dead fly and a vial of dye illuminated by a bright light accompanied the story. According to the postdoctoral research fellow who observed the phenomenon, "The flies were killed by photodynamic action, a destructive effect produced when the dye and normal light interact." The research fellow added ominously that "the wide usage of dye additives in foods, drugs and cosmetics, could result in photodynamic injury to man."[32] Rodale described Feingold's findings about food additives and hyperactivity, as well as similar observations made by Pennsylvania physician Stephen D. Lockey: "Many instances of mild psychological trauma and other weird symptoms could conceivably be caused by food chemicals. But scientists may never be able to pinpoint which ones are responsible, because of the complex interactions between all the thousands of chemicals in our environment. While researchers are busy trying to solve the puzzle, you can protect yourself by eating foods that don't contain additives."[33]

Although Rodale's business interests meant that readers might greet his concern about food additives with skepticism, the observations of investigative reporter Morton Mintz were more difficult to dismiss. Not only was Mintz a respected journalist for the *Washington Post*, he had been first to report on a number of health-related scandals, most notably the thalidomide disaster in 1962.[34] Unlike writing by McCarthy and Rodale, the tone of Mintz's front-page story was measured, and he refrained from making judgments about Feingold's theory. Mintz added how hyperactivity could also be treated with amphetamines such as Ciba-Geigy's Ritalin, mentioning that the drug "accounted for $11 million in sales," but he did not suggest explicitly that the Feingold diet might jeopardize such profits.[35] Despite the muted tenor of Mintz's article, it quickly generated significant attention. According to McCarthy, who also worked at the *Washington Post*, Mintz's story on the Feingold diet resulted in more mail being sent to him than on any other subject Mintz had covered in the twelve years since he had written about the thalidomide disaster.[36] Senator Glen Beall Jr. (1927–2006) of Maryland was so impressed by Mintz's article that, a day after it was published, he added a copy of it and a speech Feingold gave in London to the *Congressional Record*.[37] Such a response was likely due in part to Mintz's previous successes in breaking the thalidomide story, yet it also reflected the fact that public was concerned about the hidden effects of food additives on health.

While Mintz's penchant for investigative health journalism spurred him to write about the Feingold diet, other writers gravitated towards the topic because of their interest in the health food industry or holistic medicine. Writer Tom Monte, for example, described how he quit his job as a newspaper reporter in the mid-1970s because his paper refused to publish a story about macrobiotic diets.[38] He proceeded to edit *Nutrition Action*, the journal of the Center for Science in the Public Interest (CSPI), and then became a freelance writer and lecturer specializing in complementary health and macrobiotic nutrition.[39] Monte's story, "Feingold Diet: A Precious Commodity to Hyperactive Children?" was a clear endorsement of Feingold's hypothesis.[40] He began by describing a Halloween party for hyperactive children in Maryland, and expressed his surprise at how calmly the thirty children present behaved. The explanation for their good behavior was the Feingold diet. According to Monte, "Every Feingold member I spoke to at this Halloween party and in later interviews reported remarkable stories about the improved behavior of their children once they began the Feingold diet."[41] As with many articles that provided support for the Feingold diet, testimonials from families were a compelling aspect of Monte's story. Such accounts not only provided anecdotal evidence to support

Feingold's theory but also gave hope to families who were desperate to improve the behavior of their children. One family that Monte described, the Johnsons, had been told by their physician "that their son Brian, then 7, would be institutionalized because of his disruptive behavior." After a semester on the Feingold diet, however, "Brian's grades went from C's to A's. He was taken off the Ritalin and was no longer a disruptive force in school, that is, so long as he avoided artificial colors and flavors."[42]

A story in the *Los Angeles Times* further described how the Feingold diet could result in remarkable transformations. As journalist Marlene Cimons explained,

> It took a long time for Mina Otis to find out why her child was uncontrollable. Each new doctor had a different theory. "We were told he was allergic," she said. "We were told he was a screwball." Raymond Ellis Otis, 11, was neither. He was one of an estimated 5 million children in this country who are hyperactive. . . . Until this past July, Mrs. Otis had no idea what to do about her son's erratic behavior. "But now when he wakes up in the morning, his hair isn't all scruffed up from tossing and turning," Mrs. Otis said. "He doesn't grind his teeth. When you ask him a question, you get a paragraph answer instead of an 'I don't wanna.' He is able to concentrate." She looked at her son. "And he doesn't do anything dumb," she said. . . . The change in Raymond Otis, his mother said, finally occurred after she put him on a diet free of artificial colors and flavors and free of foods containing natural salicylates.[43]

Mina Otis proceeded to apologize to Cimons for the current behavior of her son; he had mistakenly eaten some corn with artificially colored butter on it. Cimons went on to criticize the use of amphetamines to treat hyperactivity, relating the story of a lawsuit filed on behalf of seventeen children from Taft, California, which alleged "that school officials forced them to take Ritalin, which, in at least one case, resulted in an epileptic seizure."[44] By contrasting the Otis story with that of the family bringing the lawsuit, Cimons insinuated that the Feingold diet was a tool that allowed parents to wrest control over their child's health back from authorities such as the school board and the medical profession. In this way, it not only served its purpose as a therapy, it empowered parents such as Mina Otis.

The theme of empowerment was also featured in a story published by *Utah Holiday*, which described two families who had successfully employed the Feingold diet. Dee and Lavon Seely had adopted three hyperactive children from another state. Their physician had recommended corporal punishment,

but this was not effective and "after a while the neighbors began to wonder
what was happening in the Seely home. . . . Finally, one neighbor reported
them for child abuse."[45] The Seelys also tried Ritalin, but "the Ritalin would
wear off in two hours and then the children would be even wilder." Eventually
Lavon found out about the Feingold diet and, within three days, her most disruptive child's behavior was improving.[46] Cleo Jeppson, the mother of another
family described by Jarvik, explained how, once her daughter Lisa started the
Feingold diet, "It was like someone peeled off an outer layer and for the first
time I saw my daughter as herself . . . I wanted to stand on the roof and shout to
the world."[47] Jeppson was so impressed that she founded the Feingold
Association of Utah.

"Another 'Miracle' Diet Cure that Failed?"

Although most newspaper stories during the 1970s were favorable towards
the Feingold diet, there were articles that reported on the findings of clinical
trials that were negative and editorials by columnists who were doubtful of
Feingold's hypothesis. Editorials that rejected the Feingold diet were typically
written by physicians and scientists who had previously expressed little sympathy for concerns about food additives. One such critic was Harvard nutrition
scientist Frederick Stare, who attacked Feingold's hypothesis from many
angles in his "Food and Your Health" column. Stare argued that Feingold had
"not reported his results in any recognized scientific journal so that other
professionals can evaluate his methods and results" and charged that this was
"not only irresponsible but a source of concern because a proscription against
additives and particular types of food would lead to the avoidance of a number
of common sources of important nutrients."[48] Although Feingold was able to
refute both of these arguments and did so in a speech to the Newspaper Food
Editors and Writers Association in 1977, he was less able to refute another one
of Stare's charges.[49] This was that the Feingold diet only elicited a placebo
effect. Stare explained,

> Unfortunately, the special diet is so drastic (no soft drinks, candy, bak-
> ery goods, ice cream, jellies and jams and so forth) that many aspects of
> family life undoubtedly change as a result. Accordingly it is possible
> that children's behavior may change (or parents' appreciation of
> children's behavior may change) as a result of increased family "togeth-
> erness" while the result is attributed to the elimination diet. There is
> no way at present to be certain that the good results apparent in
> Dr. Feingold's anecdotes are in fact more than a placebo effect due to his
> own enthusiasm and conviction.[50]

Stare's suggestion that a child's improvement on the Feingold diet was merely an example of placebo effect became one of the most common arguments leveled against Feingold, and one that was often repeated in media reports. The media typically reported arguments about placebo without questioning what this precisely meant, or what the placebo effect actually represented. One reason for this may be that, as historian Anne Harrington has described, placebo was the topic of much scientific discussion during the 1970s and 1980s, with researchers such as psychiatrists Arthur Shapiro (1922–1995), Jerome Frank (1910–2005) and Robert Ader exploring how the doctor-patient relationship and other situational factors could affect healing.[51]

Although Feingold would respond to these claims that there "may be an element of placebo, but the whole practice of medicine is placebo," contemporary interest in the phenomenon meant that there was weight to such arguments within the media and in medical literature.[52] Such critiques were reminiscent of those made of food allergists during the postwar period that stated that the symptoms of food allergy were chiefly psychosomatic. Feingold had written about psychosomatic allergy himself, but he believed that psychosomatic factors were "contributory rather than primary," exacerbating the responses to allergens instead of replacing them as the primary cause of allergic symptoms.[53] The discovery of endorphins, hormones known for their analgesic and euphoria-inducing effects, during the mid-1970s also contributed to interest in placebo since they were found to play a role in certain types of response. As Harrington states, linking endorphins with placebo meant that "placebo, an 'imaginary' treatment, had been found to have some solid flesh on its bones after all."[54] Newspapers picked up on scientific interest in placebo, and reported regularly on both its potential importance to medicine and how it could explain the effectiveness of contentious treatments such as acupuncture.[55]

Increased scientific respect for the placebo effect did not, however, help Feingold or his followers persuade physicians and food manufacturers that food additives were harmful; it did the opposite. According to a Nutrition Foundation committee that reviewed studies of the Feingold diet in 1980, "Successes reported by parents of children given an additive-free diet were most likely caused by a 'placebo effect' where the power of suggestion and hope actually produces the desired response. . . . Since the food additive-free diet has no apparent harmful effects, and since the non-specific (placebo) effects of this dietary treatment are frequently very beneficial to families, we see no reason to discourage those families who wish to pursue this type of treatment as long as they continue to follow other therapy that is helpful."[56] While the Nutrition Foundation might have accepted reluctantly that the Feingold diet was harmless, and that it might even inadvertently help families by virtue of its placebo effect, such conclusions nevertheless reinforced their claim that food additives had nothing to do with hyperactivity. Indeed, Morris Lipton, the chair of the Nutrition Foundation's investigation of the Feingold diet, charged that, far from being hazardous, food additives were a fundamental element of western society. In an article in which Lipton's assessment of the Feingold diet was juxtaposed against those of Senator George McGovern, psychologist C. Keith Conners, and Feingold himself, the psychiatrist asked, "Where would our society be without food preservatives? The shelf life of bread would be eight hours; there would be no ham, bacon, sausages, fresh vegetables, etc. How would we feed the millions in our cities? Lest we forget: Columbus discovered America seeking food preservatives and spices."[57]

Lipton's comments were misleading, since he only mentioned artificial preservatives and not the synthetic colors and flavors that Feingold also targeted. Companies did not use these additives to safeguard the food supply but rather to improve the marketability of their products. As Earl M. Handing, a marketing manager for food chemical company Warner-Jenkinson, stated in a 1976 *Los Angeles Times* story about food dyes, "Cosmetic effect is most important and it gives the competitive edge to those foods with the most appealing color. . . . People don't want gray-colored hot dogs and sausages . . . Also, how would you distinguish different flavors in gelatins all the same color?"[58] The need for bread that lasted longer than eight hours being more pressing than the need to distinguish between artificial flavors of Jell-O, Lipton sensibly limited his line of argumentation to artificial preservatives.

Lipton's arguments about the necessity of artificial preservatives were similar to those leveled against Rachel Carson a decade earlier with regards to pesticides, namely, that American society had grown dependent upon pesticides and would face a food supply disaster if the government restricted them. By delineating such harrowing scenarios, defenders of food additives were, in part, matching the dire speculations made by Carson, Feingold, and others with respect to what would occur if such substances remained in the food supply. As Feingold asserted in his section of the article, "Poor nutrition is now being closely scrutinized as a cause of juvenile delinquency, vandalism in schools and learning disabilities."[59] While Feingold's statement may not have been as polemical as Lipton's—Feingold stated that poor nutrition was "a" cause, rather than "the" cause, and referred to poor nutrition generally rather than food additives specifically—he had written at length in *Why Your Child Is Hyperactive* about how chemicals were causing an increase in antisocial behavior as well as hyperactivity.[60] As with the debates about food additives during the late 1960s and early 1970s, fearmongering based on often unsubstantiated speculation was a rhetorical strategy employed by both sides of the Feingold debate.

Criticism of the Feingold diet, however, did not have to be as heavy-handed as the pieces by Lipton or Stare to be effective. When asked in a letter about whether there was "truth to claims that food additives cause hyperactivity" in his *Chicago Tribune* health advice column, physician G. Timothy Johnson (b. 1936) answered without invective but managed to mention the difficulty of maintaining the diet, Feingold's lack of scientific evidence, the paucity of supportive trials, and a review of research into the diet found in the Nutrition Foundations' mouthpiece *Nutrition Reviews*. Responding to the writer's concerns about Ritalin, Johnson stated, "I can understand your reluctance to have your child take a drug, but I would remind you that stimulant drug therapy is a time-tested treatment."[61] In the process, Johnson not only listed many of the criticisms of the Feingold diet but insinuated that the effectiveness of stimulant drugs precluded even the need for an alternative approach to hyperactivity.

A little over a year later, Johnson addressed the Feingold diet again, stating that it was "obvious the fuss over food additives being a possible cause of hyperactivity in children will not disappear quickly. I receive many letters on the subject, and pediatricians tell me parents often ask about it."[62] Despite continued interest in the Feingold diet, Johnson downplayed the link between food additives and hyperactivity, assuring his readers that most "experts believe that if a relationship exists between diet and behavior, it is of relatively minor importance or exists only within a small subpopulation of children." Although he believed "the question deserves further study," the somewhat exasperated tone of his article, not to mention its title, "Diet-Hyperactivity Link Still Unproved," made his opinion about the Feingold diet clear.[63]

"On Nutrition" and the Feingold Diet

Other health columnists were not as decided, however, about whether the Feingold diet was a viable alternative for hyperactive children or not. The best example of this was the "On Nutrition" column written by nutrition scientist Jean Mayer and his colleagues Joanna Dwyer and Jeanne Goldberg, with whom he worked at Harvard and then Tufts Universities, respectively. One might have suspected that the Franco-American Mayer, who had significant connections to the food industry and had been a colleague of Frederick Stare, would have been highly suspicious of Feingold's hypothesis.[64] Indeed, an early newspaper feature pitted Mayer against Feingold in a debate about the danger of food additives.[65] But even this column reveals that Mayer understood that the issue of food additives and health was complicated.

Although Mayer concluded his half of the debate by stating that people were "more likely to be run over by a car than you are to be killed or harmed by an additive," not quite reassuring given the high number of traffic fatalities during the early 1970s, the bulk of his article related to the difficulty in assessing the risk of food chemicals on human health.[66] This was primarily because, as Mayer described, "we are morally opposed to testing possibly poisonous substances on human beings." To get around this moral hurdle, scientists used animals to test food chemicals, but "no matter how careful the food industry and the agencies are, some intellectual and practical problems remain," namely, that some substances, such as vitamin D, needed to be taken in near toxic doses to be effective and that "the metabolic rate varies from species to species and compound to compound." In other words, it was difficult to apply results from animal trials to humans and also to extend findings about one particular substance to another, as Mayer proceeded to argue:

> At high levels, particularly when injected, MSG causes considerable damage to animals. It can destroy certain eye and brain cells and result in abnormal growth patterns. We use MSG at much lower levels and we don't inject it into ourselves. However, since mice metabolize excess MSG at 30 times the rate for humans, it takes comparatively larger doses to build up a toxic level in mice. Given this difference and the fact that some people become quite sick when they absorb MSG (especially in clear soup on an empty stomach) can we still use the standard formula of one-hundredth the amount that causes damage in animals, to determine "safe" doses of MSG?[67]

Mayer proceeded to advise readers not to "worry unduly about additives," but "without more perfect methods of testing the best advice I can give is, use your common sense. I would use any foods about which I had doubts in strict moderation and, whenever possible, use fresh foods. They are better both nutritiously and in terms of taste. Politically, I would let your U.S. senator and representative know that you want the government's regulatory bodies to be able to investigate and enforce safety measures."[68]

Mayer's words amounted to not so much a defense of food additives as a cautionary tale about how much faith consumers should have in nutrition science, no matter whether it reflected well or poorly on food additives. Feingold, while emphasizing the validity of his observations of the effects of food additives on children, did not necessarily disagree with Mayer's assessment of evidence from animal testing but instead suggested that "the use of any compound whether as a drug or as a food additive must be determined on the basis of benefit compared with risk." Although his view would change by 1977, Feingold explained in his response to Mayer that food preservatives, for example,

> are essential to our food supply. Without preservatives our entire system of food distribution would collapse. Fortunately, adverse reactions to most preservatives seem to occur rather infrequently, which justifies their continued use. However, even these compounds should be under constant surveillance while research continues for better compounds. The experience with food colors is just the opposite. . . . the colors are not essential: they have no nutritional value. Their sole function is a cosmetic. Without them, nothing would be lost. In other words, in evaluating the synthetic colors, risk far outweighs the benefits.[69]

Feingold's lack of concern about preservatives prior to 1977, as well as other processed foods such as refined sugar, was one of the reasons that he failed to gain much support from the clinical ecology movement.[70] This, in addition to the complications raised in the debate between Mayer and Feingold, underscored the difficulties inherent in resolving the food additives dilemma. The chief difference between their positions was not so much that food additives could be dangerous but what to do about additives that did pose a threat. While Feingold's clinical experience convinced him that drastic action was warranted, Mayer's hesitance was perhaps due to his intimate knowledge of and connections to how the food industry operated and the reliance his then employer, Harvard's department of nutrition, had on corporate funding. Nevertheless, Mayer's subsequent columns about the Feingold diet, first coauthored by Joanna Dwyer and later by Jeanne Goldberg, demonstrated that he continued to wrestle with the issue among the cacophony of conflicting reports and polemical arguments.

The first of these columns, which appeared in approximately a hundred newspapers across the United States, was written in August 1976 when the first controlled trials of the Feingold diet were still underway.[71] It began by identifying the many challenges involved in determining whether or not Feingold's theory was a viable alternative for treatment of hyperactivity. The first problem noted by Mayer and Dwyer involved defining the terms used in the debate. Not only were there more than three thousand food additives being used in the food supply, but the necessity of some was deemed to be more significant than others. As Feingold had intimated in his 1974 debate with Mayer, food preservatives served a more vital role than did artificial colors and flavors, which were employed primarily to enhance the marketability of processed foods and/or

reduce the cost of their manufacture.[72] Mayer and Dwyer echoed Feingold's
notion, stating that while preservatives were "necessary," food colors and
flavors were "only added to a food to make it look or taste better."[73] One had
to distinguish between different types of food additives, therefore, in order to
analyze whether their benefits outweighed their risks.

Mayer and Dwyer also warned that the diagnosis of the hyperactive child
was difficult to determine. There was "no precise definition of hyperactivity.
What may be a hyperactive child in the eyes of some parents or teachers is a
normal, high-spirited child in the eyes of others."[74] This difficulty was despite
the fact that the authors claimed that "true hyperkinesis" was proven if a hyperactive child responded positively to stimulants such as Ritalin, a notion that
psychiatrists had begun to question.[75] Although the authors did not pursue
how such "complicating factors" might affect the research intended to determine the validity of the Feingold diet, the fact that the two primary terms of
reference concerning the diet were imprecise suggested that debates about
Feingold's hypothesis would be difficult to resolve.[76] Subsequent columns by
Mayer and Dwyer reinforced the complications inherent in drawing conclusions about the diet. In a November 1977 column, for example, the authors
responded to a question from a reader about whether or not trial results were
providing support for Feingold's hypothesis. Mayer and Dwyer responded that
evidence from the trials had been inconclusive thus far because "support for
the effectiveness of this elimination diet comes mainly from what children and
their parents themselves say," and that "studies designed to test the theory
were not well-controlled enough to permit any objective conclusion."[77] Both of
these issues would often plague researchers trying to draw conclusions about
the Feingold diet.

With respect to anecdotal reports of the Feingold diet, patient and parental
descriptions of their experiences would continue to be viewed doubtfully by
most medical researchers and scientific observers. Mayer and Dwyer's dismissal of what children and parents had to say was reinforced at the end of
their column when they reiterated the AAP's assertion that parents should not
attempt the diet because of fears about its "long-term effects," specifically,
regarding the diet's elimination of certain fruits during the early stage of the
diet, and the idea that some children might interpret the diet as punishment.[78]
Such beliefs highlighted the assumption that parental observations and patient
experiences were irrelevant in assessing the effectiveness of the Feingold diet,
in particular, and in the evaluation of child health generally, and that clinical
trials were the only meaningful arbiters of novel medical ideas. The emphasis
on the power of clinical trials to resolve medical controversies, however,

placed a great deal of faith in a process that was far from perfect. As Mayer and Dwyer admitted, not only were the trials designed to test the Feingold diet complicated to control, but it was difficult to determine which food additives were to be tested and how to assess the improvement of a child's behavior. Although they were confident that subsequent trials would be better controlled, they also cautioned that it would "be some time before a scientifically-valid assessment of the theory . . . is available."[79] Perhaps aware of their mixed message, the nutritionists concluded that "cutting down on additives and eating foods that are fresh or very lightly processed is a good idea."[80]

The next two columns by Mayer and Dwyer, written a week apart in November 1978, made matters even more complicated. The first column's headline, "Diet Changes Seem to Help," suggested that evidence had emerged that supported Feingold's theory, but the column's contents, as well as the one that followed it, revealed a murkier picture.[81] The nutritionists reported on the research conducted by a group at the University of Toronto that compared the effect of the Feingold diet with that of stimulant medication in reducing the hyperactivity of twenty-six children.[82] Although the researchers determined that stimulant medication was more effective, they agreed with Feingold that dietary changes appeared to work, especially when in combination with stimulant drugs. In attempting to explain why this was the case, Mayer and Dwyer added another factor to the equation: the possibility that it was sugar, not additives, that was the causative factor in some cases of hyperactivity. Mayer and Dwyer's suggestion about sugar was based on research done by an unidentified research group, likely led by Richard J. Walsh of the New York Institute for Child Development. The fact that they seemed to approve of the findings of both the Toronto group and the New York group was odd. This is because the Toronto group tested their subjects with chocolate cookies. While the test group received cookies containing food dyes, the other group ate dye-free cookies. Both the test and the control cookie, however, would likely have contained sugar, presumably throwing into doubt any evidence about the role of color or sugar in triggering hyperactivity.[83]

Despite possible problems with Mayer and Dwyer's interpretation of the research data, they were hitting upon a popular culprit. Sugar had been often suggested as a possible cause of hyperactivity in both the popular media and medical literature.[84] Never attaining the popularity of the Feingold diet, blaming sugar for hyperactivity nevertheless appealed to many parents and nutritionists even when research suggested that there was no such link.[85] With regard to the Feingold diet, however, the proposition that there was a link between sugar and hyperactivity not only complicated what was already a confused debate but demonstrated how Feingold's desire to devise a practical treatment for hyperactivity altered the diet itself. According to one associate, Josephine Bannister (a pseudonym), Feingold was cognizant that his diet had to appear as palatable as possible in order for it to work. Although she was able to convince Feingold during the mid-1970s that the common preservatives BHA (butylated hydroxyanisole) and BHT (butylated hydroxytoluene) could cause hyperactivity and should be added to the elimination diet's list of banned substances, Bannister was not able to convince Feingold that refined white sugar should also be added to the list. This was not so much because Feingold doubted that it was a factor; he suspected that it was, but he was concerned that families would have too much difficulty eliminating sugar from their diets. According to Bannister, "When I suggested that sugar should be added, he said, 'Oh yes, I know, but I can only suggest a few things, otherwise people will not follow any of it.' I think he was trying to be very pragmatic."[86]

It is also likely that Feingold did not want to attract the wrath of the sugar industry, which was then involved in the debates over cyclamates. This was sensible, considering the Sugar Association's powerful influence during the period. In her review of food and nutrition during the 1970s, food writer Marion Burros referred to the activism of the sugar industry numerous times. In an attempt to win over journalists, Burros wrote, "The Sugar Association was worried about sugar's bad press and put on a program at the annual Newspaper Food Editors' Conference entitled 'Exploding Myths Associated with Sugar.'"[87] Given the difficulty in eliminating refined sugar and the possible influence of the Sugar Association, sugar continues to be allowed in the Feingold diet today, in the belief that it is the synthetic additives in sugary foods that trigger hyperactivity rather than the sugar itself.[88] Nevertheless, many families on the Feingold diet took sugar out of their child's diet independently, believing that it was a contributing factor.[89]

If the suggestion that sugar, not food additives, was the key factor in rising rates of hyperactivity was not enough to confuse Mayer and Dwyer's readers, the nutritionists' following column was likely up to the task. Whereas the tenor and title of their previous column suggested that some trials were supportive of the Feingold diet, the tone of this column was significantly more negative. It is difficult to say what occurred during that week to change the authors' opinions; while it is possible that it was only then that they discovered pertinent research, it is more likely, although impossible to substantiate, that they were chastised by Feingold's detractors for the optimistic tone of their previous column. Mayer and Dwyer briefly discussed the research conducted by J. Preston Harley's team in Wisconsin as well as that led by Conners in Pittsburgh and concluded that "if diet and hyperactivity are linked, the relationship is either very slight or present only in a limited number of children."[90] Although they refused to say that diet played no role whatsoever in triggering hyperactivity, and suggested that children should eat minimally processed foods, they also emphasized that "we are able to do more for these children than we could a few years ago, thanks to the judicious use of stimulant drugs" and that "most hyperactive children outgrow the disorder."[91]

These last two comments betrayed a lack of sensitivity and understanding about the families who had attempted the Feingold diet, often as a last resort because stimulants had not been effective and because they could not simply wait for their child to outgrow their intolerable behavior. The comments also implied, however, that many medical observers were simply not interested in pursuing alternative treatments for hyperactivity. Unlike many of the families of hyperactive children, health professionals such as Mayer and Dwyer, as well as G. Timothy Johnson and others, were satisfied that prescribing stimulants was not only efficacious but an ethical practice. They did not seem to understand why parents were hesitant to see their children given a prescription for amphetamines. On the other hand, the nutritionists' repeated suggestion that parents serve fresh, unprocessed foods implied that, while the efficacy or even necessity of the Feingold diet as a treatment for hyperactivity was in question, there were inherent, yet undefined, problems with a diet high in synthetic additives.

Mayer wrote three more columns about the Feingold diet, the last two coauthored by Tufts University colleague and dietician Jeanne Goldberg instead of Joanna Dwyer. These columns, published in 1979, 1980, and 1984, continued to discuss the Feingold diet ambiguously, reflecting the mixed results that had emerged from the trials designed to test Feingold's hypothesis. In 1979 the authors were "still not sure that diet is the answer" and, reflecting on trials conducted in Toronto, Michigan, and New York in 1980, they stated that "we wish we could say that the results were clear-cut, but they're not."[92] Although the title of Mayer and Goldberg's 1984 column, "Weighing the Feingold 'Elimination' Diet on its 10th Anniversary" implied a more definitive assessment, the authors continued to be ambivalent. Accepting that the Feingold diet might help some children, Mayer and Goldberg cautioned that it was "highly restrictive" and that many of the diet's success stories could "probably be charged to the placebo effect."[93]

Unlike the glowing endorsements of the Feingold diet written by Colman McCarthy and Robert Rodale and the stinging dismissals penned by Frederick Stare and Morris Lipton, the indecisive columns by Mayer, Dwyer, and Goldberg highlighted the difficulties inherent in making objective decisions about the validity of Feingold's hypothesis and provided a more balanced interpretation of the research than most other accounts. Other columnists who wrote regularly about the Feingold diet, such as nutrition writer Jane E. Brody, also vacillated with regards to its efficacy. As Brody described in one of her later columns, one of the primary obstacles to getting clear answers was that there existed a "classic standoff between the plodding nature of rigorous scientific research and the public need for expedient answers to costly, distressing problems."[94] Journalists such as Brody who reported on the story of the Feingold diet throughout the decade when it was mainstream news could not ignore the fact that there were problems reconciling the anecdotal stories provided by parents and physicians and some of the findings reported by clinical investigators. Journalists or commentators who chose to write overwhelmingly positive or negative accounts of the Feingold diet were simply not accounting for many of the factors involved in the debate.

Brody also warned, moreover, that there was "a price to pay for misapplication of scientific research."[95] She cited the case of the "Twinkie defense," which arose in the trial of Dan White (1946–1985) for the murder of the San Francisco mayor George Moscone (1929–1978) and supervisor (city councilor) Harvey Milk (1930–1978), the first openly gay man to be elected to public office in California.[96] During the trial, Martin Blinder, a psychiatrist who testified for White, mentioned that the defendant's consumption of Twinkies and Coca-Cola (he had previously been a health food advocate), along with problems at home and at work (he had been a colleague of Milk's but had recently quit), contributed to his depression and, subsequently, diminished his responsibility for his actions. Although it is arguable how much a role the Twinkie defense actually played in the case, White was found to have diminished capacity and was only convicted of voluntary manslaughter, serving five years of his seven-year sentence before being released and committing suicide in 1985.[97] Journalists such as Brody picked up on the notion that certain foods could cause pathological behavior and linked it directly to some of Feingold's hypotheses about food additives and antisocial behavior. It was one thing to blame a child's hyperactivity on food additives; it was quite another to acquit murderers on the basis of the Twinkie defense.

Conclusion

The media that had been so captivated by Feingold's story in 1973 had become disenchanted by the time of Feingold's death in 1982. There was a sense of disappointment in some stories, for instance, when certain clinical trials found little support for Feingold's hypothesis. Joan Beck, reporting on the seemingly negative results of Harley's trial at the University of Wisconsin, stated that his conclusion "was not a popular finding in the long battles over how to identify and treat children with hyperactivity."[98] The findings, Beck continued, meant that parents, teachers, and physicians had "to rely on such controversial treatments for hyperactive children as methylphenidate (Ritalin), amphetamine, and/or behavior modification programs at home and in school."[99] Harley himself echoed such sentiments, commenting that they "would have liked nothing better than to find that hyperactivity can be cured through diet. But our study did not bear this out."[100]

Although there continued to be positive stories about the Feingold diet during the early 1980s, the tenor of the reporting became more negative, or at best neutral, during this period. Following Feingold's death on March 23, 1982, the number of stories about the Feingold diet began to diminish as well; although the occasional story surfaced during the latter part of the decade and during the 1990s about new trials, they were rare and often published in more obscure publications such as the *Brown University Child Behavior and Development Letter* or *Tufts University Diet and Nutrition Letter*.[101] Feingold's death helps to explain the waning of interest—no one with his charisma, determination, or credentials stepped forth to carry on his cause—but other factors contributed to the phenomenon as well.

For Feingold, the influence of the food, chemical, and pharmaceutical industries was paramount in influencing media coverage of the debate. Feingold believed as early as 1977 that the media was turning against him and made his concerns clear in a speech to the Newspaper Food Editors and Writers Association in June 1977. Newspapers, he argued, were reporting the findings of trials that tested his theory without critically assessing the trials for bias and, in some cases, were drawing overly negative conclusions from trial results. The explanation for such actions, according to Feingold, was industry manipulation. Feingold highlighted Harley's University of Wisconsin study, contending, "Since early January 1976, Dr. Harley has presented his data several times around the country, usually followed in almost every instance by unfavorable reports in the press of the ineffectiveness of the K-P diet."[102] Feingold charged that "an analysis of the circumstances and data of Dr. Harley's most recent presentation will illustrate how industry, with a scientific façade manipulates the situation to influence the press to report unwittingly, to industry's advantage."[103] The allergist was particularly angered by a *Los Angeles Times* story titled "Study Refutes Additive-Hyperactivity Link," which emerged out of a press conference the Dairy Council arranged for Harley at their annual nutrition conference.[104] Along with criticizing Harley's study and its conclusions,

Feingold stated, "I do not know who was responsible for this headline, but it is not only inconsistent with the facts but even with Dr. Harley's written text," something that Harley himself substantiated in a letter to the *Chicago Tribune*.[105] Moreover, Feingold added, at "no time during Dr. Harley's press briefing or in the subsequent articles was there any mention of the $600,000 support to his [Harley's] Food Research Institute from industry."[106]

The level of industry interference in media stories is difficult to gauge. Although journalists were often remiss in elucidating how specific trials were funded or the connections between investigators and various industries, many did mention that the Nutrition Foundation, for example, was a food, chemical, and pharmaceutical industry lobby group. Moreover, most stories represented both sides of the debate, including the story in the *Los Angeles Times* that Feingold criticized. Other factors, therefore, need to be considered in determining why media interest in the Feingold diet petered out.

One factor was that no resolution to the debate appeared to be on the horizon, and journalists, and possibly readers, were tiring of a story that had been running for a decade. In early 1982, for example, reports on the Feingold diet were issued by both an NIH Consensus Development Conference, whose members included the ailing Feingold as well as his critics, and the American Council on Science and Health (ACSH), a nonprofit consumer education group founded by Elizabeth Whalen and Frederick Stare and often accused of being a front for the chemical industry.[107] According to historians David Rosner and Gerald Markowitz, among others, the ACSH has received up to 40 percent of its funding from the food, chemical, and pharmaceutical industries, including companies such as American Cyanamid, Dow, Exxon, Monsanto, and Union Carbide. While the ACSH unsurprisingly concluded "that artificial food colors and flavors are not significant causes of hyperactivity," the NIH group was more circumspect.[108] Addressing a wide range of issues involved in testing the Feingold diet, the panel concluded that although "defined diets should not be universally used in the treatment of childhood hyperactivity at this time . . . initiation of a trial of dietary treatment or continuation of a diet in patients whose families and physicians perceive benefits, may be warranted."[109] In other words, the Consensus Development Conference failed to state definitively whether the Feingold diet was efficacious and, recognizing this, suggested that more research be done to test such theories. Despite the NIH's ambiguity, journalistic interpretations of its statement varied widely: while a *Washington Post* headline read "Additive-Free Diet Found Not to Curb Hyperactivity," the United Press International newswire read "Special Diet May Benefit Hyperactive Children."[110] With no end to the controversy in sight and no agreement among either physicians or journalists on how to weigh the available evidence, it was understandable that the media flocked to other stories following Feingold's death.

More generally, following 1980 public concern about food additives waned, meaning that stories demonizing such substances generated less interest than before.[111] As journalist Nancy Jenkins observed in 1984, "The whole food movement gathered strength for a while, but in the late 70s it seemed to have gone underground, along with the rest of what we used to call the counterculture."[112] Although Jenkins believed that interest in health food was waxing once again, it was "a national interest, sometimes verging on obsession, with good health and preventative medicine and the role of diet in both," that was spurring the trend, not broader ecological, political, or spiritual concerns. As Belasco and Levenstein have emphasized, the yuppies of the 1980s who were targeted by mainstream food companies as a market for healthy food were not so concerned with additive-free food as with low-fat options, as dieting and thinness became entrenched, not for the first or last time, in American culture.[113] Also suggestive of this trend was an article in the "Beauty" section of the *New York Times* that discussed how wealthy Americans were increasingly hiring nutritionists to stay slim.[114] Unlike previous food fads, establishment nutritionists such as Frederick Stare were fully supportive of this "fat-phobia" and, as Levenstein has suggested, so-called "Negative Nutrition . . . opened new windows of commercial opportunity" for food manufacturers in the form of Diet Coke, Stouffer's Lean Cuisine, and Weight Watchers' products.[115]

Concurrently with the decline in stories about the Feingold diet, the tenor of articles and editorials concerning food additives grew more critical of measures, particularly the Delaney Clause, intended to protect consumers.[116] As a 1982 story by journalist Philip M. Boffey indicated, even concern about the environmental causes of cancer, including food additives and pesticides, had faded, although when food additives did make the news during the 1980s it was usually because of their potential to cause cancer.[117] The shift mirrored the ebbing of many of the ideals of the 1960s and was made manifest in the election of right-wing Republican Ronald Reagan (1911–2004) in 1980. As Levenstein describes, "Lust for wealth displaced older ideas of public service in Washington, drove considerations of responsibility to clients, stockholders, and the public from Wall Street boardrooms."[118] Such a philosophy was reflected in the administration's support for the food, chemical, and pharmaceutical industries and successful attempts to deregulate such industries.[119]

Despite the decline in media interest, however, researchers continued to test the diet during the 1980s, albeit intermittently, and parents continued to learn about the diet through other means. Debate about Feingold's theory continued to simmer, but it did not attract the attention of the mainstream media. Although the media played a major role in publicizing the Feingold diet to millions of Americans, its overall impact on how Americans assessed Feingold's hypothesis is more difficult to determine. Depending on which story an individual happened to read, they might read a glowing endorsement, a scathing indictment, or a confounding account of a protracted debate, any of which might have accorded with what they were predisposed to think about food additives, hyperactivity, or the role of the state in regulating industry. In the case of the Feingold diet, therefore, the media as a whole did not influence public opinion as much as it reflected the complexities involved in attempting to determine whether Feingold's theory was valid or not.

Chapter 7

Testing the Feingold Diet

During the period between the publication of *Why Your Child Is Hyperactive* in 1974 and Feingold's death in 1982, researchers in the United States, Canada, and Australia designed dozens of trials that tested Feingold's theory. The prevailing opinion that emerged from these trials, reflected in the medical literature, was that the Feingold diet did not stand up to scientific scrutiny and that parents of hyperactive children should consider other treatments.[1] Despite these conclusions, FAUS and groups such as CSPI argued that tests of the Feingold diet did provide solid evidence in support of Feingold's hypothesis.[2] It is understandable that certain parties, for example, the Nutrition Foundation on one hand and FAUS on the other, would interpret the test results in manners conducive to their own vested interests, but this leaves unanswered the question of what the tests of the Feingold diet did in fact reveal.

Western society's faith in the power of scientific knowledge suggests that double-blind clinical trials of the Feingold diet should have unequivocally demonstrated whether Feingold's idea was tenable. As sociologists Harry Collins and Trevor Pinch explain, randomized controlled trials, of which double-blind trials are the most common and most accurate type, are regarded as the "gold standard for scientific medicine," the primary means to resolve medical debates.[3] Close examination of the tests of the Feingold diet reveals that they were anything but conclusive, revealing an array of positive, negative, and mixed results. What emerges from historical analysis of these trials are not definitive answers about the efficacy of the Feingold diet but more questions about how researchers designed, conducted, and most importantly, interpreted the results. The inconclusiveness of the tests not only suggests that other, nonscientific, factors were more influential in shaping the opinions of various parties regarding the Feingold diet, but it raises questions about the effectiveness of double-blind clinical trials in resolving similar debates, particularly those in the fields of psychiatry, nutrition, and allergy.

It is clear from reviews of the trials that, while Feingold's detractors were liable to ignore positive results, his supporters were inclined to downplay negative results, a tendency that was recognized in a recent review of the Feingold diet research literature.[4] The trials themselves often contained methodological problems, casting into doubt the perception that they were conclusive one way or the other. Researchers differed considerably with respect to how to interpret their results and, therefore, whether their results should be counted as being supportive or critical. While some researchers were unimpressed if large percentages of their sample reacted to food additives, other researchers were alarmed if only a few of their sample responded strongly. Finally, although Feingold's detractors consistently claimed that trial results were the basis of their critique, they also attacked the diet using arguments that had nothing to do with the trials, contending, for example, that the diet was an impractical intervention for most American families. Given all of these factors, it would therefore have been difficult for any physician, parent, or policy maker to determine whether the Feingold diet worked or not.

What to Test, How to Test, Who to Test: Methodological Difficulties

Following Feingold's presentations to the AMA in 1973 and 1974, five California-based studies were undertaken at medical centers and schools to test his idea.[5] Two studies were also carried out in Australia and published in the *Medical Journal of Australia*, prompting Feingold to visit the country on a lecturing tour in September 1976. None of the studies used control groups, however, and two of those conducted in California were carried out at Kaiser Permanente clinics with the involvement of Feingold himself. The reports from these clinical studies were generally positive and attracted the attention of the media, parents, and physicians.[6] Some members of the medical community, however, were not impressed. The Australian studies, for example, generated a considerable number of letters to the *Medical Journal of Australia*. Although most of the letters were positive, New Zealand psychiatrist John Werry's editorial (which is discussed in more detail below), was a scathing attack on Feingold's methods and motives.[7] Also concerned that no controlled studies had been conducted to assess the validity of Feingold's theory, both the FDA and the Nutrition Foundation recommended in 1975 that controlled double-blind trials be designed to test it.[8] Early in that year, the Nutrition Foundation recruited over a dozen physicians, nutrition scientists, and psychologists to form the National Advisory Committee on Hyperkinesis and Food Additives (NACHFA) to review the trials and make judgments on their findings.[9]

In setting out the rationale for their investigation of Feingold's hypothesis, NACHFA emphasized their suspicion that the benefits of the Feingold diet were due to placebo effects rather than the elimination of food additives. Placebo, they contended, could operate in three separate ways in both clinical observations and uncontrolled trials. First, dietary changes affecting the entire family could cause "alterations in family dynamics . . . related to the reported improvement in the child." Secondly, Feingold's charisma and confidence about his regimen could generate positive expectations in the patients and their families, thus affecting parental perceptions of improvement. Thirdly, "parents and teachers who rate the children know that they are on the diet and this knowledge may influence their ratings."[10] In summary, as described in a 1977 letter to the *Medical Journal of Australia*, the Feingold diet was a "very good placebo" and many "children described as hyperactive are in fact responding to their own parents' anxiety, which is alleviated at least temporarily by treatment which appears both complicated and powerful."[11] Given the numerous ways in which placebo could influence trial results and the "enormous expenditure" inherent in "producing a wide variety of dietary products in identical pairs containing, or free of, specific chemical ingredients," NACHFA recommended the use of challenge studies whereby a single food containing a particular food additive would be randomly served to participants in order to determine if it triggered increased hyperactivity.[12] Although they warned that other factors, including the compliance of participants, the validity of behavioral observations, and the large number of substances eliminated in the Feingold diet, complicated interpretation of the trials, NACHFA maintained that "data from critically designed and executed studies, free of the deficiencies noted, must be available before firm conclusions can be reached on the Feingold hypothesis."[13]

Despite the call for the Feingold diet to be tested in controlled double-blind trials and the guidelines set out by NACHFA to design such trials, methodological problems plagued nearly all of the trials conducted during the 1970s and early 1980s and, according to some researchers, discouraged others from testing the theory. Often, attempting to address the methodological weaknesses of uncontrolled trials merely led to different methodological problems. Writing in 1987, a team led by psychiatrist Mortimer D. Gross stated "a major reason for the dearth of controlled studies is the difficulty in performing them when food is involved: 1) unless the subjects are confined to a strictly controlled environment, cheating is all too easy; 2) children are difficult to persuade to stick to a prescribed diet. . . . 3) ideally the food being tested should be disguised so that the subjects are blind to what they are ingesting—and this is difficult to manage; and 4) the raters should be blind to what subjects are eating, and this, too, is difficult to arrange."[14] Gross's concern about methodological difficulties was particularly ironic since his own study, conducted at a summer camp, was itself rife with design flaws (see below).[15]

    At the heart of the methodological problems was the general perception that hyperactivity was a complex condition influenced by many factors. Although most physicians during the mid-1970s believed that the disorder was chiefly a neurological condition, NACHFA's concerns about placebo implied that a child's social, domestic, and educational environment also played a role in at least exacerbating hyperactivity. In order to establish a clear, definitive link between food additives and hyperactivity, all such factors had to be controlled. Moreover, discrepancies existed regarding how to identify the disorder and all of its constituent parts, including not only hyperactive behavior, but also distractibility, impulsivity, defiance, and aggression. Although parent and teacher questionnaires designed during the 1960s by psychologist C. Keith Conners were used in many of the Feingold trials, there was still an element of subjectivity on behalf of the person observing; what was pathological, disordered behavior to one parent or teacher, for example, could be an example of energetic play to another. As an anonymous editorial for the *Lancet* explained in 1979, Feingold's "hypothesis would be difficult to test even if the state of hyperactivity in children were a precise and readily recognisable entity. It is not . . . hyperactivity remains a clinical concept of doubtful validity."[16]

    If hyperactivity was in itself an illusive concept to define, identify, and assess, the implications of Feingold's hypothesis made comprehensive testing of the Feingold diet even more problematic. Feingold claimed that there were thousands of additives in the food supply that could trigger hyperactivity and that certain salicylate-laden fruits and vegetables could also invoke reactions. Moreover, not all children reacted to the same chemicals, as interviews with Feingold families have demonstrated. Since testing thousands of substances individually was logistically and economically impossible, many researchers limited their inquiry to a single chemical, such as the food dye tartrazine yellow, or a combination of common food dyes.[17]

    The issue of exactly what to test was a source of contention between Feingold, his supporters, and NACHFA. Although Feingold emphasized the sheer number of potentially problematic chemicals in the food supply, when he met with NACHFA in 1975 to discuss how to test his hypothesis, he recommended that initially, "in view of the complexity of the problem and the many compounds involved, studies be designed focusing on the limited list of colors, which lend themselves to better control."[18] NACHFA, therefore, advocated that artificial flavors, salicylate-laden fruits and vegetables, food preservatives, and other food additives not be tested, leaving food colors as the sole substance of interest. The advisory committee argued that there were other reasons for omitting the other substances, stating that "the chemical components of synthetic food flavorings are usually identical to the chemicals contained in natural foods," and that "such a challenge substance would have to be prepared from a list of over a thousand chemicals, and it would be impossible to disguise flavoring in the placebo food."[19] Another problem, not cited by NACHFA but elsewhere, was that there were no government guidelines on the average amount of flavorings consumed, so researchers had little idea about what dosages to test.[20] As a result, the challenge studies that NACHFA recommended were only expected to test food dyes, and the Nutrition Foundation proceeded to create a challenge cookie that contained all nine of the dyes approved by the Food, Drug and Cosmetics Act of 1938 in direct proportion to the volume of each dye sold in the United States. Chocolate was used to mask the color of the dyes, a practice that was later questioned by other researchers.[21] These cookies were provided to researchers who applied to the Nutrition Foundation for funding, having "submitted protocols containing appropriate scientific safeguards to assure the double-blind nature of their observations."[22]

The focus on food dyes alone was not what Feingold had intended; food dyes were supposed to be the starting point of a series of tests on all types of additives rather than the only substance tested. Testing dyes at the expense of other food additives, according to Feingold, meant that his hypothesis was not being fully explored and incorrectly suggested that he thought dyes were the most important factor in triggering hyperactivity. As one of Feingold's supporters, psychologist Bernard Rimland (1928–2006), exclaimed, "How researchers can claim they have tested 'the Feingold diet,' which eliminates over 3,000 additives, by conducting experiments based on fewer than 10 dyes, is beyond me."[23] On one level, such complaints were disingenuous. Feingold had recommended that testing synthetic dyes was the best place to start and colors were likely the most iconic and feared food additive. If coal-tar-based food dyes such as Brilliant Blue and Sunset Yellow could not be conclusively found to trigger hyperactivity, Feingold's hypothesis was certainly in doubt, if not theoretically, then at least in the eyes of the medical and lay community. But even if testing synthetic dyes was the key task in testing the Feingold diet, then there were still other methodological problems that made the results of dye-based trials difficult to interpret.

One important aspect, for example, was the amount of dye to be tested, or the dosage level. The amount of dye in the NACHFA cookies, for example, was based upon a calculation of the average daily per capita consumption of food dyes in the US in the years 1973 and 1974. The cookies designed by the Nutrition Foundation, and used by many researchers, contained 13 milligrams of dye, but since two cookies were intended to be consumed each day by each child in the trials, the total amount of dye ingested was 26 milligrams. This amount was calculated by adding up the entire amount of dye certified by the FDA per year and dividing it by the American population and the number of days in the year, a decidedly rough approximation and less that the FDA's estimate of average of 57.5 milligrams for average consumption. And children's habits were probably different from adults'. The advisory committee admitted that following "the first two or three challenge studies, concern was expressed that the dose of food coloring employed may be much less than the amount of coloring consumed by children. It was argued by some that children, on the average, consume a much higher proportion of artificially colored foods than do adults."[24] The FDA estimated that children at the high end of the spectrum might consume 121 milligrams of colorings up to a maximum of 315 milligrams per day.[25] Or, as Rimland put it, the "dosage levels were ridiculously small. Even if one were to accept the wholly unwarranted conclusion that seven to ten food colorings were the overwhelming important factor in the Feingold diet, one would still have to reject the bulk of the studies, since the researchers used almost trivially small doses of colorings."[26]

Rimland's hyperbole notwithstanding, there was a wide range in the doses of food dyes used by researchers, ranging from 1.2 milligrams to 150 milligrams.[27] NACHFA responded by creating a "soda-pop drink" that contained 36 milligrams for a subsequent trial.[28] A further flaw with these study foods was that the amount of each of the nine dyes was proportionate to the dye's relative use in the food supply (for example, blue number 2 only accounted for 1.7 percent of dyes in the food supply, so it only made up 1.7 percent of the dyes in the cookie), so participating children could be getting minimal amounts of the dye to which they might be particularly susceptible.[29]

Even reviews of the trials that dismissed the Feingold diet admitted that it "is conceivable that previous studies . . . used inadequate doses of food colourings."[30] Another researcher admitted that "the doses employed by us, and most of our fellow investigators, are 50 times less than the maximum allowable daily intakes (ADIs) recommended by the Food and Drug Administration."[31] Facing questions about the amount of dye used in trials, NACHFA claimed that there was "a technical limitation to the amount of food coloring that can be incorporated into a food without coloring the mouth and fingers . . . and thus preventing the disguise of the placebo challenge."[32] A number of researchers overcame this obstacle, incorporated higher levels of dye, and reported results in favor of Feingold's hypothesis.[33]

The issue of challenge materials hampered trials in other ways. In one trial, researchers expected the children to eat six cookies per day. This amount proved to be too much for one child's appetite, and too much for two parents who were alarmed by the reactions their children had after consuming what they thought was the challenge cookie. Although one of the parents correctly guessed that her child was consuming the challenge cookie, the other parent's child was consuming the placebo.[34] A similar situation occurred in one of Conners's trials; a mother took her son out of the trial when his behavior deteriorated rapidly following the ingestion of a cookie, but it turned out that the cookie was a placebo.[35] In other trials, including more recent ones, parents were wary of subjecting their children to the challenge foods and removed their children from the study.[36]

The overall compliance of children was another problem, one that made researchers question the practicality of the Feingold diet. For example, preschool-aged children in J. Preston Harley's study at the University of Wisconsin had, on average, 1.33 dietary infractions per week. Although Harley believed this to be a high rate of compliance, Feingold claimed that a single dietary infraction could affect a hyperactive child adversely for up to six days, thus compromising the results of Harley's trial.[37] In order to minimize infractions, one trial was held at a hospital and another at an Illinois summer camp for children with learning disorders.[38] The children at the camp were fed the Feingold diet during one week and then returned to an additive-rich diet the following week. Although they were better able to control what the children ate, other factors complicated how the investigators interpreted whether or not their behavior had improved: "One result was unmistakable: the children were not happy with the Feingold diet. The teachers had the feeling that there would have been a rebellion had it lasted longer than a week. They particularly disliked the colourlessness of the food, and missed the mustard and ketchup. . . . The strict Feingold diet appears to be distasteful to the typical American child."[39]

Given the rebellious attitude of the children at the camp, who were predominantly teenagers, not young children, the interpretation of behavior, which was not observed firsthand but via videotapes at four-minute intervals, was problematic. The summer camp study had other methodological problems as well. For instance, only nineteen of the thirty-nine children studied during the comparatively short two-week trial had been diagnosed with hyperactivity, and eighteen of those remained on stimulant medication throughout the trial. Moreover, three children, two of them hyperactive, were sent home for various behavioral problems during the second week when additives were reintroduced to the diet. Despite this, and the impressions of the camp director and teachers that the children had behaved worse during the second week, the researchers concluded that the Feingold diet was ineffective.[40]

Other methodological problems made interpretation a difficult task. Most researchers tested small numbers of children, usually ranging between ten and twenty, and not all children managed to complete the full trial period. Given the concerns about methodology, small sample sizes were perhaps understandable, as they made controlling many aspects of the trials easier, but then questions could be raised about the statistical significance of such small trials.[41] Another issue was when to challenge children with additives following a period on an elimination diet. While many researchers waited three to four weeks before introducing the challenges, others believed that testing four to six days after additives were eliminated from the diet was a better strategy, since this was methodologically similar to how allergists tested other food allergies.[42]

The methodological problems that plagued the trials of the Feingold diet were understandable. Hyperactivity was a diverse syndrome, characterized by many different types of behavior. Feingold's theory involved thousands of potentially harmful substances, any of which he claimed could trigger hyperactivity in a child. Children's behavior was difficult to explain, and a plethora of educational, emotional, neurological, social, and familial factors had to be eliminated before proving unequivocally that food additives were at fault. Combining all of these issues with the inherent difficulty of conducting a trial involving food made testing Feingold's hypothesis a complicated and potentially frustrating prospect.

Despite the difficulties in designing trials that would test the Feingold diet, the willingness of researchers to overcome such problems was less clear. When asked why many of the tests were so poorly constructed, for instance, one researcher, who supported Feingold, answered that many trials "were carried out by people who had the answers before they did the study. I mean that's the reason I did it. I said wait a minute, the FDA does not screen for neurotoxicity. How come? That's crazy! There were some people within it who thought it was important, but they could never get anybody to listen. So I thought, this is an important toxicology issue. It's not a question of diet and kids, but an issue for regulatory agencies. Why the hell are you not examining food additives for potential neurotoxicity?"[43] Although most other researchers were unwilling to admit that they had preconceived notions about the validity of Feingold's hypothesis prior to conducting research, the admission of this researcher suggests that many had ideas nevertheless. Discussing researchers on the other side of the debate, Canadian researchers J. Ivan Williams and Douglas M. Cram asserted that "there has been interest in testing [Feingold's hypothesis] if only to disprove it."[44] In other words, the manner in which investigators and reviewers interpreted and discussed Feingold's hypothesis may indicate that scientists who investigated the Feingold diet had strong ideas about it before they began their trials, and their opinions were not always swayed by their results.

Although methodological problems troubled many trials, a study launched by psychologist Bonnie Kaplan at the University of Calgary's Alberta Children's Hospital during the late 1980s was singled out as being particularly well-designed.[45] One key difference between Kaplan's study and most of the others was that she and her associates manipulated the entire nutrient intake of her subjects. This "dietary replacement design" was expensive and difficult to organize, but permitted "the evaluation and control of many variables not possible with the more popular challenge designs."[46] In other words, instead of testing only a limited quantity of food dyes, as most trials did, Kaplan's study tested a broader range of food additives in the quantities that they would normally be present in a child's diet. Kaplan also attempted to control what the children were eating away from home was by producing T-shirts for the children to wear that read, "Don't feed me, I'm allergic."

The other difference between Kaplan's study and many others was her rationale for conducting research into the Feingold diet. Although she had a long-standing interest in nutrition and behavior, Kaplan had not heard about Feingold's hypothesis until 1979, when Jane McNicol, a dietician working at the Children's Hospital in Calgary, brought it to her attention. McNicol "wasn't a Feingoldian, . . . She just believed she really could see improvements in children who ate a healthier diet."[47] The researchers "looked at the Feingold-stimulated research and, frankly, at that time it was pretty poor; . . . basically we decided . . . why couldn't we do a better study?"[48] Explaining the motives for the trial, one researcher stated, "I was about as open-minded as I've been about any study I've done. I hadn't seen it affect any children; I had no clinical experience. What I remember about my attitude was, 'My God, I could do a better job than some of them out there' . . . it does sound arrogant, but I saw it as a challenge in experimental research and design, but I had nothing invested in the outcome."[49] In contrast, many of the early uncontrolled studies of the Feingold diet were conducted by clinicians who had first employed the diet in their clinics and experienced success with it, possibly influencing their expectations of how their trials would turn out.[50] Equally problematic was the fact that researchers who applied to the Nutrition Foundation for funding had to submit their study design to the Foundation for approval. Although the Nutrition Foundation's stated intent was to "assure the double-blind nature of their observations," many of the trials they did fund had other methodological problems, including using the Foundation's relatively low-dosage challenge cookie.[51] The manner in which many of these researchers interpreted their findings was questionable, downplaying certain aspects of their study while stressing others.

Kaplan's interpretation of her trial's results, in contrast, was measured: "On the one hand, a much larger percentage of children responded to dietary intervention than found in previous studies. On the other hand, only half of the children who completed the study exhibited behavioral improvement, and it is safe to say that not a single parent believed that participation in this study had transformed their child into an easy to manage person. We removed everyday obstacles to compliance which practitioners regularly face: we determined the menus and provided the food at no cost to participants."[52] Despite what most observers interpreted as positive results, the "parents' attitude was almost universally: 'That's it? That's as good as it gets?' and: 'Where can I get some Ritalin to try?' And it was so discouraging."[53] Despite praise for her study, Kaplan herself eventually left the area of research, partly because her colleagues dismissed her work and partly because she found the lack of objectivity on both sides of the Feingold debate disheartening. The methodological problems of testing the diet notwithstanding, for Kaplan, creating a "superb study" was an easier task than convincing physicians and parents that there was a link between food additives and behavioral problems.[54]

"Arbitrary Negative Conclusions"?
Interpreting the Trials of the Feingold Diet

In light of the methodological problems that hampered trials of Feingold's hypothesis, one might expect that researchers, as well as those who reviewed their studies, would have been conservative with regards to interpreting their findings and making conclusive statements about the efficacy of the diet. Indeed, many researchers, in recognition of the methodological flaws present in many studies, acknowledged that their results did not resolve the debate about the Feingold diet and, accordingly, suggested that more research be done to test the effects of food additives on behavior.[55] These calls for more research notwithstanding, researchers and reviewers differed drastically with regards to how they interpreted individual trials and the body of research as a whole. While some reviewers such as psychiatrist Jeffrey Mattes contended that "no single study has reported a consistent dietary effect on the symptoms of the hyperkinetic syndrome," others such as Bernard Rimland decried the "arbitrary negative conclusions" reached by reviewers and argued that despite "anti-Feingold bias . . . all studies, without exception, do concede that some children react to additives and some children do respond to the diet."[56] Both Rimland's and Mattes's reviews were published in the same issue of *Journal of Learning Disabilities*, which at least presented their readers with both sides of the debate. Regardless, such differences in interpretation suggest that neither Feingold's supporters nor his detractors relied on science alone to make decisions about whether his hypothesis was valid or not.

One of the best examples of how investigators could differ wildly in terms of interpreting their data can be found by comparing two well-cited trials, one led by psychologist J. Preston Harley and the other led by toxicologist Bernard Weiss.[57] Harley's trial, funded by the Nutrition Foundation, compared the effects of the Feingold diet and a control diet containing typical amounts of food additives on rates of hyperactivity in forty-six boys, thirty-six of whom who were aged between six and twelve years old and ten of whom were pre-school-aged. With the Nutrition Foundation's funds (estimated at one $120 per family per week), Harley was able to design a trial that kept participants blind to the diets being tested and minimized violations.[58] Included in these measures were a number of "pseudo-dietary manipulations" that were employed in order to prevent participants from guessing which diet was being introduced, and challenge and additive-free foods were produced and packaged to appear identical.[59]

In summarizing his results, Harley stated that "the overall results do not provide convincing support for the efficacy of the experimental (Feingold) diet."[60] But the results of Harley's trial were far more ambiguous. The most obvious problem was that Harley based his overall assessment on only one of his sample populations, namely, the thirty-six school-aged boys, and downplayed the results of the smaller group of preschool-aged children. While the results from the older group were interpreted to be negative (and this was debatable), those of the younger group appeared to provide solid support for Feingold's hypothesis. According to Harley, "All ten mothers and four of the seven fathers of the preschool sample rated their children's behavior as improved on the experimental diet."[61]

Harley admitted that his interpretation was problematic, stating, "The attentive reader of this report has undoubtedly sensed, if not specifically identified, our discomfort and uncertainty in the manner of presenting the results on the preschool sample."[62] Harley went on to state that he ignored the results of the younger group because they were only based on parental, rather than parental and teacher, rating scales, and that it was more difficult to gauge hyperactivity in preschoolers. If this was the case, however, it makes one wonder why, in such a carefully designed study, younger children were included if they were so difficult to test. The discounting of the younger group becomes more troubling when one considers Feingold's observation that younger children were particularly susceptible to food additives, an observation that other researchers echoed.[63] Other observers, including Bernard Weiss and C. Keith Conners, had trouble with Harley's refusal to include the preschool sample. Conners, whose opinion about the Feingold diet during the late 1970s could be best described as ambivalent, stated, "They cannot have it both ways. If their study did indeed rigorously achieve a complete disguise of the dietary manipulations, then the parent ratings, regardless of their 'subjectivity' have to be explained. The probability of obtaining such findings by chance alone is miniscule."[64] Such criticisms notwithstanding, most later reviewers nevertheless concluded that Harley's trial yielded little evidence in favor of Feingold's hypothesis.[65]

Although the issue of the preschool data was the most questionable aspect of Harley's study, other details relating to Harley's interpretations highlight differences in how researchers described trial results. Weiss, for instance, not only disputed how Harley dealt with his preschool sample but disagreed with his interpretation of the data generated from the older group. In describing how he interpreted the overall results, Harley stated that the "few significant findings related to diet that did emerge must be conservatively interpreted for several reasons."[66] One of the reasons Harley listed for his reticence was that the most positive ratings emerged from parents, not teachers.[67] In contrast, Weiss had little trouble with the parental ratings, stating that thirteen of the thirty-six mothers and fourteen of the thirty fathers "recorded substantially improved behavior on the experimental compared to the control diet," and added that six of the thirty-six teachers reported less hyperactive behavior when the boys were on the experimental diet.[68] Weiss questioned the low frequency of observations, contending that this emphasized the relevance of dietary infractions, which occurred 0.65 times per week in the older group. He stressed that, when the entire sample of forty-six boys was considered, it had to be recognized that half of the mothers indicated that their sons had improved on the Feingold diet.[69] In explaining why he thought Harley viewed his results so negatively, Weiss suggested that to interpret them otherwise would have embarrassed his funders, and the entire situation was "a salient example of the extra-scientific barriers posed to the Feingold hypothesis."[70] Weiss proceeded to reinterpret a number of other trials which were thought to have yielded negative results and determined instead that these also lent support to Feingold's hypothesis.[71]

In order to explain why Weiss interpreted Harley's trial so differently from Harley, it is helpful to consider his conclusions regarding a trial that he himself conducted in 1980. Weiss received a grant from the FDA to test twenty-two children between two and a half and seven years old for eleven weeks, and published his results in *Science*.[72] On the surface, the toxicologist's results were even less impressive than those of Harley; only two of his subjects demonstrated reactions to the challenge. This was despite the fact that the parents of the children in Weiss's study had all previously reported using the Feingold diet successfully, thus calling into question their observations of their children's behavior and possibly Feingold's observations as well.[73]

Despite these seemingly unimpressive results, Weiss believed that his trial provided support for Feingold's hypothesis. His justification for this conclusion was partly based in his background in toxicology. Unlike other researchers who questioned Feingold's claims that a high percentage of hyperactive children reacted negatively to food additives, Weiss was only interested in whether or not such reactions were possible at all in any children. His study, therefore, was not intended to be "a group experiment, but 22 separate experiments. Our aim was not to estimate population prevalence or sensitivity, but simply to determine if behavioral sensitivity to color additives could be detected in a controlled trial."[74] The response of one of Weiss' participants, in particular, provided convincing evidence for him that food colors could indeed evoke troubling behavior in children:

> One child reacted dramatically. This 34-month-girl, weighing about 13 kg, . . . behaved significantly worse after challenge than after placebo on five of the seven aversive behaviors and on all of the global measures. One intriguing aspect of this child's response was her mother's ability to discriminate the response to color. She volunteered the information . . . that her daughter had received the challenge six times during the 77-day period. She was correct five times. . . . These data further strengthen the accumulating evidence from controlled trials, supplemented by laboratory experiments that modest doses of synthetic colors, and perhaps other agents excluded by elimination diets, can provoke disturbed behavior in children.[75]

Given the girl's young age and the fact that the other strong reactor was less than three years old, Weiss believed that his results especially highlighted the possible effects of food additives on younger children, a conclusion shared to differing degrees by many other investigators and by Feingold himself.[76]

Although Weiss believed that his trial yielded support for the Feingold diet, many of Feingold's critics counted his trial among the negative results.[77] In contrast, reviewers who supported Feingold, including Weiss, believed that Harley's results were favorable.[78] When Weiss reviewed many of the most highly regarded trials of Feingold's theory, he concluded that all of them provided some support, arguing, "The Feingold hypothesis points to new and potentially fruitful research areas for the etiology of hyperactivity and other behavior disorders which, in turn, enhance our understanding of brain-behavior relationships. . . . Specialists in child behavior should be alert to environmental contaminants as one of the potential contributors to the genesis of disturbed behavior."[79]

Weiss' assessment differed greatly from that of Jeffrey Mattes, who also reviewed the relevant literature but believed it provided little support for Feingold's hypothesis:

> This review illustrates the need for controlled objective investigation of any treatment intervention, no matter how enthusiastically endorsed. This area may well be a good example of how long research can continue on the basis of a popular "fad" and chance positive results. The popularity of the Feingold diet might be seen as an outgrowth of sociological factors (eg., the desire for "naturalness," and suspicion of an "establishment" which includes large food manufacturers) rather than true beneficial results. Clearly there is no rationale for being an advocate *for* artificial food colorings; these additives serve no function except cosmetic. But concern regarding their effects on the behavior and learning of children seems to be unwarranted.[80]

Published after most of the trials testing Feingold's hypothesis were completed and around the time of Feingold's death, these differing assessments highlight how divided many scientists remained even after the theory was tested.

It is hard to determine exactly why reviewers arrived at such different conclusions. According to one member of NACHFA, at issue for the advisory committee was the idea that the Feingold diet was a "cure," rather than a treatment for hyperactivity. This notion, which was not what Feingold originally advocated and is certainly not what FAUS claims today, nevertheless bothered many mental health professionals who worked on hyperactivity.[81] Indeed the language used by certain researchers and reviewers suggest that Feingold's hypothesis and his manner of disseminating it was galling to many. New Zealand child psychiatrist John Werry, in response to a study published in the *Medical Journal of Australia* by child psychiatrist Peter Cook and dietician Joan Woodhill, strongly expressed how

> the most chilling aspect of Feingold's work lies in the enthusiasm with which it has been embraced by the anti-medication, anti-psychiatry sec-tion of the American public and used as a cudgel to try to close down paediatric psychopharmacological research in that country. The irony is that, if research with children is shut out in America, present clinical misuse of psychotropic drugs will continue unabated and unevaluated. Furthermore, who will then know which prophet, whether it be Feingold or some other, to follow, and public and profession alike will be at the mercy of every passing medical Pied Piper.[82]

A series of letters responding to both Cook and Woodhill's study and Werry's response proceeded to inundate the *Medical Journal of Australia*, reflecting the fervor of both Feingold's supporters and detractors. Representatives of the food industry in Australia also entered the debate, calling for "a balanced view of the Feingold hypothesis" to be given to the Australian public.[83] According to the authors of a generally supportive clinical report, which Werry and another author also lambasted, Feingold's manner of promoting his diet was much to blame for the uproar: "Unfortunately Dr. Feingold must bear much of the responsibility for such reactions—as by his unusual advocacy of his dietary programme he has actively alienated those of his colleagues who are best placed to evaluate it, and Professor Werry's emotive charges of quackery and the implication that the regime may be dangerous must be seen in that light."[84] Possibly stinging from Werry's rebuke of what were merely a series of clinical observations, the authors pointedly suggested that Professor Werry was best suited to pursue the issue of the Feingold diet further in controlled trials. This suggestion was ironic given the fact that Werry was loath to spend any time or resources testing Feingold's theory.

Similarly caustic debates erupted in the pages of other journals, and observers noted how emotion had supplanted reason on both sides of the debate.[85] While reviewers in *Pediatrics* warned that "concerns about additives and hyperkinesis developed as a result of feelings, beliefs, fads, and emotions and had little to do with science," an anonymous editorial in the *Lancet* believed that passions had been aroused on both sides: "The dietary theory of hyperactivity has aroused strong emotions. Believers in the scientific method felt challenged by the speed of its public acceptance and the lack of objective evidence. The excellent results of trials in which children and parents knew the purpose of the dietary regimen had added to the enthusiasm of the proponents and the disquiet of the food industry."[86]

Finally, there was the possibility that the food, chemical, and pharmaceutical industries influenced how researchers interpreted their findings, as well as the likelihood that profound distrust of these industries on the part of certain researchers swayed those interpretations.[87] Again, Feingold's approach was considered to have affected how industry responded. *Why Your Child Is Hyperactive* was described by Bernard Weiss as "a polemic, presenting a committed position, not a tentative scientific argument, and based on one physician's experience. It hardly endeared him to the food industry, which swiftly counterattacked."[88] Weiss blamed lack of interest in Feingold's theory following Feingold's death on "an effective publicity campaign by the Nutrition Foundation, and because of their unfamiliarity with the pertinent literature."[89]

Researchers on the other side of the debate admitted that Feingold's hypothesis posed a threat to industry. Psychiatrists Morris Lipton, one of the two co-chairs of NACHFA, and James P. Mayo stated that Feingold's claims had "major implications for the public health of children and for the food industry . . . at worst, companies would be required to reveal their trade secrets."[90] Lipton and Mayo agreed with Feingold's argument that food additive manufacturers were reluctant to specify the chemicals they used, let alone restrict their use.[91] Other observers suggested that the food industry could defuse the situation considerably by voluntarily removing some of the more cosmetic additives, particularly the colors, from the food supply.[92] This suggestion, however, was not taken up, and the emotive nature of the debate continued until Feingold's death.

Although the contentious nature of the Feingold diet helps to explain differences in how the trials to test the hypothesis were interpreted, other, more subtle, reasons might have also played a role in polarizing such assessments. One factor was related to how scientists representing different disciplines conceptualized the potential risk from food additives. For Weiss, a toxicologist who often dealt with trace amounts of hazardous material and long-term pathological effects such as cancer, the positive response of 10 percent of his sample was cause for concern. Clinical psychologists and psychiatrists who believed that hyperactivity was already treatable with stimulant drugs and who might be more inclined to concentrate on associated social, educational, or familial issues as supplementary factors, in contrast, were not as concerned with the suggestion that a small proportion of the overall hyperactive population were affected by food additives. It was also possible that toxicologists were more concerned about preventative health and public health policy than most clinicians. As one toxicologist stated, "It's very hard to get practicing physicians to think about wide issues in public health and especially prevention. You know, there's no money in prevention, who's going to pay you? So that's a very big problem."[93] As historian Michelle Murphy has described, similar disciplinary differences shaped how scientists understood sick building syndrome. While industrial hygiene experts rooted their understanding of chemical exposure in terms of levels of toxicity determined by laboratory investigations, popular epidemiologists, who could be laypeople, activists, or sympathetic scientists, gathered information about chemical exposure by mapping the distribution of health problems in relation to the location of suspected pollutants. Ultimately, this led to very different perceptions of whether or not such exposures were pathological.[94]

Feingold himself admitted in his last publication that "controversy revolves around numbers. The critics of the hypothesis contend that only a small number, perhaps 5–10% of children, react adversely to food additives and salicylates rather than the 50% favourable responses reported by me."[95] But although such discrepancies might have mattered a great deal to clinicians, particularly those who disliked Feingold's populist approach, quantifying the risk of food additives was less important if you were a parent of a hyperactive child. Conners, contemplating the extremely strong reactions to food additives exhibited by one of Weiss' subjects, contended that scientists "might discount the significance for the population at large, but if the child were *my* 3-year-old, it wouldn't matter. I would still choose to eliminate the artificial colors."[96] Determining how the results of a trial should be interpreted, therefore, depended considerably on how one defined risk, and this could be influenced by both professional practices and personal situations.[97]

Although the trials undertaken to test the Feingold diet suffered from methodological problems and were interpreted in vastly different ways, most physicians and allied health professionals assumed that they provided little evidence to support Feingold's hypothesis. By 1980, NACHFA had already concluded that any positive response to the Feingold diet was evidence of placebo and that Feingold's claims had been clearly refuted.[98] Pediatrician Esther H. Wender, one of the chairs of NACHFA, added in a review that the apparent success of the diet highlighted "the power of food to function as a conditioned stimulus" and provided suggestions to clinicians on how to ease parents away from the idea that food additives triggered hyperactivity.[99] Other industry-supported groups such as ACSH also concluded that the diet did not help hyperactive children.[100] While the conclusions of the NIH Consensus Development Conference were more ambiguous, following Feingold's death, most "investigators seemed to have lost interest" in testing the hypothesis.[101] Special education specialists Kenneth A. Kavale and Mark P. Mostert, for example, have recently asserted that "the empirical evidence appears quite steadfast and suggests that artificial additives serve merely a cosmetic function with no negative effects on behavior or learning . . . the use of the Feingold K-P diet was not predicated on research evidence, which was decidedly negative, but rather on ideological factors like the desire for a nonintrusive, natural intervention."[102] It is important to note that the authors relied largely on Kavale's own "meta-analysis" of the trials of the Feingold diet. While such meta-analyses may indeed provide an indication of the direction of results in a series of trials, in the case of the Feingold diet, it appears to have been a fairly blunt instrument. This is not only because of the relatively small number of trials included in the meta-analysis—Kavale and his coauthor, Steven R. Forness, considered twenty-three studies and referred to them as a "small number of studies"—but also because the plethora of methodological and interpretative problems were not taken into consideration.[103]

The details of the trials, particularly their conclusion and discussion sections, however, indicate clearly that Feingold's detractors did not rely on empirical evidence alone to make decisions about his hypothesis. Rather, many of the most cited criticisms of the Feingold diet had more to do with other factors, including concern about how children would cope with being on a special diet, the level of nutrients in a salicylate-free diet, and, most importantly, whether or not families could actually carry out such "a difficult and exacting regimen."[104] One researcher went as far as to claim that the "nutritional deficiencies" and "social isolation and possible harm" that accompanied the diet was nearly in "the range of child abuse."[105] As the next chapter illustrates, however, many of these concerns contradicted the experiences of families on the Feingold diet.

Conclusion

In reading the medical literature associated with the Feingold diet, it is tempting to classify all researchers and reviewers as either supportive or critical. Certainly this was the case for most of those involved in the debates. Nevertheless, some researchers did change their minds about the Feingold diet. The views of child psychologist C. Keith Conners, for instance, fluctuated throughout the 1970s, and have continued to do so. Conners's interest in Feingold's hypothesis stemmed naturally from his decades of groundbreaking experience researching the diagnosis and treatment of hyperactivity, and he was among the first scientists to receive funding to test it.[106]

At first, Conners's results, published in *Pediatrics*, were in support of Feingold's hypothesis, although the psychologist cautioned that, due to "several features inherent in the present study which need further evaluation, more study was required before any firm conclusions could be reached."[107] To at least one reader, however, this was a slight underestimate of the study's limitations. James S. Miller, a physician from California, wrote to *Pediatrics*, charging that while the article was "not the worst you have published, it is surely in active competition."[108] Miller's chief complaint was that Conners's trial was not controlled, adding sarcastically that following "the same line of intellectual rigor . . . I will bet the editorial board even money that if they send me the raw data for this article, I can establish a statistically valid correlation between a major conjunction of the planets and/or Keltic divinations using the tarot."[109]

Although no other observers were so harsh, and although he defended his work against Miller's accusations, Conners designed a second trial to test Feingold's theory. The results of this trial were more ambivalent but, while Conners was again concerned about methodological problems, he nonetheless asserted that "data firmly establish that artificial colors may be partially disruptive to younger children."[110] A few years later, however, Conners's opinion about Feingold's hypothesis, represented in his book *Food Additives and Hyperactive Children*, had changed. Stressing that new "ideas in behavioral science are often difficult to track down and evaluate," Conners warned that "the 'dramatic' nature of the effects has been grossly overstated by Dr. Feingold, except insofar as placebo effects are dramatic among people who are at their wit's end with difficult and unmanageable children."[111] Despite this conclusion, Conners graciously added that Feingold was owed "a debt of gratitude for focusing attention on the research needed to advance in this area and to protect the heirs to our planet. The evidence has not been favourable to his hypothesis in our opinion, but his general advocacy on behalf of children deserves to be supported by all citizens through their support of efforts to increase research knowledge in this important area."[112]

Conners's opinion would alter yet again. He returned to the subject of the Feingold diet in his 1989 book *Feeding the Brain* and commented on how divisive the episode had been. For him, the entire controversy exemplified "the deep distrust between practitioners who believe in the power of diet and scientists who regard it as fraud but who then go on to display bias in their own handling of the issues."[113] He admitted that "I have changed my mind about the Feingold diet since the 1970s. I sympathize with pediatricians and mental health workers who find the zeal of some patients for dietary treatments to be an impediment to other good treatments. I do not want to add to their burden. But my judgement is that the evidence is strong enough, at least for preschoolers, and especially those with confirmed allergic symptoms, that one should eliminate a broad range of unnecessary and possibly harmful ingredients from these children's diets."[114] Twenty years later, Conners's position had changed for, perhaps, a final time. Retired and not completely familiar with the more recent trials of Feingold's theory, Conners believed that the effects he had witnessed were primarily due to placebo effect.[115] As a caveat and a testament to the complicated nature of Feingold's hypothesis, he nonetheless advised mothers of young children to avoid certain additives, since it was never definitively proven that such substances had no effect on preschool children.[116]

Unlike Conners, most researchers had little trouble coming to firm conclusions about the Feingold diet based on the trials and, subsequently, either praising Feingold or condemning him. Considering the litany of methodological and interpretative problems that plagued the trials, how can this be explained? On the one hand, it is apparent that researchers were influenced by a large number of ideological, epistemological, economic, and political issues that have often shaped how scientists have made decisions about contentious theories.[117] On the other hand, the history of how Feingold's theory was tested also reveals some of the limitations of using double-blind controlled trials as a tool to prove definitively the validity of some medical claims. It suggests that overreliance on such trials for epistemological proof leads physicians away from other potentially fruitful sources of evidence, sources that at least could be used in conjunction with the findings of double-blind trials in the resolution of debates. In the case of the Feingold diet, the most important of these supplementary sources of evidence was to be found in the homes of Feingold families themselves.

Chapter 8

Feingold Families

Regardless of the conclusions reached by medical researchers about Feingold's theory, the ultimate arbiters of whether the Feingold diet worked or not were hyperactive children and their parents. Parents had to decide to attempt the diet and adjust their shopping, meal planning, and cooking; monitor their children for compliance; and determine if the diet worked. Their children had to agree to the new regimen, refraining from the processed foods—particularly snacks, drinks, and desserts that they had previously enjoyed—and resisting pressure from peers to surreptitiously eat such items. In some ways, the greatest barrier to acceptance of Feingold's hypothesis was not the reluctance of physicians to support his theory but the ability of parents and children to employ it.

Why did families try the Feingold diet? What strategies did they employ to cope with its restrictions? Did they find it to be successful? Based on oral history interviews of parents who implemented the diet as well as adults who had been on the diet as children, this chapter seeks to answer these questions. Understanding the experiences of families who tried the Feingold diet not only provides insight into the validity of Feingold's hypothesis, but it tells us a great deal about the ability of patients and their families to inform debate about intractable medical controversies. For example, the experiences of Feingold families demonstrate that physicians who warned that the diet was virtually impossible to employ were incorrect. Although families found that the diet was difficult to adhere to, and many were not able to persevere with it, others did succeed, often despite the lack of support from medical professionals. Typically, though not exclusively, the more successful families were those in which the parents were married, educated, and financially secure and in which the mothers in particular demonstrated the diligence, assertiveness, and observational skills necessary to stick to the diet; ensure that school authorities, relatives, and friends of the family adhered to their dietary wishes; and determine for themselves whether the diet was effective. The success for many families, often over a period of decades, suggests that the results of double-blind trials should not have been the only way to assess the efficacy of the Feingold diet, and that improved understanding of patient experiences can inform the development of medical knowledge and health policy.

"Sounds Like a Lot of New-Age Hooey, but I'll Try Anything to Help the Boy"

There were many reasons why parents decided to try to the Feingold diet. Frustration with treatment alternatives for hyperactivity and concern about the food supply spurred numerous parents to seek out other solutions. But it is also important to note that parents who turned to the Feingold diet did so for a variety of specific reasons and in the midst of differing circumstances. While some parents found out about the Feingold diet soon after their child's behavior had become problematic, others had endured years of attempting various treatments unsuccessfully. The rationale behind the diet likewise met with different audiences: the notion that food additives could affect behavior fitted neatly into the ecological ethos of some parents, but it seemed preposterous to others. Parents learned about the diet from a wide range of sources, sometimes when they were actively looking for an alternative, and other times in a more serendipitous fashion. Although many families found out about the Feingold diet through word of mouth and chance encounters with other Feingold families, others learned about it via a variety of media sources. Not surprisingly, none of those interviewed found out about the diet through medical journals. Families could find out about some aspects of the medical debates, however, through FAUS's newsletter, *Pure Facts*, which published summaries of research conducted to test Feingold's hypothesis. These differences in how parents discovered the Feingold diet and decided to try it not only highlight how, in many respects, Feingold families were a diverse group but also how unconventional medical ideas reach patients via many different routes. It would be a mistake, in other words, to assume that Feingold families were all living an organic, bohemian lifestyle and that they all patronized alternative health practitioners. Although the families may have eventually come to share certain beliefs and values about nutrition and psychiatry, it is clear that they did not all do so when they first heard of it.

Parents differed, for instance, with regards to their experience of using other treatments to treat their children's behavioral problems. For a number of parents, stimulant drugs were simply not an acceptable treatment. Maggie Jeffries recalled fighting with her son's school authorities over whether or not her son should be prescribed Ritalin:

> Back in the early 80s when I declined the absolute orders of the school that my child be put on Ritalin, they literally threatened that he'd have to be removed from school. . . . And I just pushed right back because they just assumed that they were going to bully me like the rest of the little country girls in the small town I lived in here in Michigan. But I was not the quiet, gentle little country girl, I was a girl from over by Chicago. I just pushed them right back and said, "If you decline to have him in school then perhaps the state will reimburse me to educate him." And they just shut right up.[1]

Lynn Kitchen felt "quite uncomfortable" with the possible side effects of stimulant drugs. She and also experienced pressure from her son's teachers, who wanted him to take Ritalin, yet she resisted their demands, stating that she and her husband would "try everything we can versus doing, doing the amphetamines and the Ritalin to address his health needs."[2]

In a number of cases where the children were not of school age, parents who were hesitant about the use of amphetamines did not feel pressured by school authorities and had more time to explore their options. Although Wendy Lott described how she had prepared herself "for the possibility that he'd have to be on meds" when her son went to school, she was grateful that she discovered the diet before he was prescribed anything, and his teachers never discovered that he had been diagnosed with hyperactivity.[3] Laura Lamb was cautious about mainstream approaches to hyperactivity because of an experience involving her sister: "I had a sister that the teachers would chronically tell my mom that needed to be on medication, and they bothered her so much about it that she lied and said, 'I put her on it.' And as soon as she said it, they said, 'Oh, she's doing great!'"[4] In other situations, parents had tried other treatments, experienced limited success, and sought alternatives. Ellen Miller had noticed that Ritalin appeared to help the boy who lived next door, but found that the stimulant did not improve the behavior of her son: "For this other child it was effective. And I think that for some children it is the answer, but for [my son] it was not the answer. He lost appetite, his behavior was worse when he came off the cycle of Ritalin. I was very unhappy and I took him off."[5]

Other parents also found that hyperactivity drugs were either not helpful or had distressing side effects. Justine Ewing described how she "tried Ritalin. It didn't work. We tried Strattera. It didn't work. And I ended up ultimately putting him on Concerta, but when he was on Concerta I noticed side effects—he had a real difficulty sleeping."[6] Rosemarie Kushner did not want her son to be prescribed Ritalin, but acquiesced to the wishes of his school to have him prescribed the drug. Neither she nor the officials at her son's school were satisfied with its effects, however, and she looked for alternatives while the school officials tried to convince her to increase her son's dosage. Ironically, she was convinced to implement the Feingold diet fully—she had been casually experimenting with it—when visiting a shop in the basement of her son's therapist's office: "There was a little snack shop there and the kids were looking at the different snacks going, 'Can we have this? Can we have this? Is this for us?,' and I was saying, 'No that has color. No that has color. Yeah that would be okay.' And this woman came over and said, 'Excuse me, are you using the Feingold program?' And that was my connection with somebody who had actually used it and who could talk to me about it."[7]

As Ellen Miller declared, "when you're so desperate for help, you'll try anything."[8] Miller's greatest fear, according to her son, was that he would never finish school: "My mom had nightmares of her twenty year old son being able to drive to his own sixth-grade graduation." Her fears were never realized, since David Miller eventually earned a PhD from Cambridge University.[9] Many other parents expressed feelings of desperation and hopelessness prior to attempting the Feingold diet. For Sylvia Terry, whose ten-year-old son's behavior had regressed when he was prescribed Ritalin and who had also been receiving "continual counseling," the Feingold diet was "do or die."[10] Lesley Freeman was similarly desperate:

> He became more and more difficult to handle. He would scream at nothing. You could ask him if he wanted a scrambled egg or a fried egg, he would scream. He couldn't handle any kind of input. He couldn't handle any kind of choices. He would have tantrums from one end of the day to the next. He would roll on the floor and would scream. He'd climbed on the coffee table and I took him off and said, "No, no!" And he did that thirty-five times in a row. And I sat him down so hard and I thought, "Oh my God if I were stronger I would break his back," and I called Jewish Family Services and said "You've got to help me before I kill this child."[11]

Such desperation forced some families to embrace notions about nutrition and behavior that they would have otherwise rejected. When Trevor Davidson's wife put forward the idea of trying the Feingold diet, he recalled how "I was thinking to myself that this sort of sounds like a lot of new age hooey, but I'll try anything to help the boy."[12] As his wife Gayle described, "I was excited, [he] was the skeptic. We needed to do something to help [our son] and I was willing to try anything before medication."[13] Other parents were similarly suspicious of Feingold's theory: "The first two times I heard it, I thought it could not possibly be the case because some of the symptoms were severe. I never gave food chemicals a thought. I was raised on them. . . . I did nothing with the information for a year. I really figured it was an off-shoot of the health food movement in the 'hippy' days. However, we had no other options, so when he was about three, we tried it."[14] Liz Grossman described how she "did not in a million years think diet would change my son," and felt that medication would likely be necessary for him at some point, but she agreed to try the Feingold diet due to her husband's concerns about Ritalin.[15] Similarly, Barbara Beck, although she had never considered that food additives could cause health problems, said, "I was so desperate, I'd try anything. I would not have disregarded any solution that anyone had given me as long as it was reasonable and safe."[16]

In contrast, some parents found that Feingold's theory made sense, but they often had different reasons. Maggie Jeffries, who described herself as "a poor hippy living in the woods," had a long-standing interest in unprocessed food, shopped at a cooperative store that sold health foods such as "organic flours and cold-pressed oils," and "made a lot of stuff from scratch."[17] The fact that Jeffries suffered from numerous allergies and believed that her asthma was related to food colors predisposed her towards the Feingold diet. For other parents, such as one woman who had been raised on the Feingold diet herself, avoiding food additives was self-explanatory: "Why chance it? To the best of our understanding our brain chemistry is affected by the foods that we eat. If we're eating food with chemicals, we're affecting our brain chemistry. Why do that to a child? You want to choose foods in their most organic, natural state."[18] Greg Hewson, who had been on the diet as a child, recalled how his parents' long-standing interest in organic, home-grown food minimized the disruption of the Feingold diet to their household.[19]

Other parents had quite different reasons for questioning food additives.[20] Hanna Johnston taught allied health sciences at a university and was shocked in hindsight that her training as a histologist did not alert her to the dangers of certain chemicals. When Johnston discovered that a number of foods she was feeding her son contained tartrazine, she recalled,

> I used to use tartrazine in the lab under a fume hood. . . . Well it was like, duh? That's what I felt like. When I was reading the chemicals in some

of these foods and the colors and what their color names were, more than just Yellow number five, I read that it was tartrazine, I started thinking, we use these, these are hazardous materials in the lab. These things have MSDS [Material Safety Data Sheets] forms which I know because I used to work in histology labs and we were putting this in our mouths, we were eating this. So that's when I realized, you know, there's something wrong here and I should have known better.[21]

Johnston's husband was also appalled "that we were intelligent people that allowed this to happen, that we didn't read what we were putting into our mouths." Similarly, when Rosemarie Kushner's son, Frank Kushner, left for college to study chemistry, he became more convinced that food additives could affect his behavior and was more willing to remain on the diet.[22]

Just as the families approached Feingold's idea from a range of perspectives, they found out about the Feingold diet in a variety of ways and often did so unexpectedly. Ellen Miller, was unaware of the diet until her then-husband brought a work colleague and his wife home for a meal. She turned out to be the president of the local Feingold Association.[23] Quite often parents were told of the diet by others who had successfully used the diet themselves. Parents also heard word of the diet through relatives, friends, neighbors, magazines, television programs, and, increasingly during the last decade, the Internet.[24]

That parents learned about the Feingold diet in a wide variety of ways illustrates Feingold's success in promoting his diet directly to the general pubic after his attempts to gain the approval of his fellow physicians failed. Interestingly, only one parent interviewed found out about the diet through a health professional, specifically a chiropractor, as certain schools of chiropractics supported the use of elimination diets.[25] Instead, when most parents mentioned the Feingold diet to their general practitioner, pediatrician, or psychiatrist, they were warned that it was not recognized as an effective treatment for hyperactivity. As Rima Apple contends, while physicians may value the information provided by parents regarding some aspects of health care, for example, the side effects of drugs, they can also feel that their medical authority is threatened when parents suggest employing alternative treatments such as the Feingold diet.[26] The willingness of parents to ignore the advice of their physicians on the subject of hyperactivity illustrates Apple's findings regarding how mothers, during the last third of the twentieth century, were increasingly willing to question the advice of an "autocratic health-care practitioner."[27] By the 1970s, mothers could choose from any number of health "experts," ranging from the Boston Women's Health Book Collective to La Leche League, but then had to make difficult decisions about who to trust. For many mothers, it was difficult "to alter the authoritarian medical system they faced."[28]

Wendy Lott found that her first general practitioner was supportive of her choice to employ the Feingold diet and expressed a general interest in nutrition, but then her family had to change health insurance plans. All of the subsequent physicians they spoke to were dismissive: "They would all recite the same phrases: 'Dangerous for their nutrition,' 'Lack of Vitamin C,' 'No evidence that it works.' . . . 'It works in a very few cases.'"[29] Lynn Kitchen's first physician was supportive, but then she retired. Kitchen doubted that her "new medical doctor . . . would be open to a lot of that. I mean you have to find a pretty special medical doctor who is open to it."[30] Many parents found that they had to be assertive with medical authority figures. When Theresa McKay was told by her son's psychiatrist that he would require Ritalin, she said, "'I'm not going to use the medication, we're going to use the diet instead,' and the psychiatrist said, 'Oh well I've heard that they don't work.' I said, 'That's interesting but we're going to try anyway.' We've not been back to that psychiatrist."[31] Others, such as Rosemarie Kushner, found that their pediatricians were more concerned about the practicality of the diet, warning, "'There's not going to be anything you can eat except chicken breast and pineapple.' I knew that wasn't true. He pooh-poohed it. Eventually, he did suggest it to people as something off the wall they could try. For years and years he said it was a really stupid idea and I was quite wacko."[32] Justine Ewing, in contrast, was able to convince her physician to consider the diet: "The doctor said as long as we weren't extreme about it . . . he would go along with it, but he started to see big differences so he was impressed and wanted to use the diet on other of his patients and read all the literature about it." For the most part, however, Feingold families received little cooperation from their physicians, particularly in terms of helping them employ the diet.[33]

The willingness of Ewing to go against her physician's advice was typical of many parents who decided to try the Feingold diet. Although some physicians did not discourage parents from employing the diet, especially after it appeared to be working, others had stopped "seeing any doctors because they weren't helping."[34] In other words, many parents, often out of frustration, gave up on their physician's advice and decided that they would take primary responsibility for the health of their children. In so doing, parents demonstrated a willingness to defy medical authority and to take responsibility for their children's health. The defiant attitude of many parents was often supplemented with a resolute determination that their children follow the diet at home, at school, at birthday parties, and anywhere else their children could come in contact with food additives.

"No Big Deal" or "Very Difficult?":
Adhering to the Feingold Diet

One of the chief criticisms of the Feingold diet was that it was too difficult for the typical American family to undertake. Conversely, some of Feingold's supporters have argued that the diet was not actually that arduous and most families could cope with it. As Jane Hersey, president of FAUS explained, "The effort required will seem trivial compared to the joy of seeing your child function normally."[35] The experiences of most Feingold families, however, suggest that adhering to the Feingold diet was taxing in many aspects, and families who found success with the diet often shared a number of important attributes.

Once parents decided to attempt the Feingold diet, they were faced with a number of challenges. These included convincing their children to follow the diet, changing their shopping and cooking practices, and monitoring what their children ate and their resulting behavior. The success families had in overcoming these challenges depended on a number of factors, including the degree to which the Feingold diet differed from their previous diet; how compliant friends, family, the school system and, most importantly, their children were with regards to the diet; and how able families were to observe their child's eating and behavior, advocate for them, and adapt the diet for their specific needs. Given these challenges, it is perhaps unsurprising that two-parent families, particularly those in which the earnings of the father allowed the mother to stay at home for extended periods, experienced more success. Still, a number of single mothers were able to persevere with the diet, suggesting that, while the Feingold diet was often described by physicians as "a difficult and exacting regimen," it was by no means an impossible one.[36]

The first task all parents had in employing the Feingold diet was convincing their children, and the rest of the family, to try it. Despite the assertion made by a team of researchers that the "strict Feingold diet appears to be distasteful to the typical American child," children's responses to the prospect of a diet that eliminated food colors and flavors fluctuated from dread to optimism.[37] Some children were highly resistant to the Feingold diet. Darren Aubrey, whose family was already eating a fairly additive-free diet, declared, "I hated the diet. Tomato sauce. Ketchup. Pizza. I didn't have so many specific losses, but I remember feeling very much confined, bitter, and angry about the diet."[38]

Other children disliked having to go on the diet at first, but recognized that it might be of some benefit. Frank Kushner expressed how it was "kind of annoying, but if it was going to help then, you know, back then I think it was annoying because it set me apart from the other kids, but if it was going to help me, then it was worth it."[39] Frank's mother reiterated this stating how at "first he was like, 'I don't want to do it, I don't want to do it.' But okay, we're not going to try to do it if you're not going to buy into it because it won't work. So, he decided he was going to do it."[40] Other children were hesitant, but ultimately pliable: "I didn't want to give up all the good food that I was eating, like the dyed foods and all that. I didn't really like it, but I thought okay, I'll go with it."[41] Similarly, Jason Atwater stated how, when his mother began the Feingold diet, he "didn't know she was changing it at first, but when I found out I wasn't happy at first, but I thought it would make me better."[42]

Finally, there were children who were almost eager to try the new regimen. David Miller did not mind starting the diet, in part because it meant an alternative to Ritalin, his feelings for which he described as follows: "I hated it. I remember Mom giving me the pill when we were in the car and I started acting up and I hated the taste of it. . . . I lost my appetite and I'd be really up and then really down. I do remember not liking that pill."[43] It also helped that his mother had studied home economics in college and "was a phenomenal cook. So she was cooking things from scratch anyway because she liked doing it. So our diet was pretty good."[44] It is interesting that while Miller recalled that the effects of the diet were immediate, his mother thought they took "six to eight weeks, really working with the diet closely to see positive effects."[45]

Just as children's opinions about the Feingold diet differed at first, so too did their parents' experiences. The first stage of the diet was very restrictive, since it not only eliminated artificial colors and flavors but also fruits and vegetables, such as tomatoes, apples, and grapes, that contained high levels of salicylates. As Laura Lamb described, "stage one was very difficult because you are so limited because you are eliminating the salicylates. That was tough because that's in so many things naturally. I had to take away so many of his favorite foods."[46] Donna Larkin also found that the first stage of the diet was a challenge: "It was very difficult [sigh]. You know, three months of cleaning cupboards and not eating anything and trying to find the food you need . . . Originally . . . the meal prep was enormous. You know, making fake tomato sauce. My kids were onto me. They figured it out. So that part was tough . . . I think the hardest thing was snacks. My children had been accustomed to eating certain kinds of snacks, junk food if you will, and, you know, they still wanted a little bit of that. I felt guilty that they couldn't have that and so that was tough."[47] For Lesley Freeman, the first stage was also time-consuming, particularly determining which foods in the grocery store were acceptable: "I mostly got my information from person to person contact. I was on the phone during the first couple of days eight hours with a Feingold Association volunteer."[48] Freeman recalled spending "three hours a week at first every time I went shopping." She believed part of the difficulty parents had in the grocery store was due to brand loyalty, the idea that "people have emotional connections with certain brands and foods."[49] Other families described how their weekly shopping expanded from a half-hour excursion to a three-and-a-half-hour marathon.[50]

FAUS provided considerable support to many families during this initial stage of the diet, providing not only lists of acceptable foods but practical advice about how to cope with problematic occasions such as birthday parties and Halloween. During the second stage of the diet, parents were encouraged to reintroduce fruits and vegetables, carefully observing whether or not certain items caused problems. This process was challenging in a different way. As Donna Larkin described, "That whole trial and error process of eliminating everything, bringing back certain things, finding the brands that work for you. Because they're not the same, I don't think, for everyone . . . My son has issues with things that other people I know don't have issues with. So working that out for yourself, it takes a while. I want to say at least six months to a year, which is an awfully long time and a big commitment."[51] Other parents found that the second stage of the diet was not as difficult, but this was often due to the fact that their children did not react to the fruits and vegetables banned in stage one.[52]

For some parents, the perceived difficulties of the diet were such that they doubted their ability to persevere with it. Having read about it, Justine Ewing, whose son was taking Ritalin, described how the diet "looked like a whole lot of work, so I didn't even bother investigating it. I thought the idea of having to feed him based on no food coloring, no flavoring, and no preservatives was just going to be impossible. . . . I just thought it would be a matter of I would have to feed him things he doesn't like to eat, like fruits and vegetables and whole grains and things like that. And so the medicine at that point was working for us fine. I didn't explore it further. I just thought, 'Oh those poor people on the diet!'"[53] If Ewing, who was able to stay at home with her three children, found the diet intimidating and not a valid alternative to Ritalin, it is not surprising that the majority of families with hyperactive children decided against trying the diet, especially considering it was a treatment that most physicians did not support.

Sylvia Terry, a single mother, found the diet very challenging and was unsuccessful with it at first. For her, part of the problem was her ex-husband: "We did try the diet for the first time when he was little . . . he was five I guess, but being divorced, the other party, his dad, would not participate in the diet. He would go see him often and it was just so hard."[54] While Terry's second attempt was more successful, many other parents were not able to persevere with it. For Barbara Beck, the diet seemed to be fairly easy at first and appeared to help her daughter. She recalled how, although the diet involved "time consuming effort initially . . . looking at the chemicals on the food and hoping that they're honestly labeled," meal preparation "wasn't a huge change because I cooked dinners, proper dinners."[55] Within five days, her daughter "was a different child. The look she would get in her eyes when she was really frustrated was gone, it was just gone." Despite the improvements, other problems, particularly at school, interfered with the regimen, and Beck accepted her daughter's request to abandon the diet. Not only were the people who managed the school cafeteria unwilling to adapt their practices to help a single child, but her daughter "had all these problems with people teasing her. Other people not believing that food could change her behavior. And they would give her things and she would react. And she just didn't want to do it. And all she can remember now is that for three days all she could eat was potatoes and rice cakes."[56] Despite the fact that her daughter has not been on the diet for over twenty years, Beck's mother still receives information from FAUS. Beck continues to try to convince her daughter to consider the Feingold diet in order to wean herself off of the stimulant drugs that she currently is prescribed.

Other parents found that the process of changing their diet was relatively easy. One family adhered to a kosher diet and already spent time checking labels.[57] Others had always consumed a diet largely free of additives. For these parents, meals prepared in the home were not as problematic as snacks, drinks, and food consumed elsewhere. Ellen Miller's son, for example, reacted strongly when he ate an apple at a neighbor's house: "A neighbor called me . . . one day and said '[He] can't eat apples, can he?' And I said, 'Did you give him an apple?' She said, 'Yes, and he's on the floor laughing so hard, he doesn't know what he's doing.'"[58] For Maggie Jeffries, the problem was not only apples but cider: "Once we had been to a market in . . . this city that was close to us on a hot summer day, you know about thirty-five miles away from where we lived, and I had bought cider. And I'm drinking cider out of the jug and he's so thirsty and I said, 'Well here have some, what's the worst that will happen?' And so he got through a whole lot of cider and I'm telling you he was like a wild drunk Irishman. When we got home I ended up having to wrestle him and throw him down on the ground."[59]

For Hanna Johnston, clearing her cupboards of foods that contained additives was not particularly difficult, since she "was Italian" and "did all the cooking anyway," but some snacks and foods that she gave to her son as a treat were problematic.[60] Once she began researching the Feingold diet, Johnston discovered to her surprise that one of her son's favorite breakfast treats contained food coloring:

> I realized I was giving him waffles in the morning, and I look on the package—the waffles are the shape of zoo animals because they market it for the kids—and there was Yellow #5 on it . . . and so I was jacking him up first thing in the morning. But I always had bought him the all natural or the pure maple syrup, so I was always doing that, but never realized that the waffle itself was what was really bad. Because I just figured, well they're marketing it for kids, it must be healthy. . . . And I have learned with [him] that Yellow #5 is the worst, red comes close after, so we just avoid all artificial colors . . . that just sends him—it's like he's on crack cocaine.[61]

Although the Feingold diet helped her with his behavior at home, problems at school remained. After meeting with the school about her son's behavior, and subsequently pulling him from that school, Johnston found out that "for snacks they were giving them Goldfish [a brand of cracker]. And the regular Goldfish are okay, but the extra cheesy Goldfish, or whatever it is, has the artificial color in it. So he was having those kind of snacks during their snack-time."[62]

In general, parents found that restricting what their children ate outside of the home was one of the most difficult aspects of the Feingold diet. While the challenges involved in controlling the food their children consumed at school influenced some parents to switch schools or, in some cases, home-school their children, others found that the schools were helpful, particularly if school officials had noted improvements in behavior. In order to prevent children from eating snacks at school that contained additives, for example, many parents provided bags of additive-free snacks for the school so that their child would not feel left out during snack time, and found that the teachers cooperated willingly with this strategy.[63] Parents revealed differing levels of cooperation from friends and relatives. Although many parents expressed how supportive their family and friends were, others were not so fortunate.[64] Barbara Beck, for instance, recalled how her friends and family thought the Feingold diet was "ridiculous" and that "food couldn't possibly cause behavior problems."[65] For other parents, one side of the family was more supportive than the other. Although Jennifer Illing's parents were "awesome" about following the diet, her husband's side was not, despite the fact that they had problems with certain types of food themselves: "We have a peanut allergy with a nephew in the family, and we've had some issues with that side of the family. They put a lot more of an . . . emphasis on the peanut allergy, and haven't really cared about my kids' problems. We've had discussions about it. I've just gotten to the point where I'm sick of it and I'll bring my own food . . . They'll have only pop for the kids. Or Hi-C which is basically pop . . . My kids will say, 'No thanks, we can't have that, but Mom brought us juice boxes.'"[66]

Although Feingold families faced a good deal of skepticism, such doubts could be quelled when friends or relatives witnessed the effects of a dietary violation. When in Ontario for a family visit, for example, Hanna Johnston let her son's grandmother bring him to "the Tim Hortons [a popular Canadian donut shop chain] . . . and bought him a cinnamon bun . . . and then she took him to the grocery store and we met up with an elderly lady who was a neighbor and he started spitting in her face—that was one of the things, spitting and kicking—. . . and this was after a week of perfect behavior, just very good young boy behavior and my mother said, never again was she going to Tim Hortons."[67] For a Canadian, this was no mean feat. Founded in 1964 by Canadian hockey player Tim Horton, who died tragically in a traffic accident, the chain sponsors the Briar, the Canadian men's curling championship; funds Tim Hortons Children's Foundation, which sends disadvantaged children to camp; and has a special relationship with the Canadian Armed Forces, which asked the company to open outlets at overseas bases in order to boost morale. In other words, this grandmother did not renounce just any doughnut shop, she rejected a Canadian institution.[68]

Similarly, Theresa McKay's mother-in-law, whom she thought "would never get it," became convinced that the Feingold diet worked after witnessing improvements in her grandson's behavior herself. However, many of McKay's other friends and family bristled at her approach to her son's diet: "They think I'm the most oversensitive, obnoxious, overbearing mother there ever was, but that's okay. I'll take that. They don't get it. But they don't live with him. They don't see how much more pleasant he is to be around." In order to participate in family events, she prepared most of the food so that she was confident that her son would have acceptable foods to eat, a practice many other families followed.[69]

Parents also had to cope with other special occasions where food was involved, most notably birthday parties and Halloween. Often it was experiences with birthday parties that convinced parents that food additives were at the root of their child's hyperactivity. Justine Ewing became suspicious of food colors after

a road trip to Michigan [from Virginia] for a birthday party. . . . My mother provided this wonderfully decorated birthday cake . . . and it was full of blue food coloring. . . . Our trip home from my mom's house [the next day] was literally torture. [He] could not sit still in his car seat, he screamed the whole time home, he complained, he thrashed, he kicked—it's a nine hour trip—and he did it for the whole trip home. And the next day he was very, very unstable and very tantrummy and that was my clue, that's what made me think that there's something about this blue food coloring. I had a friend who had mentioned to me that her son is ADHD, he's on medication, and they keep him from certain colored food, too. So, I put those two together and I started researching food coloring and ADHD.[70]

An experience following a birthday party helped to convince Rosemarie Kushner that the Feingold diet was working for her son:

While he was on the Ritalin, I took him to a birthday party and we had been following this diet, and on the way to the birthday party, we sat in the car, he and I, and had a very intelligent conversation. He sat very nicely. It was like, "Wow, a calm kid." And I had made arrangements with the mom. She was going to have ice cream and cake and I had sent along a cupcake and we had heard where she was getting the ice cream and the bread and whatever and it was going to be fine. So, we're like . . . "here's your cupcake, you can have the ice cream; don't have the cake." And when I picked him up from the party, he was . . . talking a mile a minute, a different kid, and we figured out that the mom had switched ice creams. So he was told, go ahead and have the ice cream and that point I decided okay, this was really working.[71]

Many other parents also provided additive-free cupcakes to eat instead of the birthday cake, but this strategy did not always work. When Donna Larkin offered to make a cupcake for her son to bring to a party, he refused because it made him feel different from his friends.[72]

These experiences highlight not only how parents attempted to preempt dietary violations at special events by preparing special food for their children but how such preparation was not always sufficient. Although many parents developed creative ways in which to deal with Halloween, for example, by giving their children a toy in exchange for the candy they collected, they nevertheless had to trust that their children would not try to get at the confiscated candy. One Halloween, David Miller gave into temptation: "I snuck in my candy bag and I just went crazy. I ate everything in it and got really sick. I remember my parents telling me let us inspect the candy because they're some crazy people out there; sometimes they put poison in it. So all of the sudden I thought I'd got poisoned . . . I asked, 'Am I going die?' And my dad was kind of irritated with me and he said, 'If you die, you die. Go back to bed.' And I remember staying up all night crying, thinking that if I could stay awake, I wouldn't die."[73]

Perhaps because of such incidents, Miller, as with most of the other children, was usually compliant. For Miller, acquiescence equated to academic and social success. He described how, "If I kept to my good diet, I could read, I had friends, I could control myself." If he cheated, he felt guilty and was invariably caught by his mother.[74] Interestingly, Miller did not feel guilty when he had a candy bar, or another banned item, "before football games because I would go in there and just, you know, have extra energy and be all hyper because I would be hitting people in pads and beating them up." Frank Kushner also felt that he benefited from the Feingold diet, describing how when he cheated he "would feel as if I didn't have as much control . . . whatever would happen, I would react before I realized what I wanted to do."[75] Guilt, however, also played a role, as his mother recalled: "I remember when he was a little older, maybe twelve or so, we went somewhere where there was three different colors of Jell-O, and he was like, 'Can I have it?' And I said, 'You're old enough for that to be a decision that you have to make yourself, but you're responsible for your behavior if you do.' He hated that. He'd say, 'You're just trying to make me feel guilty,' and, yes, I was."[76]

Another interviewee was also reluctant to cheat, stating that when he "realized that there was an improvement, it made me want to stay on it, to keep the way I was going." It also helped that his mother "did a pretty good job of buying food that went with the Feingold diet, but was also good to eat."[77] Trevor Davidson agreed that his son's compliance was based on the recognition that it helped him to behave: "he's really good about it. I think he really knows that if he does go off the diet, how it'll make him act, you know, and he's very good at resisting temptation. If somebody brings in cupcakes to school and he's not sure if it has things in it he'll very politely say, 'You know, I don't think I can have it because I don't know what's in it and I'm not supposed to have certain things.' . . . He makes really good decisions, probably better than what I would've made at that age." Maggie Jeffries's son had a different reason for staying on the diet. According to her, food additives not only made him "extremely hyperactive," but it would also make him "urinate on himself during the day and . . . at night," a symptom that disappeared once he started the Feingold diet. He was compliant, she explained, because "urinating on yourself will make you an outcast. No one wants wet pants."[78] Lynn Kitchen also mentioned that her son's bed-wetting ceased after she put him on the diet.[79]

Other children found the Feingold diet to be a struggle and, in particular, alienated them from their peers. Bonnie Thompson, who had been on the Feingold diet and who used it with her own family, recognized how:

> there was always the group of parents who did things differently. I don't think I was as aware of it as my kids are. That was more my personality as a child, I didn't really care, but my kids have been very aware of that, that it is different. And we just recently moved . . . into a different area of town, and we noticed . . . they're feeling less different than before. It really stood out where they were before. Now there's a lot more families that are vegetarian or have different ethnic backgrounds and choose different types of food. It's not as big of a deal. Before they really did feel it made them different.[80]

Darren Aubrey felt that the diet branded him as different: "I felt like it set me apart, sort of like a Jew keeping Kosher, but without the holidays."[81] This was partly because many of the foods that he had to avoid, such as pizza, candy, or restaurant meals, were consumed during social occasions in which he could not fully participate. He recalled having primarily negative associations with the Feingold diet, stating how he resented the diet's "restrictions, doubted their efficacy, and chafed under them." Aubrey also felt bitter that, while his parents blamed his behavioral problems on dietary infractions, he was made responsible for such infractions. The diet

> was an intriguing system for compartmentalizing. If something went wrong, it was blamed on the diet and my infractions, present, past, secret or accidental. If I was being defiant, it was the food speaking. If I got a bad grade, it was either my fault because I was "off" in secret, or my fault because God was punishing me for having lied about eating something. So, the diet was mystical, sacred, mysterious, biochemical, explaining everything, explaining nothing, the will of God and the fault of society, separating me from the "normal person."[82]

Although Aubrey felt healthier while on the diet and performed better at school, he "was never sure that any of this was a benefit of the diet" and cheated on it regularly. Despite these negative feelings, Aubrey continued with the diet in college, modifying it when possible, and planned on employing it when he became a father. Nevertheless, he feared that the diet would lead to "very serious arguments" when he and his wife had children because she came from "an MSG infused culture."[83]

Modification of the diet proved to be an effective way for parents and children to make it more bearable. To a certain extent, modification was a feature of stage two of the Feingold diet, in which salicylate-laden fruits and vegetables were reintroduced, but many parents emphasized how they themselves were responsible for adapting the diet. As David Miller explained, "We basically adhered to the principles of the Feingold diet but we didn't follow the Feingold diet to a tee."[84] Others expressed how they did not always stick to the Feingold diet, but used "common sense and observation" to see if a certain food caused a change in their child's behavior.[85] While some parents modified the Feingold diet to include more foods, one mother, who was gluten and lactose intolerant and believed that sugar caused behavioral problems, restricted additional items, added vitamins, and put her son through a "heavy metal detox" in order to cleanse his system, a process that she "can't say enough about."[86] Other parents highlighted how they, too, employed observation and analysis in order to alter the diet and manage at restaurants, family events, and parties. Many of the mothers interviewed developed these skills from either university or vocational training in science, technology, or health care. Such abilities helped parents to develop coping strategies for when their children mistakenly or purposefully ate a banned substance. As Hanna Johnston described, "If he has something like that we'll just give him a bottle of water . . . Drink the water, run, and he'll just fall asleep . . . I liken it to kind of having a hangover."[87]

Parents did not rely on the Feingold diet alone to improve the behavior and learning of their children; although they typically avoided the use of stimulant drugs, other psychological and educational strategies were also employed. David Miller acknowledged the importance of the Feingold diet but also attributed his academic success to the fact that his mother found a laboratory school associated with a university that focused on, among other things, rebuilding his damaged self esteem. Miller declared, "Public school would have eaten me alive and they didn't have the resources back then to deal with kids like me."[88] Many children found that activities such as sports and cadets also provided discipline and an outlet for aggression and frustration.[89] A number of mothers home-schooled their children, which gave them more control over what their children ate, and others used yoga, behavior modification, music therapy, and a range of parenting techniques in order to assist with behavior and learning.[90] The use of such a wide range of strategies highlights how most parents took a holistic approach to their children's development, a feature that was mirrored in their approach to health in general.

The decisions parents made to adhere to the Feingold diet not only required parents to be observant, analytical, patient, diligent, flexible, and to defy conventional medical advice, but it demanded determination and assertiveness when it came to dealing with school authorities, medical professionals, and the diet itself. As Lynn Kitchen explained when her son's teachers tried to convince her to give him Ritalin, "The school tried to push us that way and you have to become a very stringent advocate for your kids in that scenario and put your boundaries down as far as what you're prepared to do."[91] Jennifer Illing's experiences with the Feingold diet also made her more assertive with medical authorities: "I'm a pretty forceful personality to begin with, but I will definitely take a greater stance with the medical field now."[92]

When it came to succeeding on the diet, nearly all parents stressed that perseverance and diligence was essential, and added that families that did not try the Feingold diet or failed in the attempt often lacked such qualities. Contemplating why his mother, who was a single parent for much of his childhood, succeeded with the diet while others failed, David Miller, who now uses the diet for his children, stated simply, "Most people are lazy and most people are followers. They want to be told the solution to their problems." He added that it was easier for parents "to give a pill, sedate him, drug him, than have to deal with the problem."[93] Theresa McKay believed drug companies also played a role, taking advantage of parents' desire for an easy solution: "it's money and laziness. The public is lazy and doesn't want to work and the drug companies want money. You put those two together and you have a nation who pops pills."[94]

Although it seems as though Feingold families shared a number of attributes that helped them successfully implement the Feingold diet, there was another essential factor that they held in common: the steadfast belief that the diet worked. All parents, including those whose children ultimately chose not to adhere to the diet, agreed that the Feingold diet had improved their children's behavior. Often such beliefs were shaped by a moment of epiphany. After attempting a wide range of treatments for her son's behavior, Lesley Freeman "talked to my child who was willing, and my husband was willing to cooperate, and we started the diet. And in four days, I'll never forget, he walked into the kitchen and said, 'Mom, I can't find my other sock.' And I just about fell to the floor because this is not something this child could've ever said. He would either have been hysterical because he wanted his other sock or he would've forgotten that he needed another sock. . . . From that point he was quite normal emotionally."[95] Justine Ewing recalled how her son's behavior also improved markedly after "about four days . . . and then he was just a dramatically different child. He wasn't crying as much; he wasn't as wild. He was sleeping through the night much better . . . I could look him in the eye and talk to him and reason with him and explain things to him."[96] Jennifer Illing found that improvements in their child's behavior occurred quickly and were not limited to behavior: "I did not expect it to have the impact on behavior that it did. I expected it to take care of rashes. I couldn't believe how much it helped with the eczema and . . . the digestive system issues. I was very amazed."[97]

While some parents had to wait longer for improvements, they were equally impressed when improvements eventually occurred. When Sylvia Terry contacted FAUS about what she should expect in terms of timing, she was told,

> If they'd been on a lot of medicine it would take six weeks ... and I am not lying when I tell you that it was six weeks to the day ... night and day difference. Everybody noticed. . . . He could sit and have a conversation without being all over the room. He would be compliant. You could ask him to do this or that and he'd just say ok and he would just do it without this huge ordeal. The teachers, I didn't get phone calls and notes and all of that just calmed down so much. There weren't problems like there were before. His aggressiveness was a big change. His aggressiveness and compliance were some of the biggest changes I saw.[98]

Laura Lamb, whose son had previously required some special education measures, found that his teachers were also impressed by his academic improvement: "he was out of the learning centre pretty much within six months. His teacher came to me and said, 'What is going on with this? He doesn't need us anymore. He's thriving and succeeding all on his own.' I said I simply changed his food."[99]

One of the chief suspicions researchers had of the Feingold diet was that its effects were only a placebo, largely due to the increased attention given to the child.[100] When parents were asked about this possibility, however, they were resolute that this was not the case: "I know this is not a placebo effect. For example last year he snuck money to school and bought school lunch (pizza). I did not know this. He ran in the house like a tornado and I just thought, 'Wow I haven't seen this in a long time.' Finally my daughter told me he had bought lunch. He was hyper the entire day and woke up the next morning still hyper. He came off the school bus that day and he was fine. He does not sneak anymore."[101] For Trevor Davidson, the times when his son went off his diet were enough to reaffirm his belief in the diet and undermine the notion that it was only a placebo: "At first you don't notice the difference in him, you know, until he goes off his diet . . . and then you're like, 'Holy cow! Now I remember why we keep him on this diet.'" Regardless of what mainstream medicine claimed about the Feingold diet, these parents had become "believers."[102] For them the diet worked.

Conclusion

It is difficult to listen to interviews of Feingold families and not feel inclined to believe, as they did, that the Feingold diet had an enormously positive impact on their children's lives. But as historical evidence, oral history interviews must be viewed as critically as any other source. Put another way, just as the few dozen trials of the Feingold diet failed to confirm conclusively that Feingold's theory was invalid, the experiences of a few dozen Feingold families did not prove that it worked. Given the small sample size, it is possible that, as many of Feingold's critics suggested, the children who responded to the Feingold diet represented an exceptional, self-selecting, and miniscule percentage of the millions of children diagnosed with hyperactivity. Although it would be remarkable for the placebo effect to have caused the improvements in behavior in all of the families interviewed, especially given the decades that had elapsed in many cases, most families employed other interventions in addition to the Feingold diet that might have resulted in improved behavior. Most importantly, medical and popular conceptualizations of hyperactivity were influenced not only by trends in medical theory and technology, but also by educational, political, cultural, economic, and demographic factors. Hyperactivity was and continues to be a disorder characterized by a mismatch of behaviors and social circumstances; behavior deemed to be pathological in one context may be seen as beneficial in another. This is not to discount the experiences of Feingold families, many of whom were deeply troubled by their children's behavior, but it nevertheless highlights how a variety of factors influenced such behavior at any given time or place.

What is safer to say, however, is that this history of Feingold families reinforces the contention of many historians, most notably Roy Porter, that physicians have not always been the primary agents of health care, that people sought their own cures before seeking medical advice, and, when physicians were found wanting, they looked elsewhere.[103] In the case of Feingold families, one could go even further: parents, particularly mothers, became the medical experts regarding many aspects of the health of their children. When conventional medical solutions were unacceptable, parents conducted research, weighed the available evidence, and then experimented with the Feingold diet, observed its effects, modified it according to their requirements, and made the decision to persevere with it. Although they believed that physicians were required for some interventions, parents nevertheless took responsibility for most aspects of their children's health. As Laura Lamb explained,

> I think that there is a time and place for everything. . . . My son would have died ten years ago if they didn't have the drugs and technology to

perform his heart surgery. However, that doesn't mean that every time he has an ear infection or something like that they should constantly be putting him on antibiotics . . . It's a band aid. They don't want to take the time to find out what's really bothering this child. Let's drug him. And then you have all of these pharmaceutical companies, they're making a fortune, and the food companies the same thing. The meat market, they pump the cow with steroids to get another twenty extra steaks out of it. Well who eats that hormone? We do. Why are little girls getting breasts at ten years old and getting their period at ten?[104]

Overall, parents tended to express more anger at pharmaceutical companies and the food industry than they did at mainstream physicians for downplaying Feingold's theory. Physicians, most thought, simply lacked a more holistic education, particularly when it came to nutrition. As Ellen Miller described, "We do have doctors that are really interested in nutrition, but the majority of them have not had a lot of training in medical school on nutrition and I think that's a serious problem."[105] Feingold families found that they could not trust their physicians as completely as they might have wished and so educated themselves about what they believed best for their child's health.

If parents can be seen as experts in certain aspects of their children's health, then it seems clear that medical historians should increasingly regard parents as an essential and important feature in the history of medical debates concerning children. The experiences of Feingold families suggest that parent and patient accounts could have played a much larger role in informing the debate about the Feingold diet itself. Or as Rima Apple argues more generally, there is a "need to ensure that scientific and medical professionals and mothers have the resources necessary to learn from each other."[106] Patient and parent experiences, in conjunction with the results of the double-blind trials, might not have resolved the debate about the Feingold diet but would likely have encouraged researchers to continue exploring the link between food additives and behavior, perhaps in more innovative ways, such as a longitudinal study of Feingold families.[107] Instead, the experiences of families were largely dismissed as unhelpful anecdotes that muddied the supposedly incontrovertible evidence emerging from the trials. Given the litany of problems that plagued these trials, it is ironic how unimportant the parental accounts were seen to be by most researchers.

Despite being excluded from official debates, parents were nevertheless able to keep Feingold's idea alive when most physicians had rejected it. Through FAUS and informal networking, a small but significant number of parents whose children had been diagnosed with hyperactivity continued to discover the Feingold diet. Most of the parents who were interviewed, as well as their grown-up children, recommended the diet to others, sharing not only their success stories but the challenges of avoiding food additives and how they overcame them. By continuing to employ and promote the Feingold diet, parents have encouraged a handful of researchers in the twenty-first century to consider Feingold's hypothesis once again.

Chapter 9

Conclusion

From the manner in which Feingold depicted the origins of his theory to the reasons why it became a popular phenomenon and the way decisions were made about it, the history of the Feingold diet demonstrates how novel medical ideas have had to serve the interests of numerous parties. Physicians, politicians, industries, the media, and patients and their families came to understand the Feingold diet in disparate ways and for different reasons, and this complicated the debates that Feingold's idea generated. While the media saw the Feingold diet as an exciting story that would sell newspapers, the food and chemical industries saw it as a threat to how it conducted business. Although Feingold families found that the diet gave them hope, many physicians and medical researchers viewed it with suspicion, believing that it discouraged families from accessing reliable treatments for hyperactivity. The history of the Feingold diet suggests that, during the late twentieth century in the United States, medical knowledge was not a steadily growing body of unquestioned information and practices that were universally accepted, but instead a mutable and fluid series of explanations and understandings that vied with each other for legitimacy. The reason an idea appealed to a particular party could have as much to do with politics, ideology, or economics as it had to do with the weight of scientific evidence that supported it or the way it helped patients.

An undercurrent to this story has been the use of history as a way to analyze and assess the outcomes of medical debates. Historians bring critical and contextual perspective to understanding why certain medical theories achieved legitimacy and others did not and, as such, are in a position to help inform public health policy. While some historians have begun to address such issues with reference to the history of medicine and health, such accounts have often failed to deconstruct how scientific knowledge is made authoritative or, conversely, have applied social theories too bluntly in an attempt to explain the uptake of particular medical ideas. The history of the Feingold diet suggests that the development of psychiatric and immunological knowledge has been a subtle, complex, and often contradictory process, one that reveals as much about the elements of the society involved as it does about science. It provides not only a case study about an unusual explanation for hyperactivity but shows how changes in the ways Americans understood and dealt with mental illness and allergy during the twentieth century reflected broader debates about the education of children, the testing of scientific ideas, the use of psychoactive drugs, the presence of chemicals in the food supply, and the role of parents in determining which medical treatments were best for their children. It suggests that, as society evolves, attitudes to medical notions once presumed to be incorrect can also change.

In 2004, an article appeared in the *Archives of Disease in Childhood* that put Feingold's theory to the test yet again. Bowing to public pressure, the British Food Standards Agency (FSA) had issued a call for proposals to test whether the behavior of children in the general population was affected by food additives.[1] The research group that was awarded the funding was from the University of Southampton and was led by psychologist Jim Stevenson. The group designed a double-blind trial that tested the behavioral responses of 277 three-year-old children from the Isle of Wight to challenges of artificial food colorings and the preservative sodium benzoate.[2] The team's focus on the Isle of Wight was interesting because that jurisdiction was also studied by prominent British child psychiatrist Michael Rutter in one of the first epidemiological studies of childhood mental health during the mid-1960s. Rutter later compared the rates of mental illness of children on the Isle of Wight with that of children from inner London in 1970. He found that the London children had twice the rate of mental illness as those from the Isle of Wight, and posited that higher levels of stress affecting not only the children but their parents were responsible for the higher rates. Such findings accorded with the social psychiatry prominent during the 1960s and reflected how social psychiatry had a greater and more enduring impact in Britain than it did in the United States.[3]

Four decades later the focus was on not the children's social environment but what they were consuming. Although formal testing did not confirm that the additive-free diet reduced hyperactivity, parental rating scales did, and the researchers concluded that "significant changes in children's hyperactive behaviour could be produced by the removal of artificial colourings and sodium benzoate from their diet" and that "benefit would accrue for all children if artificial food colours and benzoate preservatives were removed from their diet."[4] Two letters to the editor that appeared on the journal's web site soon after, however, indicated that, thirty years after Feingold had published *Why Your Child Is Hyperactive*, his idea continued to divide opinion.

The first letter, from a physician who worked in private medical practice was enthusiastic:

I remember the days of cramming for exams, working part-time and checking off the remaining days to the end of the torture in my diary. I am talking about the seventies, when petrol crises alternated with political disasters like the Nixon Gate. It was then that we first heard of Dr Feingold's revolutionary findings: Apparently, colourings and other chemicals in food and environment could cause behaviour problems and learning difficulties. A very sexy and down to earth psychology professor persuaded many of us to forego the Hostess Twinkies, the Hot Dogs and the beautifully coloured licorice twists, fig Newtons and Oreo cookies. Of course, being mature beyond our years, we aimed to please and soon found other staples. And there was no doubt about it, the therapy was effective. Having only read the abstract I can't say whether credit was given where credit is due but suffice it to say that Feingold was ahead of his time. May he rest snugly.[5]

The other letter, written by a medical professor at the University of North Carolina, was less enthusiastic:

Having been an interested observer to the Feingold Hypothesis many years ago, I was startled to see *it rise from the dead* [highlighted in many medical excerpting services]. I eagerly downloaded this article, and shortly thereafter, my thoughts could be paraphrased in a well-done American advertisement: "Where's the meat?" Figure 3 screamed at me one obvious conclusion: "Parents are sensitive to knowing something was to be changed in their child's environment." The withdrawal phase, placebo phase, and challenge phase ALL seemed to cause identical responses in both experimental orders. Imagine if the two groups (e.g., placebo-challenge vs challenge-placebo) had instead been a repeat experiment done at a different time. For a clinical study, the obvious conclusion was "wow, really tight, repeatable findings." Instead, some manner of statistics has overwhelmed common sense, leading to wide publicity of a "toxic effect." Most people will never read this manuscript, and the reviewers and editors owed us careful thought before opening up this Pandora's Box. The field will not Find-Gold with Feingold.[6]

The two letters suggest that the dilemma at the heart of debates about the Feingold diet has persisted: although Feingold's hypothesis seemed sensible to many people, and although his diet appeared to work, it was nevertheless difficult to prove, largely because its effects could be attributed to placebo effect rather than dietary change. Although the second letter questioned whether the trial was actually blind, an editorial that accompanied the article described it as "a meticulously performed, double-blind, placebo controlled trial," stating that it was "unlikely" that parents detected which diet their children were consuming and "congratulated" the authors "for tackling a complicated subject, in a rigorous manner."[7] The editorial also addressed the issue of whether the parental rating scales should be considered more valid than formal tests of hyperactivity. This was an issue that the study's authors also contemplated:

> Parental ratings might be more sensitive to changes in behaviour in that parents experience their child's behaviour over a longer period of time, in more varied settings and under less optimal conditions. The tests conducted in clinic are liked by the majority of children who see them as an entertaining game; they are given when the children are optimally alert and engaged. In contrast, parents will observe the child's behaviour when they are competing with siblings for attention; at times when the child is hungry or tired; when the child has less devoted attention from one adult; when the child is interacting with other children; or in a constraining setting such as on public transport or in a supermarket queue.[8]

Although the editorial itself was hesitant to endorse unconditionally the validity of parental ratings, it nonetheless implied that physicians should reconsider how they perceived parental observations of childhood behavior, and acknowledged that the study would "fuel the debate that there are environmental causes of hyperactivity, and that prior to medicating children we need to aggressively eliminate them."[9]

In 2007, Stevenson led another study that compared the effect of an additive-free diet on 153 three-year-old and 144 eight- and nine-year-old children. Their findings, which were published in the *Lancet*, provided "strong support for the case that food additives exacerbate hyperactive behaviours . . . in children at least up to middle childhood" and showed that such increases were "not just seen in children with extreme hyperactivity (ie, ADHD) but also can be seen in the general population and across the range of severities of hyperactivity."[10]

The authors added that the "implications of these results for the regulation of food additive use could be substantial," and the FSA proceeded to revise their advice to parents about the safety of food colors.[11] Ultimately, however, the FSA was limited in how it could curtail the use of such additives because of European Union regulations, which were still in the process of being reviewed.[12]

Unlike the 2004 study, which attracted little media attention, the 2007 trial and subsequent revisions of the FSA's advice to parents generated a flood of reports in print and on television, radio, and the Internet, much to the surprise of the researchers, who nevertheless thought that the prestige of the *Lancet* played a considerable role in promoting their research.[13] Journalistic interest was matched by that of the general public. Andrew Wadge, the FSA's chief scientist, for example, commented on the FSA web site that he could not "think of another topic that's generated so much feedback so quickly, expressed with a strength of feeling that I don't think we've seen on the blog before."[14] It also garnered attention from the AAP, which published a summary of the research results in *AAP Grand Rounds*, a digest of the pediatric research most relevant to clinicians. The commentary, written by Alison Schonwald, stated that the researchers' findings gave "practitioners . . . a reasonable option to offer parents."[15] The editor's note that followed the commentary stated that not only was the trial "a carefully conducted study in which the investigators went to great lengths to eliminate bias and rigorously measure outcomes" but "the overall findings of the study are clear and require that even we skeptics, who have long doubted parental claims of the effects of various foods on the behavior of their children, admit we might have been wrong."[16] Other physicians also altered their views about Feingold's hypothesis. Although Swiss pediatricians Phillipe Eigenmann and Charles Haenggeli criticized the Southampton group's 2004 research, stating that they "strongly believe that unnecessary diets should not be instituted for hyperactivity," following the 2007 *Lancet* article they admitted that physicians "taking care of children with hyperactivity could advise parents who wish to do so to start an elimination diet of artificial colourings and additives."[17]

Thirty-five years after Feingold presented his research to the AMA and failed to publish his findings in *JAMA*, the AAP statement represented a major reversal in how at least one major American medical association perceived the connection between food additives and hyperactivity. Despite its acknowledgement that the 2007 study lent support to Feingold's hypothesis, however, it would be a mistake to attribute their change of stance to the results of the study alone. Both of the Stevenson studies certainly had fewer methodological problems and involved a larger number of participants than nearly all of the trials that occurred during the 1970s and early 1980s. But most studies that emerged during the late 1980s and 1990s, while they failed to attract much media or medical attention, also tended to be better designed and yielded results that supported Feingold's theory. Bonnie Kaplan's trial was one such, but there were a handful of others that provided supportive evidence.[18]

Despite having addressed some of the methodological problems, the 2004 and 2007 trials were not flawless, however, and critics questioned how the researchers defined hyperactivity, controlled their trials, and interpreted their results.[19] The AAP's reversal, as well as the increase in media interest, had less to do with the emergence of a convincing, decisive study as it did with cultural, technological, and political developments that made the Feingold diet appear, once again, to be a viable alternative to conventional treatments for hyperactivity. In particular, dynamics such as concern about the health of the food supply, growing consumer wariness about drugs, and new information technologies had intervened to reinvigorate interest in the Feingold diet. Furthermore, the center for research and debate regarding Feingold's hypothesis had shifted from the United States to other jurisdictions, particularly Britain.

One compelling aspect of the media storm that followed the results of Stevenson's 2007 study was that the majority of media interest emanated from Britain, rather than the United States. This was opposite to the media response that accompanied Feingold's research during the 1970s, and indicated how medical and media interest in the Feingold diet had relocated from one side of the Atlantic to the other. While American families continued to discover and attempt the Feingold diet, American researchers were no longer leading investigations into Feingold's hypothesis. In fact, this trend had begun during the mid-1980s, following Feingold's death, as most of the small number of trials conducted during the late 1980s and 1990s were British, along with a few Australian and Canadian studies.[20]

Growing interest in the Feingold diet in Britain paralleled increased British interest in hyperactivity more generally. Although hyperactivity was the most common American childhood mental health issue by the late 1960s, it took longer for the disorder to become widespread in Britain. The first mention about hyperactivity in the *Lancet*, for example, did not appear until 1970. It consisted of a letter to the editor, along with a description of research, written by American psychiatrists. The only response to the letter was also by an American psychiatrist.[21] One of the reasons why hyperactivity became predominant in American child psychiatry during the late 1950s involved how it was described and defined by Maurice Laufer, Eric Denhoff, and Gerald

Solomons in 1957. "Hyperkinetic Impulse Disorder," which was truncated to hyperkinesis or, more commonly, hyperactivity, was a broad category that encapsulated a wide range of childhood behaviors.[22] British physicians and educators, however, were reluctant to embrace the term and, instead, employed a range of other labels to describe children with behavioral and learning problems. While British schoolchildren were often described by educators as "maladjusted" or "medium educational subnormal," British psychiatrists might diagnose them with "conduct disorder," "school phobia," "emotional disorder," or even "autism."[23] When British psychiatrists such as Michael Rutter did diagnose children with hyperactivity, the symptoms were much more severe than those described in diagnoses of hyperactivity made in North America.[24]

Although British psychiatrists seemed reluctant to emulate their American colleagues in diagnosing millions of children with hyperactivity and prescribing amphetamines for treating the disorder, there was debate about which approach was preferable. A 1973 editorial in the *Lancet*, for instance, asked, "Are the Americans ahead of the British, or behind them, or do their children's brains dysfunction in such an ostentatiously exotic transatlantic fashion that they require drug therapy?"[25] By the end of the 1970s, British physicians were still wary of the American approach:

> hyperactivity ought to mean nothing more than increased (or excessive) activity, but all too often the word is used to describe a neurobehavioural disturbance which should be treated with potent drugs. In the U.S.A. at least 5% of all normal schoolchildren are thought to be victims of the hyperactivity syndrome, and many of them are given treatment. The position in the U.K., though less alarming, is not negligible and could become worse. Fortunately, over the years Rutter and his colleagues have been painstakingly studying behavioural symptomatology and now conclude that "there is *no* evidence for the validity of a broader concept of hyperkinetic syndrome."[26]

By the mid-1980s, however, British physicians were less confident about their proclivity to disregard the American approach to defining and treating hyperactivity. Another *Lancet* editorial described how "British paediatricians, family practitioners and child psychiatrists are far less ready than their colleagues in the USA to diagnose and treat a syndrome of hyperactivity," but warned that "severe and pervasive hyperactivity is a risk factor and can handicap social development" and "British medicine and education will need to make its modification a higher priority."[27] Such warnings were heeded, as amphetamine prescriptions in Britain rose from 183,000 in 1991 to 1.58 million in 1995.[28] Despite the increase, British prescription rates remained much lower than in North America and British physicians continued to debate whether or not the disorder was underdiagnosed.[29]

Perhaps because of their reluctance to embrace an American-style biomedical approach to hyperactivity, British physicians came to understand hyperactivity in a more pluralistic manner. This was reflected not only in Rutter's holistic approach to childhood mental illness, and his work on its social causes in particular, but also in the fact that many of the first articles written about hyperactivity in British medical journals focused on alternative explanations for the disorder, in particular, theories about lead exposure and, indeed, food additives.[30] Although there were exceptions, particularly the commentaries of Thomas Jukes, who worked for a chemical company and had a history of supporting the use of food additives, most editorials about the Feingold diet were supportive and seemed to be more concerned about how to define hyperactivity than the possibility that chemicals in food could cause behavioral problems.[31] British parents were eager to consider the link between additives and hyperactivity, and looked to organizations such as the Hyperactive Children's Support Group, founded in the late 1970s by Sally Bunday, for assistance in planning an additive-free diet. One of the publications of Bunday's group was a collection of success stories entitled *The Proof of the Pudding*, which provided inspiration to parents.[32]

Increased concern about and a pluralistic approach to hyperactivity were not the only factors, however, that contributed to British interest in the Feingold diet. Many of the developments that made the Feingold diet popular in United States during the early 1970s, particularly concern about food safety and fears about psychiatric drugs, became prevalent for different reasons in Britain during the 1990s and 2000s, and encouraged both British parents and medical researchers to consider the link between food additives and hyperactivity. Moreover, the British food industry and government believed such a link might be valid, unlike their counterparts in the United States, and took proactive steps to reduce the amount of additives in food, especially foods commonly consumed by children.

Although the British organic food movement dated back to the 1930s and has always attracted both right- and left-wing adherents, a number of specific events related to the food and pharmaceutical industries during the 1990s and 2000s created a context in which the Feingold diet was seen as a sensible alternative to stimulant drugs.[33] The British BSE and Creutzfeldt-Jakob disease (CJD) epidemic of the mid-1990s, which killed approximately eighty Britons and resulted in the culling of nearly 5 million cattle, raised questions not only about how cattle were reared but about the safety of the food supply more generally. Britons increasingly considered organic food alternatives following the epidemic, and organic food activists employed it to garner support for their cause.[34] Similarly, concerns about genetically modified foods, pesticides, food poisoning, and diet-related chronic diseases such as obesity and diabetes, combined with often enthusiastic reporting of such "food crises," reduced British consumers' faith in the food supply and made theories such as Feingold's appear more plausible.[35]

Increased interest in the Feingold diet paralleled other developments that highlighted British dissatisfaction with the state of the food supply. In 2005, for example, a documentary starring celebrity chef Jamie Oliver was broadcast on British television. It documented the nutritional content of cafeteria food fed to children in a borough of London. Finding the food to be processed, lacking in nutrition, and high in saturated fat and chemicals, Oliver launched a campaign called "Feed Me Better" to provide additive-free, organic, and seasonal food in school cafeterias and collected over 270,000 signatures on a petition that was delivered to 10 Downing Street. Later that year, the Tony Blair government pledged £280 million of support.[36] On his web site, Oliver listed "poor concentration," "hyperactivity and behavioural problems," and "mood swings," as effects of the "processed junk foods" served in schools, thus underlining a link between nutrition and mental health.[37]

Although the campaign was seen to be successful, it was also clear that there were many obstacles to changing how British children were fed, including financing; educating parents, teachers, principals, and school cafeteria workers and; perhaps most importantly, convincing children to eat healthier food.[38] Oliver even backed a plan proposed by a school in North Wales to lock school gates at lunchtime in order to prevent children from leaving school grounds to buy junk food.[39] Nevertheless, the "Feed Me Better" campaign indicated that the British public as well as the government was willing to make nutrition a public health policy priority.

In addition, many large companies in the British food industry decided to preempt legislative action and changed the production and packaging of their products to accord with nutrition concerns. Although some of the measures were designed to avoid accidental contact with peanuts and other food allergens, many addressed fears about food additives, particularly colors. Marks and Spencer, for example, removed 99 percent of the artificial colors and flavors found in their foods, and other supermarkets followed suit.[40] Nestlé pledged to remove all artificial colors from Smarties, resulting in the demise of the blue Smartie, and Burton Foods, the makers of Jammie Dodger cookies, followed suit.[41] Other food manufacturers and supermarkets, often responding to pressure from parents, began to use natural dyes such as beetroot instead of those made from petrochemicals and emphasized on the packaging of certain products that they were free of artificial additives.[42] Such actions, which did not occur to the same extent in the United States, indicate how a combination of celebrity-driven publicity, parent pressure, and the findings of medical research created an environment in which it was feasible to change the production, packaging, and marketing of food products to reduce the amount of artificial additives. Although American supermarkets have not been as responsive as their British counterparts in switching to natural dyes, a number of organic supermarkets, such as Trader Joes and Whole Foods Market, have become more visible in the United States, providing American consumers with additive-free products. Many of the Feingold families reported relying almost exclusively on these supermarkets for their groceries, even though it could require an extra hour of travel time and cost up to a third more.[43]

Running parallel to fears about the food supply were concerns about pharmaceutical products, which led parents in the United States, Britain, and elsewhere to consider alternative treatments for hyperactivity. American parents were worried about the use of stimulant drugs as early as the late 1960s, and this was one of the chief reasons why they turned to alternatives such as the Feingold diet. Nevertheless, prescriptions for drugs such as Ritalin continued to increase in the decades that followed. During the 1990s and 2000s, however, a number of reports emerged that raised suspicions about the makers of hyperactivity drugs, as well as the pharmaceutical industry in general. In 1996, for example, CNN.com reported that scientists had shown how Ritalin caused cancer in mice.[44] A year later the Canadian Broadcasting Corporation described how scientists at a NIH conference that addressed the use of Ritalin "expressed concerns about a lack of data on the long-term effects of the drug."[45]

The short-term health risks of Ritalin also made headlines during the late 1990s when the American Heart Foundation issued guidelines for the monitoring of children prescribed Ritalin and other stimulants after a number of children and adolescents taking such drugs died suddenly from cardiovascular problems.[46] One well-publicized case was that of Matthew Smith, a fourteen-year-old whose fatal heart failure was attributed to long-term Ritalin use.[47] Although the percentage of children thought to be at risk from sudden death caused by stimulants was believed to be low, health authorities in North America were nonetheless alarmed. Health Canada, for example, temporarily removed the hyperactivity drug Adderall from the marketplace in 2005 after reports of twenty deaths.[48] Although the American FDA did not follow suit, an

FDA advisory committee recommended in 2006 that guidelines and warnings be strengthened to reflect such risks. Steven E. Nissen, a consultant for the advisory committee, believed that the risk of serious cardiovascular problems "warranted strong and immediate action" and argued that hyperactivity drugs be subject to "more selective and restricted use."[49] In response, the FDA "directed the manufacturers of all ADHD medicines to add a 'black box' warning to their products, pointing to the potential cardiovascular risks."[50] The risks were believed to be higher if children were engaged in strenuous exercise; indeed, Matthew Smith was skateboarding when he suffered his fatal heart problems. Ironically, exercise had been mentioned as one of the ways children could burn off excess energy and alleviate their hyperactive symptoms.[51]

Concerns about hyperactivity drugs were matched by concerns about the side effects of other drugs, as well as the motives of the pharmaceutical industry in general. While the cardiovascular health risks of pain reliever Vioxx led to U.S. Senate investigations, antidepressant Zoloft was linked to suicidal and homicidal behavior.[52] In Britain, a report from the University of Hull announced in 2008 that the commonest antidepressant drugs, including Prozac, had little effect in all but the most severely depressed patients, prompting Health Minister Allan Johnson to announce plans to train 3,600 more therapists able to provide "talk therapy," rather than drugs.[53]

Perhaps the most extreme example of public distrust of drug companies and conventional medical knowledge, however, was the furor over the measles, mumps, and rubella vaccine (MMR) that emerged during the late 1990s when British surgeon Andrew Wakefield (b. 1957) alleged a possible connection between MMR and autism.[54] Although Wakefield continued to advise parents to vaccinate their children against measles, mumps, and rubella using single, separately administered vaccines, he suggested that the combined MMR vaccine could be a cause of autism and, as did Feingold, voiced his concerns at a press conference before he had gathered much supporting evidence.[55] Many other features of the debates about MMR help to explain why Feingold's theory also experienced a renaissance during the same period and, indeed, many parents who employed the Feingold diet were concerned about vaccines.[56]

The controversy that erupted over MMR pitted the majority of the medical profession against parents, anti-vaccination activists, and a small number of unorthodox medical professionals. Whereas the risks of employing the Feingold diet were comparably nonexistent, decline in the use of MMR resulted in an increase in cases of measles in both Britain and North America.[57] Despite the lack of scientific evidence to support the association of MMR and autism, ethical questions about how Wakefield designed his investigations, and the fact that the public health risks of decreased vaccination could be severe, many parents grew alarmed that in attempting to prevent one disease they might trigger another, perhaps even more frightening, affliction.

Even if there was an association between MMR and autism, it could be argued that the dangers posed by a widespread measles epidemic outweighed the risks of increased cases of autism. Sociologists Harry Collins and Trevor Pinch describe this issue as the "prisoner's dilemma": "Think of vaccination as equivalent to a year in prison and catching the disease in question as equivalent to ten years. If everyone vaccinates, then everyone gets one year. If no one vaccinates, then everyone gets ten years. If everyone else vaccinates and you do not, you go free." Ironically, the resolution of this ethical quandary threatened the previously successful writing partnership of Collins and Pinch when the latter decided to hold off vaccinating his child against whooping cough (pertussis) using the conventional American vaccine in order to obtain what he believed to be a safer vaccine from Japan. Collins disagreed with Pinch's rationale for this decision and their resulting debate is described at length in *Dr. Golem*.[58] It is possible that the decision made by many parents to accept the greater likelihood of their child contracting measles, a potentially fatal disease, in the belief that this would prevent their child from developing autism also indicated how fear of infectious disease in developed nations had been replaced by fear of chronic diseases and, especially, mental illness. Certainly, the notion that the specter of infectious disease had been replaced by the threat of mental illness was expressed as early as 1963 by President Kennedy in his speech to Congress on mental illness and retardation. Nevertheless, measles remains a major public health risk in the developing world and in countries such as Japan where vaccination is relatively low.[59]

Public fears about MMR reflected doubts about the safety of pharmaceutical products, but they also showed how concern could be stoked by the media and activist groups through the Internet, the medium through which many Feingold families during the late 1990s and onward found out about the Feingold diet. For Feingold families, the Internet provided not only practical advice and information, including increasingly long lists of Feingold-friendly products, but it also afforded moral support for parents in the form of online support forums and chat rooms. Similarly, by 2002 there were twenty-two web sites promoting the anti-MMR campaign, and the Internet became the medium through which parents could research MMR, analyze the countless debates, perhaps contribute to them themselves, and make decisions about their children's vaccination.[60] In Britain, where the MMR controversy was most vociferous, largely due to the fact that vaccination was not compulsory as it was in the

United States, the public's lack of confidence in what the medical profession, the pharmaceutical industry, and the government had to say about MMR also reflected the perception that these authorities had recently made mistakes with respect to other public health controversies, most notably the BSE outbreak. The vitriolic nature of the British debate about MMR was evident in the first pages of Richard Horton's book on the subject. Horton, currently the editor in chief of the *Lancet*, participated in the debates himself and described what followed Wakefield's press conference as "a cascade of bizarre and catastrophic events."[61]

That parents in both North America and Britain were convinced to forego MMR vaccination, despite the fact that doing so was unsupported by scientific evidence, was possibly unethical and left their children vulnerable to previously widespread and potentially fatal infectious diseases. The situation highlighted the apprehension with which many people viewed medicine, the industries associated with it, and the governing bodies designed to regulate it during the late 1990s and 2000s. In the midst of this anxiety, it is not surprising that parents and researchers, particularly those in Britain, also considered alternatives to conventional hyperactivity treatment. Although the Feingold diet became the most discussed alternative, parents at the turn of the millennium also considered others, including fish oils, biofeedback, and even increasing the amount of playtime allowed to their children.[62] Just as conditions were appropriate for parents and physicians to consider the Feingold diet in the United States during the 1970s, they were ripe for a resurgence of interest in the diet during the 2000s. Whether this shift in opinion will result in a watershed in how hyperactivity is researched, understood, and treated remains to be seen and will similarly depend on a wide range of cultural, economic, political, and scientific factors. Although a recent German report associating hyperactivity and eczema suggests that the link between allergic disease and behavioral disorders is becoming more concrete, increased unemployment might convince a wider range of people to try amphetamines in an effort to improve their vocational performance and lead to renewed acceptability for their use in children.[63] The reasons for the ultimate acceptance or rejection of the Feingold diet, or, possibly more likely, its continued positioning on the margins of medicine, will be determined not only by double-blind trials but also by how well it accords with the prevailing scientific trends, societal conditions, and ideological beliefs.

In order to comprehend the changing fortunes of Feingold's hypothesis, it has been essential to analyze the broader historical contexts into which such ideas have emerged. The corollary to this argument is that other medical debates can and, perhaps, should be informed by discussions about the histories of these debates. It is important to understand, however, that historical context is not a fixed, indivisible concept that can be easily ascertained. Part of the reason why the Feingold diet was so contested was that, while it appeared logical to some Americans, particularly parents frustrated with conventional hyperactivity treatments, it seemed suspicious to others, most notably physicians who had long held suspicions about food allergy. Feingold's attempt to present the origins of his diet in *Why Your Child Is Hyperactive* in a manner that would be palatable to both conservative physicians and desperate parents suggests that, as a previously orthodox pediatric allergist, he understood that his theory had to operate under multiple paradigms at once.

Similarly, the way in which word about the Feingold diet spread from San Francisco to the rest of the United States and elsewhere also spotlights the gaps between popular and medical understandings and concerns about food additives and hyperactivity. Although Feingold's intent was to publish his theory conventionally, in medical journals such as *JAMA*, the medical establishment, wary of associating themselves with such a controversial claim, rebuffed his overtures. In contrast, the American media and the general public provided Feingold with a forum from which to present his ideas since they found Feingold's hypothesis addressed both dissatisfaction with conventional explanations and treatments of hyperactivity and worries about food additives. This shift in focus, from trying to convince orthodox physicians to concentrating on parents, the media, and the general public, had crucial ramifications for the fate of the Feingold diet; while it alienated many physicians, it empowered Feingold families and FAUS to become medical experts in their own right and ensured the survival of Feingold's theory long after Feingold's death and the subsequent dwindling of medical research into his idea.

Finally, in order to understand why different parties, including the media, physicians, and parents, made decisions about the efficacy of the Feingold diet, it is vital to analyze carefully the basis on which such opinions were formed. While the judgments of both Feingold's supporters and detractors in the media and the medical community were characterized by prejudice—with some notable exceptions, including Jean Mayer, C. Keith Conners, and Bonnie Kaplan—Feingold families were more concerned with analyzing whether or not the diet worked for them. And it must be said that the diet did work for most of them. Given this and the positive results from the Southampton studies, the role of parents and their children in the resolution of medical debates is a subject that requires further study from medical historians, medical researchers, and health policy makers.

Although it has been commonly asked, I have not attempted to answer the question, "Did the Feingold diet work?" This is an important query and one that can be confidently answered in the affirmative with respect to many of the Feingold families, but it is a query that requires deconstruction. What is meant by "the Feingold diet"? Is it simply a list of acceptable foods or, instead, a lifestyle choice that encompasses not only dietary change but a family's determination to understand their children's behavior in a broader social, educational, emotional, and ecological context and respond to it accordingly? If so, does it not also imply that parents take up the role of medical experts, not only becoming canny observers and experimenters but the arbiters of their children's health care in the process? What exactly is meant by "work?" Did it work for every family, at every time, in every circumstance? The answer to this is clearly no, but when the reasons for why the diet was not effective are picked apart, it becomes evident that many other factors—availability of Feingold-friendly products; support from school authorities, medical professionals, family, and friends; as well as the willingness of both children and parents to persevere on the diet—must be also considered. Addressing whether the Feingold diet worked is a complicated task and, although opinions about food additives and hyperactivity are changing somewhat, there are still numerous barriers in place that will hamper many families' attempts to employ it successfully.

Instead of asking "did the Feingold diet work?" I have questioned why the efficacy of the Feingold diet became such a divisive subject and what factors led to such debate. What is revealed in the answers to this question is that medical controversies are about more than academic disputes over matters of scientific truth. The points of view represented on various sides of the debate also reflect the ideals, desires, experiences, and beliefs of those who hold them. To a certain degree, there is nothing wrong with this and, regardless, it is probably impossible to filter such factors out of any medical controversy. But what is problematic is that when such debates have occurred, the opinions and experiences of patients and their families, as well as unorthodox medical professionals, have been downgraded and ignored, attenuating any resolution that has eventually emerged. This does not imply that unorthodox or popular beliefs should not be rigorously critiqued. In the case of MMR, medical authorities were correct that the link between the vaccine and autism was tenuous and, even if a link could be proven, the morality of refusing vaccination is questionable. But during debates about the Feingold diet, the experiences of parents were overlooked as physicians tallied, not particularly carefully, the results of double-blind controlled trials. As the Feingold diet once again becomes a contentious issue, it is my hope that physicians and policy makers will take note of the history of the initial debates and reconsider how they judge the opinions and experiences of patients and their families.

Bibliography

Archival Sources

American Academy of Allergy, Asthma and Immunology. "American Academy of Allergy, Asthma and Immunology Records, 1923– (Ongoing)." UMW Manuscript Collection 139, University of Wisconsin–Milwaukee Libraries, Archives Department.

Beatrice Trum Hunter Collection. Howard Gotlieb Archival Research Center at Boston University.

Theron G. Randolph Papers: 1935–1991, H MS c183. Harvard Medical Library in the Francis A. Countway Library of Medicine, Center for the History of Medicine.

Oral History Interviews (all pseudonyms)

Anderson, Marilyn. December 10, 2007.

Atwater, Janice. January 26, 2008.

Atwater, Jason. February 7, 2008.

Aubrey, Darren. May 20, 2008.

Aubrey, Sharon. January 29, 2008.

Bannister, Josephine. March 2, 2007.

Bannister, Josephine. December 9, 2007.

Beck, Barbara. January 17, 2008.

Bright, John. January 14, 2009.

Davidson, Gayle. January 20, 2008.

Davidson, Trevor. December 6, 2007.

Drake, Alex. April 1, 2008.

Ewing, Justine. February 5, 2008.

Freeman, Lesley. January 28, 2008.

Grossman, Liz. February 19, 2008.

Hawking, Desmond. May 22, 2007.

Hewson, Greg. February 4, 2009.

Illing, Jennifer. February 12, 2008.

Jeffries, Maggie. February 17, 2008.

Johnson, Kristine. November 5, 2007.

Johnston, Hanna. February 4, 2008.

Kahn, Alice. November 6, 2006.

Kitchen, Lynn. November 5, 2007.

Kushner, Frank. April 22, 2008.

Kushner, Rosemarie. April 8, 2008.

Lamb, Laura. April 17, 2008.

Larkin, Donna. February 25, 2008.

Lopes, Phillip. February 19, 2007.

Lott, Wendy. July 24, 2008.

McKay, Theresa. February 13, 2008.

Miller, David. May 19, 2008.

Miller, Ellen. May 20, 2008.

Osmond, Kevin. October 8, 2007.

Parker, Jane. February 3, 2009.
Ridge, Mark. March 16, 2009.
Terry, Erik. April 1, 2008.
Terry, Sylvia. March 29, 2008.
Thompson, Bonnie. January 28, 2008.
Unger, Stuart. March 23, 2007.
Zimmerman, Gina. February 17, 2009.

Primary Sources

Adams, Paul L. "Review of *Hyperactivity: Research, Theory, and Action* by Dorothea M. Ross and Sheila A. Ross." *American Journal of Psychiatry* 134 (1977): 833–34.

Altman, Lawrence K. "Physicians Urged to Widen Understanding of Placebo." *New York Times*, July 2, 1975.

Alvarez, Walter C. "Puzzling 'Nervous Storms' Due to Food Allergy." *Gastroenterology* 7 (1946): 241–52.

American Council on Science and Health. *Food Additives and Hyperactivity*. Summit, NJ: American Council on Science and Health, 1984.

———. "CSPI vs. ACSH." http://www.acsh.org/about/pageID.86/default.asp (accessed October 22, 2008).

American Medical Association. "Historical Health Fraud and Alternative Medicine." http://www.ama-assn.org./ama/no-index/about-ama/17954.shtml (accessed March 3, 2009).

American Psychiatric Association: Committee on Nomenclature and Statistics. *Diagnostic and Statistical Manual of Mental Disorders*, 2nd ed. Washington, DC: American Psychiatric Association, 1968.

———. "Position Statement on *Crisis in Child Mental Health: Challenge for the 1970s*, Final Report of the Joint Commission on Mental Health of Children." *American Journal of Psychiatry* 125 (1969): 1197–1203.

Amster, Linda. "Saturday News Quiz." *New York Times*, April 5, 1980.

Anderson, Camilla. *Society Pays the High Cost of Minimal Brain Damage in America*. New York: Walker, 1972.

Andreatta, David. "Food Additives Found to Fuel Hyperactivity." *Globe and Mail*, 6 September 2007, http://www.theglobeandmail.com/servlet/story/RTGAM.20070906 .whyperkids06/BNStory/specialScienceandHealth/home (accessed March 9, 2009).

Anonymous. Personal correspondence to Oprah Winfrey. July 2005.

"Anti-Depressants, Little Effect." February 26, 2008, http://www.news.bbc.co.uk/1/hi/ health/7263494.stm (accessed March 20, 2009).

Arnold, L. Eugene. "Alternative Treatments for Adults with Attention-Deficit Hyperactivity Disorder (ADHD)." *Annals of the New York Academy of Sciences* 931 (2001): 310–41.

Barclay, Dorothy. "A Turn for the Wiser." *Pediatrics* 23 (1959): 759–60.

Baron-Faust, Rita. "Biofeedback Widens Its Role in Medicine." February 17, 2000, http://www.edition.cnn.com/2000/HEALTH/alternative/02/17/neuro.feedback.wmd/ index.html (accessed March 23, 2009).

Bateman, B., J. O. Warner, E. Hutchinson, T. Dean, P. Rowlandson, C. Grant, J. Grundy, C. Fitzgerald, and J. Stephenson. "The Effects of a Double-blind, Placebo Controlled, Artificial Food Colourings and Benzoate Preservative Challenge on Hyperactivity in a General Population Sample of Preschool Children." *Archives of Disease in Childhood* 89 (2004): 506–11.

Bateman, Barbara. "Learning Disorders." *Review of Education Research* 36 (1966): 93–119.

Battle, Esther S., and Beth Lacey. "A Context for Hyperactivity in Children over Time." *Child Development* 43 (1972): 757–73.

Bauchner, Howard. "Food Colourings and Benzoate Preservatives: Do They Change Behaviour?" *Archives of Disease in Childhood* 84 (2004): 499.

Baughman, Fred A., Jr. *The ADHD Fraud: How Psychiatry Makes "Patients" Out of Normal Children.* Victoria, BC: Trafford, 2006.

Beck, Joan. "Another 'Miracle' Diet Cure that Failed." *Chicago Tribune*, July 11, 1977.

Benjamini, E. Ben, F. Feingold, and L. Kartman. "Allergy to Flea Bites. III. The Experimental Induction of Flea Bite Sensitivity in Guinea Pigs by Exposure to Flea Bites and by Antigen Prepared from Whole Flea Extracts of Ctenocephalides Felis Felis." *Experimental Parasitology* 10 (1960): 214–22.

Berlin, Irving N. "Some Models for Reversing the Myth of Child Treatment in Community Mental Health Centers." *Journal of the American Academy of Child Psychiatry* 14 (1975): 76–94.

Berlin, I. N., and S. A. Szurek. *Learning and Its Disorder: Clinical Approaches to Problems of Childhood.* Palo Alto, CA: Science and Behavior Books, 1965.

Berman, Sidney. "Techniques of Treatment of a Form of Juvenile Delinquency, the Antisocial Character Disorder." *Journal of the American Academy of Child Psychiatry* 3 (1964): 24–52.

Bierer, Joshua. "Introduction to the Second Volume." *International Journal of Social Psychiatry* 2 (1956): 1–11.

Bierman, C. Warren, and Clifton T. Furukawa. "Food Additives and Hyperkinesis: Are There Nuts among the Berries?" *Pediatrics* 61 (1978): 932–33.

Birchard, Karen. "Europe Tackles Consumer Fears over Food Safety." *Lancet* 357 (2001): 1276.

"The Bitter Verdict against Saccharin." *New York Times*, March 11, 1977.

Black, Jonathan. "The Speed that Kills." *New York Times*, June 21, 1970.

Blain, Daniel. "The Presidential Address; Novalescence." *American Journal of Psychiatry* 122 (1965): 1–12.

Blakeslee, Sandra. "Food Safety a Worry in Era of Additives." *New York Times*, November 9, 1969.

———. "Challenge to Food Tests." *New York Times*, November 10, 1969.

Blank, Charles H. "The Delaney Clause: Technical Naïveté and Scientific Advocacy in the Formulation of Public Health Policies." *California Law Review* 62 (1974): 1084–1120.

Boffey, Philip M. "Cancer Experts Lean towards Steady Vigilance, but Less Alarm, on Environment." *New York Times*, March 2, 1982.

Boris, M., and F. S. Mandel. "Foods and Additives Are Common Causes of the Attention Deficit Hyperactive Disorder in Children." *Annals of Allergy* 72 (1994): 462–68.

Boyden, Stephen. "The Environment and Human Health." *Medical Journal of Australia* 1 (1972): 1229–34.

Bradley, Charles. "The Behavior of Children Receiving Benzedrine." *American Journal of Psychiatry* 94 (1937): 577–685.

Branch, C. H. Hardin. "Presidential Address: Preparedness for Progress." *American Journal of Psychiatry* 120 (1963): 1–11.

Breggin, Peter. *Talking Back to Ritalin: What Doctors Aren't Telling You about Stimulants for Children.* Monroe, ME: Common Courage Press, 1998.

Brenner, Arnold. "A Study of the Efficacy of the Feingold Diet on Hyperkinetic Children: Some Favorable Personal Observations." *Clinical Pediatrics* 16 (1977): 652–56.

Brody, Jane E. "If the Child Seems to Be 'Bad,' He Could Have Hyperkinesis." *New York Times*, December 1, 1976.

———. "How Diet Can Effect Mood and Behavior." *New York Times*, November 17, 1982.

———. "Diet Therapy for Behavior Is Criticized as Premature." *New York Times*, December 4, 1984.

Brosin, Henry A. "Response to the Presidential Address." *American Journal of Psychiatry* 124 (1967): 7–8.

———. "The Presidential Address: Adaptation to the Unknown." *American Journal of Psychiatry* 125 (1968): 1–16.

Brown, Ethan Allan. "American Academy of Allergy: The Changing Picture of Allergy." *Journal of Allergy* 28 (1957): 365–73.

Brown, R. T. "Perceived Family Functioning, Marital Status, and Depression in Parents of Boys with Attention Deficit Disorder." *Journal of Learning Disabilities* 22 (1989): 581–87.

Buckely, Robert. "Hyperkinetic Aggravation of Learning Disturbance." *Academic Therapy* 13 (1977): 153–60.

Bunyan, Nigel. "Jamie Oliver Supports School Lunch Lock-Ins." *Daily Telegraph*, September 6, 2007, http://www.telegraph.co.uk/news/main.jhtml;jsessionid=AOOQCMF2RSGZJQFIQMGCFF4AVCBQUIV0?xml=/news/2007/09/06/njamie106.xml (accessed March 13, 2009).

Burros, Marian. "Coloring Food: Who Suffers?" *Washington Post*, January 23, 1975.

———. "Eating Well May Be the Best Revenge; The '70s: A Decade of Concern; Looking Back Through the Consumer '70s." *Washington Post*, December 30, 1979.

Call, Justin M. "Some Problems and Challenges in the Geography of Child Psychiatry." *Journal of the American Academy of Child Psychiatry* 15 (1976): 139–60.

"Can Dye-Hyped Foods Cause Hyperactivity?" *Chicago Tribune*, February 17, 1977.

Cantwell, Dennis P. "Genetic Factors in the Hyperkinetic Syndrome." *American Journal of Psychiatry* 15 (1976): 214–23.

Cantwell, Dennis P, Lorian Baker, and Richard E. Mattison. "The Prevalence of Psychiatric Disorder in Children with Speech and Language Disorder: An Epidemiologic Study." *Journal of the American Academy of Child Psychiatry* 18 (1979): 450–61.

Carson, Rachel. *Silent Spring*. London: Folio Society, 2000.

Carter, C. M., M. Urbanowicz, R. Hemsley, L. Mantilla, S. Strobel, P. J. Graham, and E. Taylor. "Effects of a Few Food Diet in Attention Deficit Disorder." *Archives of Disease in Childhood* 69 (1993): 564–68.

"The Case of the Useful Carcinogen." *New York Times*, December 7, 1978.

Cassel, Elaine. "Did Zoloft Make Him Do It?" February 7, 2005, http://www.edition.cnn.com/2005/LAW/02/07/cassel.pittman/index.html (accessed March 20, 2009).

"Catered Health Foods, for Washingtonians, 'More Curious than Committed.'" *New York Times*, March 6, 1972.

Cavett, Dick. "When that Guy Died on My Show." *New York Times*, May 3, 2007, http://www.cavett.blogs.nytimes.com/2007/05/03/when-that-guy-died-on-my-show/ (accessed June 12, 2008).

CBS Evening News. November 8, 1970, http://www.tvnews.vanderbilt.edu/diglib-fulldisplay.pl?SID=20080613905212402&code=tvn&RC=207475&Row=19 (accessed June 13, 2008).

Center for Science in the Public Interest. "Non-Profit Organizations Receiving Corporate Funding." http://www.cspinet.org/integrity/nonprofits/american_council_on_science_and_health.html (accessed October 22, 2008).

Cermak, S. A., F. Stein, and C. Abelson. "Hyperactive Children and an Activity Group Therapy Model." *American Journal of Occupational Therapy* 27 (1973): 311–15.

Channel 4. *Jamie's School Dinners.* http://www.channel4.com/life/microsites/J/jamies_school_dinners/index.html (accessed March 13, 2009).

Chess, Stella, Alexander Thomas, Michael Rutter, and Herbert G. Birch. "Interaction of Temperament and Environment in the Production of Behavioral Disturbances in Children." *American Journal of Psychiatry* 120 (1963): 142–48.

Chess, Stella, Alexander Thomas, and Herbert G. Birch. "Behavior Problems Revisited: Findings of an Anteroperspective Study." *Journal of the American Academy of Child Psychiatry* 6 (1967): 321–31.

"Child's Brain Cited in Ills." *Science News* 90 (1966): 55.

"Children and Artificial Food." *Washington Post*, September 14, 1975.

Christie, D., and E. Tansey. *Environmental Toxicology: The Legacy of Silent Spring.* Wellcome Witnesses to Twentieth Century Medicine 19 (2004). Wellcome Trust Centre for the History of Medicine at UCL, London, http://www.ucl.ac.uk/silva/histmed/downloads/c20th_group/wit19 (accessed 2 March 2009).

Ciampa, Linda. "Ritalin Abuse Scoring High on College Illegal Drug Circuit." January 8, 2001, http://www.edition.cnn.com/2001/HEALTH/children/01/08/college.ritalin/index.html (accessed March 23, 2009).

Cimons, Marlene. "Hyperactivity and Food Additives." *Los Angeles Times*, September 15, 1975.

Clark, Matt, Dan Shapiro, Mary Hager, Janet Huck, and Pamela Abramson. "The Curse of Hyperactivity." *Newsweek*, June 23, 1980, 59.

Clarke, T. Wood. "Neuro-Allergy in Childhood." *New York State Journal of Medicine* 42 (1948): 393–97.

———. "The Relation of Allergy to Character Problems in Children: A Survey." *Annals of Allergy* 8 (1950): 175–87.

"Classroom Pushers." *Time*, February 26, 1973, http://www.time.com/time/magazine/article/0,9171,910580,00.html?promoid=googlep (accessed March 23, 2009).

Clouston, T. S. "Stages of Overexcitability, Hypersensitiveness, and Mental Explosiveness and Their Treatment by the Bromides." *Scottish Medical and Surgical Journal* 4 (1899): 481–90.

Coca, Arthur C. *Familial Nonreaginic Food-Allergy.* Springfield, IL: Charles C. Thomas, 1943.

Cohen, Carl I., Joel S. Feiner, Charles Huffine, H. Steven Moffic, and Kenneth S. Thompson. "The Future of Community Psychiatry." *Community Mental Health Journal* 39 (2003): 459–71.

Colamosca, Anna. "Health Foods Prosper Despite High Prices." *New York Times*, November 17, 1974.

Conant, James Bryant. *Slums and Suburbs.* New York: McGraw-Hill, 1961.

Conners, C. Keith. *Food Additives and Hyperactive Children.* New York: Plenum, 1980.

———. *Feeding the Brain: How Foods Affect Children.* New York: Plenum, 1989.

Conners, C. Keith, and Leon Eisenberg. "The Effects of Methylphenidate on Symptomology and Learning in Disturbed Children." *American Journal of Psychiatry* 120 (1963): 458–64.

Conners, C. Keith, Charles H. Goyette, Deborah A. Southwick, James M. Lees, and Paul A. Andrulonis. "Food Additives and Hyperkinesis: A Controlled Double-Blind Experiment." *Pediatrics* 58 (1976): 154–66.

Cook, Peter S., and Joan M. Woodhill. "The Feingold Dietary Treatment of the Hyperkinetic Syndrome." *Medical Journal of Australia* 2 (1976): 85–89.

Cott, Allan. "A Reply." *Academic Therapy* 13 (1977): 161–71.

Council of Australian Food Technology Association, Inc. "Dr. Benjamin Feingold—Hyperactivity." *Food Technology in Australia* 29 (1977): 433.

Crook, William G. "Food Allergy: The Great Masquerader." *Pediatric Clinics of North America* 22 (1975): 227–38.

———. "Adverse Reactions to Food Can Cause Hyperkinesis." *American Journal of Diseases of Childhood* 132 (1978): 819–20.

———. "More on Food Additives and Hyperkinesis." *American Journal of Diseases of Children* 133 (1979): 1080–81.

———. "Diet and Hyperactivity." *Journal of Learning Disabilities* 17 (1984): 66.

Crook, William G., Walton W. Harrison, Stanley E. Crawford, and Blanche S. Emerson. "Systematic Manifestations Due to Allergy: Report of Fifty Patients and a Review of the Literature on the Subject (Sometime Referred to as Allergic Toxemia and Allergic Tension-Fatigue Syndrome)." *Pediatrics* 27 (1961): 790–99.

Cruz, Narlito V., and Sami L. Bahna. "Do Foods or Additives Cause Behavior Disorders?" *Pediatric Annals* 35 (2006): 744–54.

David, Oliver J. "Association between Lower Level Lead Concentrations and Hyperactivity in Children." *Environmental Health Perspectives* 7 (1974): 17–25.

David, T. J. "Reactions to Dietary Tartrazine." *Archives of Disease in Childhood* 62 (1987): 119–22.

Davids, Anthony, and Jack Sidman. "A Pilot Study: Impulsivity, Time Orientation, and Delayed Gratification in Future Scientists and in Underachieving High School Students." *Exceptional Children* 29 (1962–1963): 170–74.

Davidson, Henry A. "Comment: The Reversible Superego." *American Journal of Psychiatry* 120 (1963): 192–93.

———. "The Image of the Psychiatrist." *American Journal of Psychiatry* 121 (1964): 329–34.

Davison, H. M. "Cerebral Allergy." *Southern Medical Journal* 42 (1949): 712–16.

De Witt, Karen. "Challenging the Additive Rule." *New York Times*, December 10, 1980.

———. "Just a Regulated Day in the Life of an Ordinary Citizen." *New York Times*, April 12, 1981.

DeGrandpre, Richard J. *Ritalin Nation: Rapid-Fire Culture and the Transformation of Human Consciousness*. New York: W. W. Norton: 1999.

"Deleterious Food." *Brooklyn Daily Eagle*, September 20, 1885.

"Diet and Hyperactivity: Any Connection?" *Nutrition Reviews* 34 (1976): 151–58.

"Diet Can Ease Behaviour Problems." February 13, 2002, http://www.news.bbc.co.uk/1/hi/health/1816938.stm (accessed March 23, 2009).

Diller, Lawrence H. *Running on Ritalin: A Physician Reflects on Children, Society, and Performance in a Pill*. New York: Bantam Books, 1999.

Dobbs, Lou. "Promote Safety not Profits." January 14, 2005, http://www.edition.cnn.com/2005/US/01/13/fda.safety/index.html (accessed March 20, 2009).

"Does Hyperactivity Matter?" *Lancet* 327 (1986): 73–74.

Dorhenwend, A. B., and B. S. Dorhenwend. *Social Status and Psychological Disorder: A Causal Inquiry*. New York: John Wiley, 1969.

Dosti, Rose. "Study Refutes Additive-Hyperactivity Link." *Los Angeles Times*, April 14, 1977.

"Drugs Seem to Help Hyperactive Children." *JAMA* 214 (1970): 2260–62.

Duffy, Judith. "Hyperactive Children 'Need Exercise, Not Drugs.'" *Sunday Herald*, November 12, 2006.

Duke, William Waddell. *Allergy, Asthma, Hay Fever, Urticaria, and Allied Manifestations of Reaction.* London: Henry Klimpton, 1925.

Dwyer, Joanna, Patricia Harper, Charles H. Goyette, and C. Keith Conners. "Nutrient Intakes of Children on the Hyperkinesis Diet." *Journal of the American Dietetic Association* 73 (1980): 515–20.

Ebaugh, Franklin G. "Neuropsychiatric Sequelae of Acute Epidemic Encephalitis in Children." *American Journal of Diseases of Children* 25 (1923): 89–97.

———. "Comment: The Case of the Confused Parent." *American Journal of Psychiatry* 116 (1960): 1136–38.

"Editor's Note." *AAP Grand Rounds* 19 (2008): 17.

"Editorial Statement." *Social Psychiatry* 1 (1966): 1.

Egger, J., C. M. Carter, P. J. Graham, D. Gumley, and J. F. Soothill. "Controlled Trial of Oligoantigenic Treatment in the Hyperkinetic Syndrome." *Lancet* 325 (1985): 540–45.

Eigenmann, Philippe A., and Charles A. Haenggeli. "Food Colourings and Preservatives: Allergy and Hyperactivity." *Lancet* 364 (2004): 823–24.

———. "Food Colourings, Preservatives, and Hyperactivity." *Lancet* 370 (2007): 1524–25.

Eisenberg, Leon. "Discussion of Dr. Solnit's Paper 'Who Deserves Child Psychiatry? A Study in Priorities.'" *Journal of the American Academy of Child Psychiatry* 5 (1966): 17–23.

Eisenberg, Leon, Anita Gilbert, Leon Cytryn, and Peter A. Molling. "The Effectiveness of Psychotherapy Alone and in Conjunction with Perphenazine or Placebo in the Treatment of Neurotic and Hyperkinetic Children." *American Journal of Psychiatry* 116 (1960): 1088–93.

Elliot, Valerie. "Food Alert as Every Additive Comes Under Suspicion." *The Times*, September 6, 2009, http://www.timesonline.co.uk/tol/news/uk/health/article2395623.ece (accessed March 9, 2009).

Ettelson, L. N., and Louis Tuft. "The Value of the Coca Pulse-Acceleration Method in Food Allergy." *Journal of Allergy* 32 (1961): 514–24.

Ewalt, Jack R. "Presidential Address." *American Journal of Psychiatry* 121 (1964): 1–8.

Federal Food and Drugs Act of 1906 (Wiley Act). Public Law Number 59–384, June 30, 1906.

Feingold Association of the United States. "Diet and ADHD." http://www.feingold.org/pg-research.html (accessed January 21, 2009).

———. "The Feingold Program." http://www.feingold.org/pg-faq.html (accessed October 9, 2008).

Feingold, Ben F. "Tonsillectomy in the Allergic Child." *California Medicine* 71 (1949): 341–44.

———. "Infection in the Allergic Child." *Annals of Allergy* 8 (1950): 718–33.

———. "Treatment of Allergic Disease of the Bronchi." *JAMA* 146 (1951): 319–23.

———. "Recognition of Food Additives as a Cause of Symptoms of Allergy." *Annals of Allergy* 26 (1968): 309–13.

———. *Introduction to Clinical Allergy.* Springfield, IL: Charles C. Thomas, 1973.

———. "Food Additives and Child Development." *Hospital Practice* 8 (1973): 11–21.

———. "The Arguments Con." *Washington Post*, September 19, 1974.

———. "Food Additives in Clinical Medicine." *International Journal of Dermatology* 14 (1975): 112–14.

———. "Hyperkinesis and Learning Disabilities Linked to Artificial Food Flavors and Colors." *American Journal of Nursing* 75 (1975): 797–803.

———. "A Critique of 'Controversial Medical Treatments of Learning Disabilities.'" *Academic Therapy* 13 (1977): 173–83.

———. "A View from the Other Side." Speech to the Newspaper Food Editors and Writers Association, Milwaukee, Wisconsin, June 1977, http://www.feingold.org/pg-aboutus.html (accessed March 4, 2009).

———. "Behavioral Disturbances Linked to the Ingestion of Food Additives." *Delaware Medical Journal* 49 (1977): 89–94.

———. "Can Food Chemical Additives Have Any Effect on Behavior?" *Hartford Courant*, August 3, 1977.

———. "Food Additives in Dentistry." *Journal of the American Society for Preventive Dentistry* 7 (1977): 13–15.

———. "Hyperkinesis and Learning Disabilities Linked to the Ingestion of Artificial Food Colors and Flavors (Speech to the American Academy of Pediatrics)." New York, November 8, 1977, http://www.feingold.org/pg-aboutus.html (accessed 28 January 2009).

———. "Dietary Management of Juvenile Delinquency." *International Journal of Offender Therapy and Comparative Criminology* 23 (1979): 73–84.

———. "The Role of Diet in Behaviour." *Ecology of Disease* 1 (1982): 153–65.

———. *Why Your Child Is Hyperactive*. New York: Random House, 1996.

Feingold, Ben F., and Eli Benjamini. "Allergy to Flea Bites: Clinical and Experimental Observations." *Annals of Allergy* 19 (1961): 1275–89.

Feingold, Ben F., Eli Benjamini, and M. Shimizu. "Induction of Delayed and Immediate Types of Skin Reactivity in Guinea Pigs by Variation in Dosages of Antigens." *Annals of Allergy* 22 (1964): 543–75.

Feingold, Ben F., Frank J. Gorman, Margaret Thaler Singer, and Kurt Schlesinger. "Psychological Studies of Allergic Women: The Relation between Skin Reactivity and Personality." *Psychosomatic Medicine* 24 (1962): 195–202.

Feingold, Ben F., and Helene S. Feingold. *The Feingold Cookbook for Hyperactive Children*. New York: Random House, 1979.

Feingold, Ben F., Margaret T. Singer, Edith H. Freeman, and A. Deskins. "Psychological Variables in Allergic Disease: A Critical Appraisal of Methodology." *Journal of Allergy* 38 (1966): 143–55.

"Feingold's Regimen for Hyperkinesis." *Lancet* 2 (1979): 617–18.

Felix, Robert H. "The Image of the Psychiatrist: Past, Present, and Future." *American Journal of Psychiatry* 121 (1964): 318–22.

Firestone, Philip, Jean Davey, John T. Goodman, and Susan Peters. "The Effects of Caffeine and Methylphenidate on Hyperactive Children." *Journal of the American Academy of Child Psychiatry* 17 (1978): 445–56.

Fischer, Howard. "Fifty Years Ago in the *Journal of Pediatrics*: Hyperkinetic Behavior Syndrome in Children." *Journal of Pediatrics* 150 (2007): 520.

Fitzpatrick, Michael. *MMR and Autism: What Parents Need to Know*. New York: Routledge, 2004.

"Food Additives Tied to Child Behavior." *Hartford Courant*, June 28, 1973.

"Food Watchdog Condemned for 'Totally Inadequate' Response to Harmful Food Additives." *This Is London*, September 6, 2007, http://www.thisislondon.co.uk/

news/article-23411169-details/Parents+warned:+additives+in+food+DO+harm+ our+children/article.do (accessed March 13, 2009).

Fox, Maggie. "Food Additives May Cause Hyperactivity: Study." September 5, 2007, http://www.reuters.com/article/healthNews/idUSN0520103220070905 (accessed September 7, 2007).

Franks, David J. "Ethnic and Social Status Characteristics of Children in EMR and LD Classes." *Exceptional Children* 37 (1970–1971): 537–38.

Franks, Lucinda. "F.D.A., in Shift, Tests Pediatrician's Diet for Hyperactivity." *New York Times*, February 9, 1975.

"Frederick Stare." *The Economist*, April 18, 2002, http://www.economist.com/ obituary/displaystory.cfm?story_id=E1_TDRGGRJ (accessed June 17, 2008).

Freeman, Edith H., Ben F. Feingold, Kurt Schlesinger, and Frank J. Gorman. "Psychological Variables in Allergic Disorders: A Review." *Psychosomatic Medicine* 26 (1964): 543–75.

Freeman, Edith H., Frank J. Gorman, Margaret T. Singer, Marilyn T. Affelder, and Ben F. Feingold. "Personality Variables and Allergic Skin Reactivity: A Cross-Validation Study." *Psychosomatic Medicine* 29 (1967): 312–22.

Freud, Anna. *Normality and Pathology in Childhood.* New York: International Universities Press, 1965.

Friedman, Alice D. "Management with the Elimination Diet." In *Introduction to Clinical Allergy*, by Ben F. Feingold, 162–70. Springfield, IL: Charles C. Thomas, 1973.

———. *History of the Kaiser Permanente Medical Care Program.* Regional Oral History Office, Bancroft Library, University of California, Berkeley, 1986, http://www.bancroft.berkeley.edu/ROHO/projects/kaiser/index.html (accessed on 23 February 2009).

Friend, J. C. M. "The Syndrome of Childhood Hyperactivity." *Medical Journal of Australia* 1 (1977): 819–23.

Fritz, Gregory K. "Dietary Intervention for Hyperactive Children Supported in New Study." *Brown University Child Behavior and Development Letter* 5 (1989): 5.

Gardner, George E. "Aggression and Violence: The Enemies of Precision Learning in Children." *American Journal of Psychiatry* 128 (1971): 445–50.

Garfield, Sidney R. "A Report on Permanente's First Ten Years." *Permanente Foundation Medical Bulletin* 10 (1952): 1–11.

Garfinkel, Barry D., Christopher D. Webster, and Leon Sloman. "Methylphenidate and Caffeine in the Treatment of Children with Minimal Brain Dysfunction." *American Journal of Psychiatry* 131 (1974): 723–28.

Gibson, R. M. "Hyperkinesis—Revisited." *University of Michigan Medical Center Journal* 34 (1968): 213.

Ginzberg, Eli, and Marcia Freedman. "Problems of Educational and Vocational Development in Adolescence." In *The Psychopathology of Adolescence*, ed. Joseph Zubin and Alfred M. Freedman, 79–85. New York: Grune and Stratton, 1970.

Golden, Gerald S. "Nonstandard Therapies in the Developmental Disabilities." *American Journal of Diseases of Children* 134 (1980): 487–91.

Goyette, C. H., C. K. Conners, T. A. Petti, and L. E. Curtis. "Effects of Artificial Colors on Hyperkinetic Children: A Double-Blind Challenge Study." *Psychopharmacological Bulletin* 14 (1978): 39–40.

Greene, Wade. "Guru of the Organic Food Cult." *New York Times*, June 6, 1971.

Grootenboer, E. A. "The Relation of Housing to Behavior Disorder." *American Journal of Psychiatry* 119 (1962–1963): 469–72.

Gross, Mortimer D., Ruth A. Tofanelli, Sharyl M. Butzirus, and Earl W. Snodgrass. "The Effects of Diets Rich in and Free from Additives on the Behaviour of Children with Hyperkinetic and Learning Disorder." *Journal of the American Academy of Child and Adolescent Psychiatry* 26 (1987): 53–55.

"'Growing Fears' over Mad Cow Disease." *BBC News*, October 19, 2000, http://www .news.bbc.co.uk/1/hi/scotland/979103.stm (accessed March 13, 2009).

Guru-Murthy, Krishnan. Channel 4 News, September 6, 2007.

Harding, Anne. "Study: Kids with Eczema More Likely to Have ADHD." February 18, 2009, http://www.edition.cnn.com/2009/HEALTH/02/18/healthmag.eczema.adhd/ index.html (accessed March 23, 2009).

Harley, J. Preston. "Diet for Hyperactivity." *Chicago Tribune*, August 29, 1977.

Harley, J. Preston, C. G. Matthews, and P. Eichman. "Synthetic Food Colors and Hyperactivity in Children: A Double-Blind Challenge Experiment." *Pediatrics* 62 (1978): 975–83.

Harley, J. Preston, Roberta S. Ray, Lawrence Tomasi, Peter L. Eichman, Charles G. Matthews, Raymond Chun, Charles S. Cleeland, and Edward Traisman. "Hyperkinesis and Food Additives: Testing the Feingold Hypothesis." *Pediatrics* 61 (1978): 818–28.

Hegsted, D. Mark. "Frederick John Stare (1910–2002)." *Journal of Nutrition* 134 (2004): 1007–9.

Hersch, Charles. "The Clinician and the Joint Commission Report: A Dialogue." *Journal of the American Academy of Child Psychiatry* 10 (1971): 406–17.

Hersey, Jane. *Why Can't My Child Behave?* 1996; Williamsburg, VA: Pear Tree Press, 2006.

Hewitt, Jean. "Organic Food Fanciers Go to Great Lengths for the Real Thing." *New York Times*, September 7, 1970.

———. "Buying Health Foods Is Easier Now." *New York Times*, June 19, 1971.

Hindle, R. C., and Janelle Priest. "The Management of Hyperkinetic Children: A Trial of Dietary Therapy." *New Zealand Medical Journal* 88 (1978): 43–45.

———. "Dietary Control of Hyperkinesis." *New Zealand Medical Journal* 88 (1978): 344–45.

Holden, Constance. "Amphetamines: Tighter Controls on the Horizon." *Science* 194 (1976): 1027–28.

Hollingshead, A. B., and F. C. Redlich. *Social Class and Mental Illness: A Community Study.* New York: John Wiley, 1958.

Hoobler, B. Raymond. "Some Early Symptoms Suggesting Protein Sensitization in Infancy." *American Journal of Diseases of Children* 12 (1916): 129–35.

Horton, Richard. *MMR: Science and Fiction: Exploring a Vaccine Crisis.* London: Granta Books, 2004.

"Hot Dogs and Hyperkinesis." *Newsweek*, July 9, 1973.

"House Passes a Delay of Ban on Saccharin." *New York Times*, July 25, 1979.

Hoyt, Palmer. "What Is Ahead for Our Schools." *Grade Teacher* 76 (1958–1959): 20–21.

Hudson, B. W., Ben F. Feingold, and L. Kartman. "Allergy to Flea Bites II: Investigations of Flea Bite Sensitivity in Humans." *Experimental Parasitology* 9 (1960): 264–70.

Huestis, Robert D., L. Eugene Arnold, and Donald J. Smeltzer. "Caffeine versus Methylphenidate and d-Amphetamine in Minimal Brain Dysfunction: A Double-Blind Comparison." *American Journal of Psychiatry* 132 (1975): 868–70.

Huey, Leighton Y., Mark Zetin, David S. Janowsky, and Lewis L. Judd. "Adult Minimal Brain Dysfunction and Schizophrenia." *American Journal of Psychiatry* 134 (1977): 1563–65.

Hunter, Beatrice Trum. *The Natural Foods Cookbook.* New York: Pyramid, 1961.

———. *Consumer Beware! Your Food and What's Been Done to It.* New York: Simon and Schuster, 1970.

———. *The Mirage of Safety: Food Additives and Federal Policy.* Brattleboro, VT: Stephen Greene Press, 1982.

Hyperactive Children's Support Group. "Our Publications." http://www.hacsg.org.uk/ HACSG%20PUBLICATIONS.htm (accessed March 16, 2009).

"Hyperactivity." *Lancet* 312 (1978): 561.

"Hyperactivity Drug under Scrutiny." November 18, 1998, http://www.cbc.ca/health/ story/1998/11/18/ritalin981118a.html (accessed March 13, 2009).

"The Importance of Food Coloring." *Los Angeles Times,* June 24, 1976.

"The Importance of Not Being Earnest." November 6, 1998, http://www.news.bbc.co.uk/ 1/hi/health/208729.stm (accessed March 23, 2009).

"Is Diet Making Your Child Hyper?" *Tufts University Diet and Nutrition Letter* 7 (1989): 5.

Jacobson, Michael F., and David Schardt. *Diet, ADHD, and Behavior: A Quarter Century Review.* Washington, DC: Center for Science in the Public Interest, 1999.

Jarvik, Elaine. "The Calming of the Hyperactive." *Utah Holiday,* May 1978, 48–50, 63.

Jenkins, Nancy. "Health Food and the Change in Eating Habits." *New York Times,* April 4, 1984.

Jenkins, Richard L. "Classification of Behavior Problems of Children." *American Journal of Psychiatry* 125 (1969): 1032–39.

Jenson, Peter S., Stephen P. Hinshaw, James M. Swanson, Laurence L. Greenhill, C. Keith Conners, L. Eugene Arnold, Howard B. Abikoff, Glen Elliot, Lily Hechtman, Betsy Hoza, John S. March, Jeffrey H. Newcorn, Joanne B. Severe, Benedetto Vitiello, Karen Wells, and Timothy Wigal. "Findings from the NIMH Multimodal Treatment Study of ADHD (MTA): Implications and Applications for Primary Care Providers." *Developmental and Behavioral Pediatrics* 22 (2001): 60–73.

Johnson, Adelaide M., and S. A. Szurek. "The Genesis of Antisocial Acting Out in Children and Adults." In *Learning and Its Disorder: Clinical Approaches to Problems of Childhood,* ed. I. N. Berlin and S. A. Szurek, 120–38. Palo Alto, CA: Science and Behavior Books, 1965.

Johnson, G. Timothy. "Food Additive Link to Hyperactivity Unproven." *Chicago Tribune,* June 24, 1977.

———. "Diet-Hyperactivity Link Still Unproved." *Chicago Tribune,* September 21, 1978.

Jones, Ita. *The Grubbag: An Underground Cookbook.* New York: Random House, 1971.

Jukes, Thomas H. "Food Additives." *Science* 134 (1961): 798, 869.

———. "Language in Action." *Nature* 264 (1976): 602.

———. "Friedrich Wöhler RIP." *Nature* 273 (1978): 421.

Kahn, E., and L. H. Cohen. "Organic Drivenness: A Brain-Stem Syndrome and an Experience with Case Reports." *New England Journal of Medicine* 210 (1934): 748–56.

Kal, Edmund F. "Organic versus Functional Diagnoses." *American Journal of Psychiatry* 125 (1969): 1128.

Kallet, Arthur, and F. J. Schlink. *100,000,000 Guinea Pigs: Dangers in Everyday Foods, Drugs, and Cosmetics.* New York: Vanguard, 1933.

Kanner, Leo. *Child Psychiatry.* 1st ed. Springfield, IL: Charles C. Thomas, 1935.

———. *Child Psychiatry.* 2nd ed. Springfield, IL: Charles C. Thomas, 1949.

———. *Child Psychiatry.* 3rd ed. Springfield, IL: Charles C. Thomas, 1957.

Kaplan, Bonnie J. "The Relevance of Food for Children's Cognitive and Behavioural Health." *Canadian Journal of Behavioural Science* 20 (1988): 359–73.

Kaplan, Bonnie J., Jane McNicol, Richard A. Conte, and H. K. Moghadam. "Dietary Replacement in Preschool-Aged Hyperactive Boys." *Pediatrics* 83 (1989): 7–17.

Kavale, Kenneth A., and Steven R. Forness. "Hyperactivity and Diet Treatment: A Meta-Analysis of the Feingold Hypothesis." *Journal of Learning Disabilities* 16 (1983): 324–30.

Kennedy, John F. "Message from the President of the United States Relative to Mental Illness and Mental Retardation." *American Journal of Psychiatry* 120 (1964): 729–37.

Kernberg, Paulina F. "The Problem of Organicity in the Child: Notes on Some Diagnostic Techniques in the Evaluation of Children." *Journal of the American Academy of Child Psychiatry* 8 (1969): 517–41.

Kewley, Geoffrey D. "Personal Paper: Attention Deficit Hyperactivity Disorder Is Underdiagnosed and Undertreated in Britain." *BMJ* 316 (1998): 1594–96.

"Key Scientist Favors Elimination of Saccharin Use within Three Years." *New York Times*, April 12, 1979.

Kinberg, Olof. "Reply to the Foregoing." *American Journal of Psychiatry* 116 (1959): 84.

Kirsch, Irving, Brett J. Deacon, Tania B. Huedo-Medina, Alan Scoboria, Thomas J. Moore, and Blair T. Johnson. "Initial Severity and Anti-Depressant Benefits: A Meta-Analysis of Data Submitted to the Food and Drug Administration." *PLoS Medicine* 5 (2008): 260–67.

Kittler, Fred J., and Deane G. Baldwin. "The Role of Allergic Factors in the Child with Minimal Brain Dysfunction." *Annals of Allergy* 28 (1970): 203–6.

Knopf, Irwin Jay. *Childhood Psychopathology: A Developmental Approach*. Englewood Cliffs, NJ: Prentice-Hall, 1979.

Knowles, Asa S. "For the Space Age: Education as an Instrument of National Policy." *Phi Delta Kappa* 39 (1958): 305–10.

Koch, William H. *Chiropractic: The Superior Alternative*. Calgary: Bayeux Arts, 1995.

Kotulak, Ron. "Find Food Tie to Child Behavior." *Chicago Tribune*, June 27, 1973.

Kwok, Ho Man. "Chinese Restaurant Syndrome." *New England Journal of Medicine* 278 (1968): 796.

Langdell, John I. "Phenylketonuria: Some Effects of Body Chemistry on Learning." *Journal of the American Academy of Child Psychiatry* 6 (1967): 166–73.

Lappé, Frances Moore. *Diet for a Small Planet*. New York: Ballantine, 1991.

Laufer, M. W., and E. Denhoff. "Hyperkinetic Behavior Syndrome in Children." *Journal of Pediatrics* 50 (1957): 463–74.

Laufer, M. W., E. Denhoff, and G. Solomons. "Hyperkinetic Impulse Disorder in Children's Behavior Problems." *Psychosomatic Medicine* 19 (1957): 38–49.

Leary, Warren E. "Report Sees No Relationship between Hyperactivity, Diet." *Associated Press*, October 16, 1980.

Levy, F., S. Dumbrell, G. Hobbes, M. Ryan, N. Wilton, and J. M. Woodhill. "Hyperkinesis and Diet: A Double-Blind Crossover Trial with a Tartrazine Challenge." *Medical Journal of Australia* 1 (1978): 61–64.

Levy, Harold B. "Amphetamines in Hyperkinetic Children." *JAMA* 216 (1971): 1864–65.

Lichtenstein, Grace. "'Organic' Food Study Finds Pesticides." *New York Times*, December 2, 1972.

Lieber, B. "Letter to the Editor." *International Journal of Social Psychiatry* 2 (1956): 235–37.

Lipton, Morris. "Can Food Chemical Additives Have Any Effect on Behavior?" *Hartford Courant*, August 3, 1977.

Lipton, Morris A., and James P. Mayo. "Diet and Hyperkinesis: An Update." *Journal of the American Dietetic Association* 83 (1983): 132–34.

Lockey, Stephen D. "Allergic Reactions Due to F. D. and C. Yellow No. 5, Tartrazine, an Aniline Dye Used as a Coloring and Identifying Agent in Various Steroids." *Annals of Allergy* 17 (1959): 719–21.

Lofgren, L. Borje. "A Comment on 'Swedish Psychiatry.'" *American Journal of Psychiatry* 116 (1959): 83–84.

Lowell, Francis C., and Irving W. Schiller. "Editorial: It Is So—It Ain't So." *Journal of Allergy* 25 (1954): 57–59.

Lucas, Alexander R., and Morris Weiss. "Methylphenidate Hallucinosis." *JAMA* 217 (1971): 1081–91.

Lyons, Richard D. "Congressman Says Actress's Speech Helped Bar Cyclamates." *New York Times*, October 22, 1969.

———. "Saccharin Ban Causes Storm of Complaints." *New York Times*, March 11, 1977.

Mackarness, Richard. *Not All in the Mind: How Unsuspected Food Allergy Can Affect Your Body and Your Mind.* London: Pan Books, 1976.

Mahler, Don. "Review of the Film: *The Hyperactive Child.*" *Exceptional Children* 38 (1971–1972): 161.

Mailman, Richard B. "Where's the Effect?" *Archives of Disease in Childhood* 89 (2004), http://www.adc.bmj.com.login.ezproxy.library.ualberta.ca/cgi/eletters/89/6/506#927 (accessed March 6, 2009).

Malone, Charles A. "Some Observations on Children of Disorganized Families and Problems of Acting Out." *Journal of the American Academy of Child Psychiatry* 2 (1963): 22–49.

Mattes, Jeffrey A. "The Feingold Diet: A Current Reappraisal." *Journal of Learning Disabilities* 16 (1983): 319–23.

Mattes, J. A., and R. Gittelman. "Effects of Artificial Food Colorings in Children with Hyperactive Symptoms." *Archives of General Psychiatry* 38 (1981): 714–18.

May, Charles D. "Food Allergy: A Commentary." *Pediatric Clinics of North America* 22 (1975): 217–20.

Mayer, Jean. "The Arguments Pro." *Washington Post*, September 19, 1974.

Mayer, Jean, and Jeanne Goldberg. "Hyperactive Children: When the Food Dye Is Cast." *Los Angeles Times*, August 28, 1980.

———. "Weighing the Feingold 'Elimination' Diet on Its Tenth Anniversary." *Los Angeles Times*, September 27, 1984.

Mayer, Jean, and Joanna Dwyer. "Food Additives, Hyperactivity, and Dr. Feingold's Diet." *Washington Post*, August 5, 1976.

———. "Nutrition." *Washington Post*, November 17, 1977.

———. "Diet Changes Seem to Help." *Chicago Tribune*, November 16, 1978.

———. "The Latest Tally on Diets for Hyperactive Kids." *Chicago Tribune*, November 24, 1978.

———. "Diet May Help Hyperactive Children." *Chicago Tribune*, August 9, 1979.

Maynard, Robert. "Omaha Pupils Given 'Behavior' Drugs." *Washington Post*, June 29, 1970.

Mayron, L. W. "Hyperactivity from Fluorescent Lighting—Fact or Fancy: A Commentary on the Report by O'Leary, Rosenbaum, and Hughes." *Journal of Abnormal Child Psychology* 6 (1978): 291–94.

McCabe, S. E., John R. Knight, Christian J. Teter, and Henry Wechsler. "Non-Medical Use of Prescription Stimulants among U.S. College Students: Prevalence and Correlates from a National Survey." *Addiction* 100 (2005): 96–106.

McCann, Donna, Angelina Barrett, Alison Cooper, Debbie Crumpler, Lindy Dalen, Kate Grimshaw, Elizabeth Kitchin, Kris Lok, Lucy Porteous, Emily Prince, Edmund Sonuga-Barke, John O. Warner, and Jim Stevenson. "Food Additives and Hyperactive Behaviour in Three-Year-Old and Eight/Nine-Year-Old Children in the Community: A Randomised, Double-Blinded, Placebo-Controlled Trial." *Lancet* 370 (2007): 1560–67.

McCarthy, Colman. "Color It Dangerous." *Washington Post*, January 23, 1975.

"Measles Fears Prompt MMR Campaign.". August 7, 2008, http://www.news.bbc.co.uk/1/hi/health/7545151.stm (accessed March 23, 2009).

Merrill, Richard A. "Food Safety Regulation: Reforming the Delaney Clause." *Annual Review of Public Health* 18 (1997): 313–40.

Mettler, F. A. "Morphologic Correlates of Azide-Induced Hyperkinesis and Hypokinesis." *Transactions of the American Neurological Society* 93 (1968): 141–44.

Miller, James S. "The Diet Wasn't Controlled." *Pediatrics* 61 (1978): 326–27.

"Millions Turn to Organic Food." *BBC News*, February 8, 2000, http://www.news.bbc.co.uk/1/hi/health/634371.stm (accessed March 13, 2009).

Minde, K., D. Lewin, Gabrielle Weiss, H. Lavigueur, Virginia Douglas, and Elizabeth Sykes. "The Hyperactive Child in Elementary School: A Five-Year, Controlled, Followup." *Exceptional Children* 38 (1971–1972): 215–21.

"Minimal Brain Dysfunction." *Lancet* 302 (1973): 487–88.

Mintz, Morton, "'Heroine' of FDA Keeps Bad Drug Off of Market." *Washington Post*, July 15, 1962.

———. *The Therapeutic Nightmare.* Boston: Houghton Mifflin, 1965.

———. "Study Links Food Additives to Hyperactive Children." *Washington Post*, October 29, 1973.

Monte, Tom. "Feingold Diet: A Precious Commodity to Hyperactive Children?" *Chicago Tribune*, January 5, 1980.

Moore-Colyer, Richard, and Philip Conford. "A 'Secret Society'? The Internal and External Relations of the Kinship in Husbandry." *Rural History* 15 (2004): 189–206.

Morris, Kelly. "A Danger at My Table?" *Lancet* 354 (1999): 1565.

Myers, Jerome K., and Lee L. Bean. *A Decade Later: A Follow-Up of Social Class and Mental Illness.* New York: John Wiley, 1968.

National Advisory Committee on Hyperkinesis and Food Additives. *Report to the Nutrition Foundation.* New York: Nutrition Foundation, 1975.

———. *Final Report to the Nutrition Foundation.* New York: Nutrition Foundation, 1980.

National Center for Health Statistics. "Live Births, Birth Rates, and Fertility Rates, by Race: United States, 1909–1994." *Vital Statistics of the United States, 1994, Volume I, Natality.* Washington, DC: U.S. Department of Health and Human Services, 2007, http://www.cdc.gov/nchs/datawh/statab/unpubd/natality/natab94.htm (accessed February 18, 2008).

National Institutes of Health. "Defined Diets and Childhood Hyperactivity." *NIH Consensus Statement Online* 4 (January 13–15, 1982) http://www.consensus.nih.gov/1982/1982DietHyperactivity032html.htm (accessed October 22, 2008).

Nehrlich, Herbert H. "Feingold Revisited and Acknowledged." *Archives of Disease in Childhood* 89 (2004), http://www.adc.bmj.com.login.ezproxy.library.ualberta.ca/cgi/eletters/89/6/506#927 (accessed March 6, 2009).

Nelson, Harry. "Hyperactive Children and Diet: Is There a Link?" *Los Angeles Times*, April 19, 1976.

Nigg, Joel T., G. Knottnerus, M. Martel, K. Cavanagh, W. Karmaus, and M. Rappley. "Low Blood Levels Associated with Clinically Diagnosed Attention-Deficit/Hyperactivity Disorder and Mediated by Weak Cognitive Control." *Biological Psychiatry* 63 (2008): 325–31.

Nissen, Steven E. "ADHD Drugs and Cardiovascular Risk." *New England Journal of Medicine* 354 (2006): 1445–48.

O'Leary, K. D., A. Rosembaum, and P. C. Hughes. "Fluorescent Lighting: A Purported Source of Hyperactive Behavior." *Journal of Abnormal Child Psychology* 6 (1978): 285–89.

"Obituary of Arthur Fernandez Coca." *Journal of Allergy* 31 (1960): 382.

"Oliver's School Meal Crusade Goes On." *BBC News*, September 4, 2006, http://www.news.bbc.co.uk/1/hi/uk/5313882.stm (accessed March 13, 2009).

Orford, Eileen. "Commentary: Diagnosis Needs Tightening." *BMJ* 316 (1998): 1594–96.

Ormiston, Susan. "Will Heavyweight Krispy Kreme Step on Tim's Toes?" *Marketplace*, March 20, 2002, http://www.archives.cbc.ca/lifestyle/food/clips/15211/ (accessed February 24, 2009).

Palmer, Sushma, Judith L. Rapoport, and Patricia O. Quinn. "Food Additives and Hyperactivity." *Clinical Pediatrics* 14 (1975): 956–59.

"Paperback Bestsellers." *New York Times*, June 24, 1979.

"Parents Warned of Additives Link." September 6, 2009, http://www.news.bbc.co.uk/1/hi/health/6979976.stm (accessed March 9, 2009).

Park, Madison. "Autism Ruling Fails to Convince Many Vaccine-Link Believers." February 14, 2009, http://www.edition.cnn.com/2009/HEALTH/02/12/court.autism.reactions/index.html (accessed March 23, 2009).

Penney, Alexandra. "The Year of the Nutritionist." *New York Times*, July 1, 1979.

Pew Internet and American Life Project. "Vital Decisions: How Internet Users Decide What Information to Trust When They or Their Loved Ones are Sick." http://www.pewinternet.org/~/media//Files/Reports/2002/PIP_Vital_Decisions_May2002.pdf.pdf (accessed April 14, 2009).

Piness, George, and Hyman Miller. "Allergic Manifestations in Infancy and Childhood." *Archives of Pediatrics* 42 (1925): 557–62.

Pluenneke, Geraldine. "Food Chemicals: Eat, Drink, and Be Wary?" *Business Week*, January 13, 1975, 12.

Pogash, Carol. "The Myth of the 'Twinkie Defense.'" *San Francisco Chronicle*, November 23, 2003.

Pollock, I., and J. O. Warner. "Effects of Artificial Food Colours on Childhood Behaviour." *Archives of Disease in Childhood* 65 (1990): 74–77.

Randolph, Theron G. "Allergy as a Causative Factor of Fatigue, Irritability, and Behavior Problems of Children." *Journal of Pediatrics* 31 (1947): 560–72.

———. "Human Ecology and Susceptibility to the Chemical Environment." *Annals of Allergy* 19 (1961): 518–40, 657–77, 779–99, 908–29.

Randolph, Theron G., and Ralph W. Moss. *An Alternative Approach to Allergies: The New Field of Clinical Ecology Unravels the Environmental Causes of Mental and Physical Ills.* New York: Lippincott and Crowell, 1980.

Rapoport, J. L., I. T. Lott, D. F. Alexander, and A. U. Abramson. "Urinary Noradrenaline and Playroom Behaviour in Hyperactive Children." *Lancet* 296 (1970): 1141.

Rapoport, Judith, Alice Abramson, Duane Alexander, and Ira Lott. "Playroom Observations of Hyperactive Children on Medication." *Journal of the American Academy of Child Psychiatry* 10 (1971): 524–34.

Rapp, Doris J. *Allergies and the Hyperactive Child*. New York: Simon and Schuster, 1979.

Reeves, Katherine. "Each in His Own Good Time." *Grade Teacher* 74 (1956–57): 8, 117.

Reinhold, Robert. "Learning Parley Divided on Drugs." *New York Times*, February 6, 1968.

———. "Rx for Children's Learning Malady." *New York Times*, July 3, 1970.

———. "Drugs that Help Control the Unruly Child." *New York Times*, July 5, 1970.

Reiser, David E. "Observations of Delinquent Behavior in Very Young Children." *Journal of the American Academy of Child Psychiatry* 2 (1963): 50–71.

Rensberger, Boyce. "Doctors Consider Pledge to Curb Amphetamine Prescriptions." *New York Times*, June 18, 1971.

———. "Acupuncture Likened to Placebo." *New York Times*, June 19, 1975.

Rexford, Eveoleen N. "Child Psychiatry and Child Analysis in the United States." *Journal of the American Academy of Child Psychiatry* 1 (1962): 365–84.

———. "A Developmental Concept of the Problem of Acting Out." *Journal of the American Academy of Child Psychiatry* 2 (1963): 6–21.

Richard, Randall. "Drugs for Children: Miracle or Nightmare?" *Providence Journal*, February 8, 1972.

Rickover, H. G. *American Education—A National Failure: The Problem of Our Schools and What We Can Learn from England*. New York: E. P. Dutton, 1963.

Rimland, Bernard. "The Feingold Diet: An Assessment of the Reviews by Mattes, Kavale, and Forness and Others." *Journal of Learning Disabilities* 16 (1983): 331–33.

Rinkel, Herbert J., Theron G. Randolph, and Michael Zeller. *Food Allergy*. Springfield, IL: Charles C. Thomas, 1951.

Roan, Maura, and Jessica Roan. "ADHD and Chiropractic." *Aspire Magazine* (August/ September 2007), http://www.aspiremag.net/articles/parenting/childrenshealth/ adhdandchiropractic.html (accessed February 23, 2009).

Rochlin, Gregory. "Discussion of David E. Reiser's 'Observations of Delinquent Behavior in Very Young Children.'" *Journal of the American Academy of Child Psychiatry* 2 (1963): 66–68.

Rockmore, Milton. "Can Food Chemical Additives Have Any Effect on Behavior?" *Hartford Courant*, August 3, 1977.

Rodale, Robert. "Food Additives Sometimes Cause Strange Effects." *Hartford Courant*, May 29, 1974.

———. "Can Pure Food Be a Reality?" *Hartford Courant*, February 26, 1975.

Rodgers, William H., Jr. "The Persistent Problem of the Persistent Pesticides: A Lesson in Environmental Law." *Columbia Law Review* 70 (1970): 567–611.

Rogers, George A. "Methylphenidate Interviews in Psychotherapy." *American Journal of Psychiatry* 117 (1960): 549–50.

Rose, Terry L. "The Functional Relationship between Artificial Food Colors and Hyperactivity." *Journal of Applied Behavior Analysis* 11 (1978): 439–46.

Ross, Dorothea M., and Sheila A. Ross. *Hyperactivity: Research, Theory, and Action*. New York: John Wiley, 1976.

Rossiter, Al, Jr. "Feingold Diet Disputed." *United Press International*, October 16, 1980.

———. "Does Diet Affect Rambunctious Behavior?" *United Press International*, January 13, 1982.

———. "Special Diet May Benefit Hyperactive Children." *United Press International*, January 15, 1982.

Rowe, Albert H. *Clinical Allergy Due to Foods, Inhalants, Contactants, Fungi, Bacteria, and Other Causes: Manifestations, Diagnosis, and Treatment*. London: Baillière, 1937.

————. *Elimination Diets and the Patient's Allergies: A Handbook of Allergy.* 2nd ed. London: Henry Klimpton, 1944.

Rowe, Albert H., and Albert Rowe, Jr. *Food Allergy: Its Manifestations and Control and the Elimination Diets, a Compendium with Important Consideration of Inhalant (Especially Pollen), Drug, and Infectant Allergy.* 2nd ed. Springfield, IL: Charles C. Thomas, 1972.

Rowe, Albert H., Albert Rowe Jr., Kahn Uyeyama, and E. James Young. "Diarrhea Caused by Food Allergy." *Journal of Allergy* 27 (1956): 424–36.

Rowe, Albert H., Jr., Albert Rowe, and E. James Young. "Bronchial Asthma Due to Food Allergy Alone in Ninety-Five Patients." *Allergy Abstracts* 24 (1959): 1158.

Rowe, K. S. "Synthetic Food Colourings and 'Hyperactivity': A Double-Blind Crossover Study." *Australian Paediatric Journal* 24 (1988): 143–47.

Rowe, K. S., and K. J. Rowe. "Synthetic Food Coloring and Behavior: A Dose Response Effect in a Double-Blind, Placebo-Controlled, Repeated-Measures Study." *Journal of Pediatrics* 125 (1994): 691–98.

Russell, Cristine. "Additive-Free Diet Found Not to Curb Hyperactivity." *Washington Post* January 15, 1982.

Rutter, Michael. "Isle of Wight Revisited: Twenty-Five Years of Child Psychiatric Epidemiology." In *Annual Progress in Child Psychiatry and Child Development*, ed. Stella Chess and Margaret E. Hertzig, 131–79. New York: Psychology Press, 1990.

Rutter, Michael, J. Tizard, W. Yule, P. Graham, and K. Whitmore. "Research Report: Isle of Wight Studies, 1964–1974." *Psychological Medicine* 6 (1976): 313–32.

Rutz, Dan. "Ritalin Comes under Scrutiny after Cancer Found in Mice." January 14, 1996, http://www.edition.cnn.com/HEALTH/9601/ritalin/index.html (accessed March 20, 2009).

"Saccharin Held Free of Risk." *New York Times*, November 8, 1985.

Sachs, Jessica Snyder. "Vaccines: Separating Facts from Fiction." December 9, 2008, http://www.edition.cnn.com/2008/HEALTH/family/11/05/par.vaccine.kids/index.html (accessed March 23, 2009).

Salvatore, Steve. "Group Issues Guidelines for Monitoring Ritalin in Children." November 9, 1998, http://www.edition.cnn.com/HEALTH/9811/09/hearts.ritalin/index.html (accessed March 20, 2009).

Salzman, Louis K. "Allergy Testing, Psychological Assessment and Dietary Treatment of the Hyperactive Child Syndrome." *Medical Journal of Australia* 2 (1976): 248–51.

Sanders, Jacquin. "Organic Food: A Growing Market." *Washington Post*, June 28, 1970.

Sauerhoff, M. W., and I. A. Michaelson. "Hyperactivity and Brain Catecholamines in Lead-Exposed Developing Rats." *Science* 182 (1973): 1022–24.

Schab, David W., and Nhi-Ha T. Trinh. "Do Artificial Food Colors Promote Hyperactivity in Children with Hyperactive Syndromes? A Meta-Analysis of Double-Blind Placebo-Controlled Trials." *Journal of Developmental and Behavioral Pediatrics* 25 (2004): 423–34.

Schauss, Alexander G. "Nutrition and Behaviour: Complex Interdisciplinary Research." *Nutrition and Behavior* 3 (1984): 9–37.

Schmeck, Harold M., Jr. "Tighter Controls Asked on Two Drugs." *New York Times*, July 17, 1971.

Schnackenberg, Robert. "Caffeine as a Substitute for Schedule II Stimulants in Hyperkinetic Children." *American Journal of Psychiatry* 130 (1973): 796–98.

Schneider, Wilmot F. "Psychiatric Evaluation of the Hyperkinetic Child." *Journal of Pediatrics* 26 (1945): 559–70.

Schonwald, Alison. "ADHD and Food Additives Revisited." *AAP Grand Rounds* 19 (2008): 17.

Schrager, Jules, Janet Lindy, Saul Harrison, John McDermott, and Paul Wilson. "The Hyperkinetic Child: An Overview of the Issues." *Journal of the American Academy of Child Psychiatry* 5 (1966): 526–33.

Schworm, Peter. "Can Exercise Help Hyperactivity?" *International Herald Tribune*, May 31, 2006, http://www.iht.com/articles/2006/05/10/news/snalt.php (accessed March 4, 2009).

Selye, Hans. *Stress without Distress.* Philadelphia: J. B. Lippincott, 1974.

Settipane, Guy A., and F. H. Chafee. "Asthma Caused by F. D. and C. Approved Dyes." *Journal of Allergy* 40 (1967): 65–72.

Shannon, W. Ray. "Neuropathic Manifestations in Infants and Children as a Result of Anaphylactic Reaction to Foods Contained in Their Dietary." *American Journal of Disease of Children* 24 (1922): 89–94.

Shelley, W. B. "Birch Pollen and Aspirin Psoriasis: A Study in Salicylate Hypersensitivity." *JAMA* 189 (1964): 985–88.

Sieben, Robert L. "Controversial Medical Treatments of Learning Disabilities." *Academic Therapy* 13 (1977): 133–47.

Silbergeld, E. K., and A. M. Goldberg. "Hyperactivity: A Lead-Induced Behavior Disorder." *Environmental Health Perspectives* 7 (1974): 227–32.

Silver, Larry B. "The Playroom Diagnostic Evaluation of Children with Neurologically Based Learning Disabilities." *Journal of the American Academy of Child Psychiatry* 15 (1976): 240–56.

Sinclair, Upton. *The Jungle.* 1906; Harmondsworth: Penguin, 1974.

"A Skirmish Involving a Pacifist." *New York Times*, November 17, 1986.

Smyth, Jeannette. "Stores Do a Healthy Business in Natural Food." *Washington Post*, February 28, 1971.

Sobotka, T. J. "Estimates of Average, 90th Percentile and Maximum Daily Intakes of FD & C Artificial Food Colors in One Day's Diets among Two Age Groups of Children." *Food and Drug Administration Memorandum*, July 1976.

Solnit, Albert J. "Who Deserves Child Psychiatry? A Study in Priorities." *Journal of the American Association of Child Psychiatry* 5 (1966): 1–16.

Spain, W. C. "Book Review of *Food Allergy* by Herbert J. Rinkel, Theron G. Randolph, and Michael Zeller." *Quarterly Review of Biology* 28 (1953): 97–98.

Speer, Frederic. "Food Allergies." In *The Allergic Child*, ed. Frederic Speer, 106–37. New York: Harper and Row, 1963.

Spiegel, John P. "Social Change and Unrest: The Responsibility of the Psychiatrist." *American Journal of Psychiatry* 125 (1969): 1581–82.

Spurlock, Morgan. *Supersize Me.* Kathbur Pictures, 2004.

Srole, Leo, Thomas S. Langner, Stanley T. Michael, Marvin K. Opler, and Thomas A. C. Rennie. *Mental Health in the Metropolis: The Midtown Manhattan Study.* New York: McGraw-Hill, 1962.

Stare, Frederick. "Placebo Effect No Substitute for Research." *Hartford Courant*, March 27, 1975.

———. "Do Additives Make Your Child Hyperactive?" *Hartford Courant*, December 30, 1975.

Steer, C. R. "Managing Attention Deficit/Hyperactivity Disorder: Unmet Needs and Future Directions." *Archives of Disease in Childhood* 90 (2005): i19–i25.

Stevens, Tara, and Miriam Mulsow. "There Is No Meaningful Relationship between Television Exposure and Symptoms of Attention-Deficit/Hyperactivity Disorder." *Pediatrics* 117 (2006): 665–72.

Stewart, Mark A. "Correspondence: Dynamic Orientation." *American Journal of Psychiatry*, 117 (1960): 85.

———. "Urinary Noradrenaline and Playroom Behaviour in Hyperactive Children." *Lancet* 297 (1971): 140.

Stewart, Mark A., and B. H. Burne. "Minimal Brain Dysfunction." *Lancet* 302 (1973): 852.

Still, George F. "The Coulstonian Lectures on Some Abnormal Psychical Conditions in Children. Lectures I-II." *Lancet* 159 (1902): 1008–12, 1077–82.

Strain, Gladys Witt. "Nutrition, Brain Function, and Behavior." *Psychiatric Clinics of North America* 4 (1981): 253–68.

Strauss, Alfred A., and Heinz Werner. "Disorders of Conceptual Thinking in the Brain-Injured Child." *Journal of Nervous and Mental Disease* 96 (1942): 153–72.

Strauss, Stephen. "Linking Vaccines, Autism Tantamount to Crying 'Fire' When There Isn't One." March 12, 2009, http://www.cbc.ca/technology/story/2009/03/11/f-strauss-autism-vaccines.html (accessed April 1, 2009).

"Study Ties Food Dye to Erratic Behavior." *Chicago Tribune*, October 9, 1977.

"Subclinical Lead Poisoning." *Lancet* 301 (1973): 87.

Swain, Ann, Velencia Soutter, Robert Loblay, and A. Stewart Truswell. "Salicylates, Olioantigenic Diets, and Behaviour." *Lancet* 326 (1985): 41–42.

Swanson, James W., and Marcel Kinsbourne. "Food Dyes Impair Performance of Hyperactive Children on a Laboratory Learning Test." *Science* 207 (1980): 1485–87.

Swindler, Marsha. "Feingold—Swindler Family." Unpublished essay written for Azusa Pacific University, 1999.

Taylor, Charlotte C. "Chemical Toxicity and Mental Disorder." *American Journal of Psychiatry* 131 (1974): 609.

Thomas, Alexander, Herbert Birch, Stella Chess, and Lillian C. Robbins. "Individuality in Responses of Children to Similar Environmental Situations." *American Journal of Psychiatry* 116 (1960): 798–803.

Thorley, Geoffrey. "Pilot Study to Assess Behavioural and Cognitive Effects of Artificial Food Colours in a Group of Retarded Children." *Developmental Medicine and Child Neurology* 26 (1984): 56–61.

Tryphonas, Helen, and Ronald Trites. "Diet and Hyperactivity." *Nutrition Bulletin* 9 (1984): 24–31.

U.S. Congress. *Congressional Record* 119 (October 30, 1973): S19736–42.

Vaughan, Warren Taylor. *Allergy: Strangest of All Maladies*. London: Hutchinson's Scientific and Technical Publications, 1942.

Von Hoffman, Nicholas. "Concerning Hyperkinesis, Food Additives, and Crime." *Washington Post*, September 11, 1974.

Wadge, Andrew. "Colours and Hyperactivity." http://www.fsascience.net/2007/09/06/colours_and_hyperactivity (accessed March 9, 2009).

Waggoner, Raymond W., Sr. "The Presidential Address: Cultural Dissonance and Psychiatry." *American Journal of Psychiatry* 127 (1970): 1–8.

Wakefield, A. J., S. H. Murch, A. Anthony, J. Linnell, D. M. Casson, M. Malik, M. Berelowitz, A. P. Dhillon, M. A. Thomson, P. Harvey, A. Valentine, S. E. Davies, and J. A. Walker-Smith. "Ileal-Lymphoid-Nodular Hyperplasia, Non-Specific Colitis, and Pervasive Developmental Disorder in Children." *Lancet* 351 (1998): 637–41.

Walsh, Edward R. "Why Are We Poisoning Our Children?" *New York Times*, December 26, 1976.

Walters, Ray. "Paperback Talk." *New York Times*, May 27, 1979.

"We've Been Asked How Healthful Is 'Health Food?'" *U.S. News and World Report*, July 21, 1975, 64.

Weinreb, J., and R. M. Counts. "Impulsivity in Adolescents and Its Therapeutic Management." *Archives of General Psychiatry* 2 (1960): 548–58.

Weiss, Bernard. "Food Additives and Environmental Chemicals as Sources of Childhood Behavior Disorders." *Journal of the American Academy of Child Psychiatry* 21 (1982): 144–52.

——. "Food Additives as a Source of Behavioral Disturbance in Children." *Neurotoxicology* 7 (1986): 197–208.

Weiss, Bernard, J. Hicks Williams, Sheldon Margen, Barbara Abrams, Bette Caan, L. Jay Citron, Christopher Cox, Jane McKibben, Dale Ogar, and Stephen Schultz. "Behavioural Responses to Artificial Food Colours." *Science* 207 (1980): 1487–89.

Wellford, Harrison, and Samuel Epstein. "The Conflict over the Delaney Clause." *New York Times*, January 13, 1973.

Wells, Patricia. "An Ire Fed by Fabricated Foods." *New York Times*, June 24, 1978.

Wender, Esther H. "Food Additives and Hyperkinesis." *American Journal of Diseases of Children* 131 (1977): 1204–6.

——. "The Food Additive-Free Diet in the Treatment of Behavior Disorders: A Review." *Journal of Developmental and Behavioral Pediatrics* 7 (1986): 35–42.

Werry, John S. "Food Additives and Hyperactivity." *Medical Journal of Australia* 2 (1976): 281–82.

——. "The Use of Psychotropic Drugs in Children." *Journal of the American Academy of Child Psychiatry* 16 (1977): 446–68.

——. "An Overview of Pediatric Psychopharmacology." *Journal of the American Academy of Child Psychiatry* 21 (1982): 3–9.

Werry, John S., and M. G. Aman. "Dietary Control of Hyperkinesis," *New Zealand Medical Journal* 88 (1978): 297–98.

Whalen, Elizabeth M., and Frederick J. Stare. *Panic in the Pantry: Food Facts, Fads, and Fallacies.* New York: Atheneum, 1975.

"Why Cyclamates Were Banned." *Lancet* 295 (1970): 1091–92.

Wilens, Thomas E., Jefferson B. Prince, Thomas J. Spencer, and Joseph Biederman. "Stimulants and Sudden Death: What Is a Physician to Do?" *Pediatrics* 118 (2006): 1215–19.

Williams, J. Ivan, and Douglas M. Cram. "Diet in the Management of Hyperkinesis: A Review of the Tests of Feingold's Hypotheses." *Canadian Psychiatric Association Journal* 23 (1978): 241–48.

Williams, J. Ivan, Douglas M. Cram, Frances T. Tausig, and Evelyn Webster. "Relative Effects of Drugs and Diet on Hyperactive Behaviors: An Experimental Study." *Pediatrics* 61 (1978): 811–17.

Winfrey, Carey. "A Controversial Theory Links Hyperactivity to Nutrition." *New York Times*, January 14, 1980.

Wright, Robert A. "Health Foods: Only a Fad?" *New York Times*, October 15, 1972.

Zimmerman, Frederic T., and Bessie B. Burgemeister. "Action of Methyl-Phenidylacetate (Ritalin) and Reserpine in Behavior Disorders of Children and Adults." *American Journal of Psychiatry* 115 (1959): 323–28.

Zimmerman, Frederick J., and Dimitri A. Christakis. "Associations between Content Types of Early Media Exposure and Subsequent Attentional Problems." *Pediatrics* 120 (2007): 986–92.

Zwi, Morris, Paul Ramchandani, and Carol Joughin. "Evidence and Belief in ADHD." *BMJ* 321 (2000): 975–76.

Secondary Sources

Anderson, Warwick, Myles Jackson, and Barbara Gutmann Rosenkrantz. "Toward an Unnatural History of Immunology." *Journal of the History of Biology* 27 (1994): 575–94.

Apple, Rima D. *Vitamania: Vitamins in American Culture.* New Brunswick, NJ: Rutgers University Press, 1996.

———. *Perfect Motherhood: Science and Childrearing in America.* New Brunswick, NJ: Rutgers University Press, 2006.

Aronowitz, Robert A. *Making Sense of Illness: Science, Society, and Disease.* Cambridge: Cambridge University Press, 1998.

Beck, Ulrich. *Risk Society: Towards a New Modernity.* London: Sage, 1992.

Belasco, Warren. *Appetite for Change: How the Counterculture Took on the Food Industry.* Ithaca: Cornell, 2007.

Berlivet, Luc. "'Association or Causation?' The Debate on the Scientific Status of Risk Factor Epidemiology, 1947–c. 1965." In *Making Health Policy: Networks in Research and Policy after 1945*, ed. Virginia Berridge, 39–74. Amsterdam: Rodopi, 2005.

Berridge, Virginia, and Kelly Loughlin, eds. *Medicine, the Market, and the Mass Media: Producing Health in the Twentieth Century.* London: Routledge, 2005.

Bivins, Roberta. *Alternative Medicine? A History.* New York: Oxford University Press, 2007.

Box, Steven. Preface to *The Myth of the Hyperactive Child: And Other Means of Child Control*, by Peter Schrag and Diane Divoky, 7–30. New York: Penguin, 1982.

Boyce, Tammy. *Health, Risk, and News: The MMR Vaccine and the Media.* New York: Peter Lang, 2007.

Brancaccio, Maria Teresa. "Educational Hyperactivity: The Historical Emergence of a Concept." *Intercultural Education* 11 (2000): 165–77.

Brander, Michael. *Eve Balfour: Founder of the Soil Association and Voice of the Organic Movement: A Biography.* Haddington: Glenneil Press, 2003.

Brumberg, Joan Jacobs. *Fasting Girls: The History of Anorexia Nervosa.* Cambridge: Harvard University Press, 1989.

Brynner, Rock, and Trent D. Stephens. *Dark Remedy: The Impact of Thalidomide and Its Revival as a Vital Medicine.* Cambridge: Perseus, 2001.

Burnett, John. *Plenty and Want: A Social History of Diet in England from 1815 to the Present Day.* London: Scolar Press, 1966.

Carslaw, Nicola. "Communicating Risks Linked to Food: The Media's Role." *Trends in Food Science and Technology* 19 (2008): S14–S17.

Carstairs, Catherine. "Look Younger, Live Longer: Gayelord Hauser and the Campaign for a Healthy Old Age." Paper presented to the Canadian Society for the History of Medicine, Vancouver, Canada, June 1, 2008.

Chen, Wai. "The Laboratory as Business: Sir Almroth Wright's Vaccine Programme and the Construction of Penicillin." In *The Laboratory Revolution in Medicine*, ed. Andrew Cunningham and Perry Williams, 245–92. Cambridge: Cambridge University Press, 1992.

Collins, Harry, and Trevor Pinch. *Dr. Golem: How to Think about Medicine.* Chicago: University of Chicago Press, 2005.

Conford, Philip. "The Alchemy of Waste: The Impact of Asian Farming on the British Organic Movement." *Rural History* 6 (1995): 103–14.

———. *Origins of the Organic Movement.* Edinburgh: Floris Books, 2001.

Conrad, Peter. "The Discovery of Hyperkinesis: Notes on the Medicalization of Deviant Behavior." *Social Problems* 23 (1975): 12–21.

————. *Identifying Hyperactive Children: The Medicalization of Deviant Behavior.* Toronto: Lexington Books, 1976.

Cooter, Roger, and Stephen Pumfrey. "Separate Spheres and Public Places: Reflections on the History of Science Popularization and Science in Popular Culture." *History of Science* 32 (1994): 237–67.

Diack, Lesley, and David Smith. "The Media and the Management of a Food Crisis: Aberdeen's Typhoid Outbreak in 1964." In *Medicine, the Market, and the Mass Media: Producing Health in the Twentieth Century,* ed. Virginia Berridge and Kelly Loughlin, 79–94. London: Routledge, 2005.

Diller, Lawrence. "The Run on Ritalin: Attention Deficit Disorder and Stimulant Treatment in the 1990s." *Hastings Center Report* 26 (1996): 12–18.

Dyck, Erika. *Psychedelic Psychiatry: LSD from Clinic to Campus.* Baltimore: Johns Hopkins University Press, 2008.

Ehrenreich, Barbara, and Deirdre English. *For Her Own Good: 150 Years of the Experts' Advice to Women.* Garden City, NY: Anchor Books, 1979.

Epstein, Steven. *Impure Science: AIDS, Activism, and the Politics of Knowledge.* Berkeley: University of California Press, 1996.

Fitzgerald, Michael. "Wolfgang Amadeus Mozart: The Allegro Composer." *Canadian Journal of Diagnosis* 17 (2000): 61–64.

————. "Did Lord Byron Have Attention Deficit Hyperactivity Disorder?" *Journal of Medical Biography* 9 (2001): 31–33.

Fitzgerald, Michael, and W. Flannery. "Did Cromwell Have Hyperkinetic Syndrome?" Paper presented to the Royal College of Psychiatrists, Child and Adolescent Meeting, Harrogate, UK, September 20, 2002.

Goldin, Claudia. "America's Graduation from High School: The Evolution and Spread of Secondary Schooling in the Twentieth Century." *Journal of Economic History* 58 (1998): 345–74.

Grob, Gerald N. *Mental Illness and American Society, 1870–1940.* Princeton: Princeton University Press, 1983.

————. *From Asylum to Community: Mental Health Policy in Modern America.* Princeton: Princeton University Press, 1991.

Hacking, Ian. "Making Up People." In *The Science Studies Reader,* ed. Mario Biagioli 161–171. New York: Routledge, 1999.

Hale, Nathan. *The Rise and Crisis of Psychoanalysis in the United States.* New York: Oxford University Press, 1995.

Harrington, Anne, ed. *The Placebo Effect: An Interdisciplinary Exploration.* London: Harvard University Press, 1997.

Healy, David. *The Antidepressant Era.* Cambridge: Harvard University Press, 1997.

————. *Let Them Eat Prozac: The Unhealthy Relationship between the Pharmaceutical Industry and Depression.* New York: New York University Press, 2004.

Herzberg, David. *Happy Pills in America: From Miltown to Prozac.* Baltimore: Johns Hopkins University Press, 2009.

Iversen, Leslie. *Speed, Ecstasy, Ritalin: The Science of Amphetamines.* Oxford: Oxford University Press, 2008.

Jackson, Mark. *Allergy: The History of a Modern Malady.* London: Reaktion, 2006.

————. "'Allergy con Amore': Psychosomatic Medicine and the 'Asthmogenic Home' in the Mid-Twentieth Century." In *Health and the Modern Home,* ed. Mark Jackson, 153–74. New York: Routledge, 2007.

————. "The Pursuit of Happiness: The Social and Scientific Origins of Hans Selye's Natural Philosophy of Life." *History of the Human Sciences* 23 (2010).

Jakle, John A. "Roadside Restaurants and Place-Product Packaging." In *Fast Food, Stock Cars, and Rock 'n' Roll*, ed. George O. Carney, 97–117. London: Rowman and Littlefield, 1995.

Johnson, Hilary. *Osler's Web: Inside the Labyrinth of the Chronic Fatigue Syndrome Epidemic*. New York: Crown, 1996.

Keirns, Carla. "Better than Nature: The Changing Treatment of Asthma and Hay Fever in the United States, 1910–1945." *Studies in History and Philosophy of Biological and Biomedical Sciences* 34 (2003): 511–31.

Kenner, Robert, *Food, Inc.* Magnolia Pictures, 2008.

King, Martin, and Clare Street. "Mad Cows and Mad Scientists: What Happened to Public Health in the Battle for the Hearts and Minds of the Great British Beef Consumer?" In *Representing Health: Discourses of Health and Illness in the Media*, ed. Martin King and Katherin Watson, 115–32. New York: Palgrave Macmillan, 2005.

Krimsky, Sheldon. *Hormonal Chaos: The Scientific and Social Origins of the Environmental Endocrine Hypothesis*. Baltimore: Johns Hopkins University Press, 2000.

Kroll-Smith, Steve, and H. Hugh Floyd. *Bodies in Protest: Environmental Illness and the Struggle over Medical Knowledge*. New York: New York University Press, 1997.

Kutchins, Herb, and Stuart A. Kirk. *Making Us Crazy: DSM: The Psychiatric Bible and the Creation of Mental Disorders*. New York: Free Press, 1997.

Lakoff, Andrew. "Adaptive Will: The Evolution of Attention Deficit Disorder." *Journal of the History of the Behavioral Sciences* 36 (2000): 149–69.

Latour, Bruno. *The Pasteurization of France*. Trans. Alan Sheridan and John Law. London: Harvard University Press, 1988.

Lear, Linda. *Rachel Carson: Witness for Nature*. London: Allen Lane, 1998.

Leveille, John J. "Jurisdictional Competition and the Psychoanalytic Dominance of American Psychiatry." *Journal of Historical Sociology* 15 (2002): 252–80.

Levenstein, Harvey. *Revolution at the Table: The Transformation of the American Diet*. Oxford: Oxford University Press, 1988.

———. *Paradox of Plenty: A Social History of Eating in Modern America*. Oxford: Oxford University Press, 1993.

Ley, Barbara. *From Pink to Green: Disease Prevention and the Environmental Breast Cancer Movement*. New Brunswick, NJ: Rutgers University Press, 2009.

Löwy, Ilana. "The Strength of Loose Concepts: Boundary Concepts, Federative Experimental Strategies and Disciplinary Growth—The Case of Immunology." *History of Science* 30 (1992): 371–96.

Matless, David. "Bodies Made of Grass Made of Earth Made of Bodies: Organism, Diet, and National Health in Mid-Twentieth-Century England." *Journal of Historical Geography* 27 (2003): 355–76.

Mayes, Rick, and Adam Rafalovich. "Suffer the Restless Children: The Evolution of ADHD and Paediatric Stimulant Use, 1900–1980." *History of Psychiatry* 18 (2007): 435–57.

McLaughlin, Terrence. *A Diet of Tripe: The Chequered History of Food Reform*. London: David and Charles, 1978.

Metzl, Jonathan Michel. *Prozac on the Couch: Prescribing Gender in the Era of Wonder Drugs*. Durham: Duke University Press, 2003.

Mintz, Steven, and Susan Kellogg. *Domestic Revolutions: A Social History of Family Life*. New York: Free Press, 1988.

Mitman, Gregg. *Breathing Space: How Allergies Shape Our Lives and Landscapes*. London: Yale University Press, 2007.

Moore-Colyer, Richard. "Towards 'Mother Earth': Jorian Jenks, Organicism, the Right, and the British Union of Fascists." *Journal of Contemporary History* 39 (2004): 353–71.

Mosby, Ian. "'That Won-Ton Soup Headache': The Chinese Restaurant Syndrome, MSG, and the Making of American Food, 1968–1980." *Social History of Medicine* 22 (2009): 133–51.

Murphy, Michelle. *Sick Building Syndrome and the Problem of Uncertainty: Environmental Politics, Technoscience, and Women Workers.* Durham: Duke University Press, 2006.

Nestle, Marion. *Food Politics: How the Food Industry Influences Nutrition and Health.* Berkeley: University of California Press, 2002.

Oddy, Derek J. *From Plain Fare to Fusion Food: The British Diet from the 1890s to the 1990s.* Woodbridge: Boydell, 2003.

Pennington, Hugh T. *When Food Kills: BSE, E. coli, and Disaster Science.* Oxford: Oxford University Press, 2003.

Pol, Hans. "Anomie in the Metropolis: The City in American Sociology and Psychiatry." *Osiris* 18 (2003): 194–211.

Porter, Roy. "The Patient's View: Doing Medical History from Below." *Theory and Society* 14 (1985): 175–98.

Pressman, Jack D. *Last Resort: Psychosurgery and the Limits of Medicine.* Cambridge: Cambridge University Press, 1998.

Prior, Lindsay. *The Social Organization of Mental Illness.* London: Sage, 1993.

Radetsky, Peter. *Allergic to the Twentieth Century.* Boston: Little, Brown, 1997.

Rafalovich, Adam. "The Conceptual History of Attention-Deficit/Hyperactivity Disorder: Idiocy, Imbecility, Encephalitis, and the Child Deviant, 1877–1929." *Deviant Behavior* 22 (2001): 93–115.

———. *Framing ADHD Children: A Critical Examination of the History, Discourse, and Everyday Experience of Attention Deficit/Hyperactivity Disorder.* Lanham, MD: Lexington Books, 2004.

Rasmussen, Nicolas. *On Speed: The Many Lives of Amphetamine.* New York: New York University Press, 2008.

Rosenberg, Charles E. *Explaining Epidemics and Other Studies in the History of Medicine.* Cambridge: Cambridge University Press, 1992.

———. "Pathologies of Progress: The Idea of Civilization at Risk." *Bulletin of the History of Medicine* 72 (1998): 714–30.

Rosner, David, and Gerald Markowitz. "Industry Challenges to the Principle of Prevention in Public Health: The Precautionary Principle in Historical Perspective." *Public Health Reports* 117 (2002): 501–12.

Rothstein, William G. *Public Health and the Risk Factor: A History of an Uneven Medical Revolution.* Rochester: University of Rochester Press, 2003.

Rusnock, Andrea. "Catching Cowpox: The Early Spread of Vaccination, 1798–1810." *Social History of Medicine* 83 (2009): 17–36.

Schlosser, Eric. *Fast Food Nation: The Dark Side of the All-American Meal.* New York: Houghton Mifflin, 2001.

Schrag, Peter, and Diane Divoky. *The Myth of the Hyperactive Child: And Other Means of Child Control.* New York: Penguin Books, 1982.

Schurman, Rachel. "Fighting 'Frankenfoods': Industry Opportunity Structures and the Efficacy of the Anti-Biotech Movement in Western Europe." *Social Problems* 51 (2004): 243–68.

Seale, Clive. *Media and Health.* London: Sage, 2002.

Sellers, Christopher. "Discovering Environmental Cancer: Wilhelm Hueper, Post–World War II Epidemiology, and the Vanishing Clinician's Eye." *American Journal of Public Health* 87 (1997): 1824–35.

Shorter, Edward. *A History of Psychiatry.* New York: John Wiley, 1997.

Siddiqui, A., and Michael Fitzgerald. "Did Sir Winston Churchill Have Hyperkinetic or Bipolar Affective Disorder?" *European Journal of Child and Adolescent Psychiatry* 12 (2003): 219.

Singh, Ilina. "Bad Boys, Good Mothers, and the Miracle of Ritalin." *Science in Context* 15 (2002): 577–603.

———. "Biology in Context: Social and Cultural Perspectives on ADHD." *Children and Society* 16 (2002): 360–67.

———. "Boys Will Be Boys: Fathers' Perspectives on ADHD Symptoms, Diagnosis, and Drug Treatment." *Harvard Review of Psychiatry* 11 (2003): 308–16.

———. "Doing Their Jobs: Mothering with Ritalin in a Culture of Mother-Blame." *Social Science and Medicine* 59 (2004): 1193–1205.

———. "Will the 'Real Boy' Please Behave: Dosing Dilemmas for Parents of Boys with ADHD." *American Journal of Bioethics* 5 (2005): 34–47.

Smith, David F., and Jim Phillips. "Food Policy and Regulation: A Multiplicity of Actors and Experts." In *Food, Science, Policy, and Regulation in the Twentieth Century,* ed. David F. Smith and Jim Phillips, 1–16. London: Routledge, 2000.

Smith, Matthew. "Into the Mouths of Babes: Hyperactivity, Food Additives, and the Rise and Fall of the Feingold Diet." In *Health and the Modern Home,* ed. Mark Jackson, 304–21. London: Routledge, 2007.

———. "The Uses and Abuses of the History of Hyperactivity." In *(De)Constructing ADHD: Critical Guidance for Teachers and Teacher Educators,* ed. Linda J. Graham. New York: Peter Lang, 2010.

———. "Putting Hyperactivity in Its Place: Cold War Politics, the Brain Race, and the Origins of Hyperactivity in the United States." *Locating Health,* ed. Erika Dyck and Christopher Fletcher. London: Pickering and Chatto, 2011.

———. "Psychiatry Limited: Hyperactivity and the Evolution of American Psychiatry, 1957–1980." *Social History of Medicine* 21 (2008): 541–59.

Söderqvist, Thomas. *Science as Autobiography: The Troubled Life of Niels Jerne.* Trans. David Mel Paul. London: Yale University Press, 2003.

Steuter, Erin. "Pedalling Skepticism: Media Representations of Homeopathy as 'Junk Science.'" *Journal of American and Comparative Cultures* 24 (2001): 1–10.

Szreter, Simon. "History, Policy, and the Social History of Medicine." *Social History of Medicine* 22 (2009): 235–44.

Tauber, Alfred I. *The Immune Self: Theory or Metaphor?* Cambridge: Cambridge University Press, 1994.

Tomes, Nancy. "The Great American Medicine Show Revisited." *Bulletin of the History of Medicine* 79 (2005): 627–63.

Viner, Russell. "Putting Stress in Life: Hans Selye and the Making of Stress Theory." *Social Studies of Science* 29 (1999): 391–410.

Young, Allan. *The Harmony of Illusions: Inventing Posttraumatic Stress Disorder.* Princeton: Princeton University Press, 1995.

Young, James Harvey. "The Pig that Fell into the Privy: Upton Sinclair's *The Jungle* and the Meat Inspection Amendments of 1906." *Bulletin of the History of Medicine* 59 (1985): 467–80.

Notes

Chapter 1

1. Ben F. Feingold, *Why Your Child Is Hyperactive* (New York: Random House, 1996). In most publications, Feingold's birth is listed as 1900, and this is the year in which Feingold thought he was born. A recently discovered census document, however, indicates that he was actually born on June 9, 1899. Feingold Association of the United States (FAUS), http://www.feingold.org/pg-aboutus.html (accessed March 31, 2009).

2. Hyperactivity is used here throughout to denote what physicians now call attention-deficit/hyperactivity disorder (ADHD), partly because it was the most common term for the disorder during the 1970s, but also because it continues to be the term most patients, parents, and physicians recognize and understand. Hyperactivity has been otherwise known as minimal brain damage, minimal brain dysfunction, acting out, hyperkinesis, and attention deficit disorder (ADD). The disorder shared similarities to other childhood disorders, including learning disorder and oppositional conduct disorder. For a study on the prevalence of hyperactivity during the 1970s, see Dennis P. Cantwell, Lorian Baker, and Richard E. Mattison, "The Prevalence of Psychiatric Disorder in Children with Speech and Language Disorder: An Epidemiologic Study," *Journal of the American Academy of Child Psychiatry* 18 (1979): 50–461.

3. Peter Conrad, *Identifying Hyperactive Children: The Medicalization of Deviant Behavior* (Toronto: Lexington Books, 1976); Peter Schrag and Diane Divoky, *The Myth of the Hyperactive Child: And Other Means of Child Control* (New York: Penguin, 1982).

4. "Hot Dogs and Hyperkinesis," *Newsweek*, July 9, 1973, 53; Lucinda Franks, "F.D.A., in Shift, Tests Pediatrician's Diet for Hyperactivity," *New York Times*, February 9, 1975; Edward R. Walsh, "Why Are We Poisoning Our Children?," *New York Times*, December 26, 1976; Ray Walters, "Paperback Talk," *New York Times*, May 27, 1979.

5. "Paperback Bestsellers," *New York Times*, June 24, 1979; letter from Ben F. Feingold to Beatrice Trum Hunter, October 2, 1979, from the Beatrice Trum Hunter Collection, Howard Gotlieb Archival Research Center at Boston University, box 47; Ben F. Feingold and Helene S. Feingold, *The Feingold Cookbook for Hyperactive Children* (New York: Random House, 1979).

6. Camilla Anderson, *Society Pays the High Cost of Minimal Brain Damage in America* (New York: Walker, 1972), 214–16, 219.

7. This is similar to an argument made by journalist Peter Radetsky with respect to people with multiple chemical sensitivity. Peter Radetsky, *Allergic to the Twentieth Century* (Boston: Little, Brown, 1997), 18.

8. Marion Nestle, *Food Politics: How the Food Industry Influences Nutrition and Health* (Berkeley: University of California Press, 2002), 31–33.

9. Geraldine Pluenneke, "Food Chemicals: Eat, Drink, and Be Wary?" *Business Week*, January 13, 1975, 12.

10. Matthew Smith, "Psychiatry Limited: Hyperactivity and the Evolution of American Psychiatry, 1957–1980," *Social History of Medicine* 21 (2008): 541–59.

11. Narlito V. Cruz and Sami L. Bahna, "Do Foods or Additives Cause Behavior Disorders?" *Pediatric Annals* 35 (2006): 744; Philippe A. Eigenmann and Charles A. Haenggeli, "Food Colourings and Preservatives: Allergy and Hyperactivity," *Lancet* 364 (2004): 823–24; C. R. Steer, "Managing Attention Deficit/Hyperactivity Disorder: Unmet Needs and Future Directions," *Archives of Disease in Childhood* 90 (2005): i22.

12. Forty-one oral history interviews have been used as primary source material, in addition to archival, medical, media, and online sources. Interviews were semi-structured and conducted and transcribed by the author. Many of the interviews were made possible by the Feingold Association of the United States who kindly allowed me to put an advertisement in their newsletter, *Pure Facts*. The rest I contacted myself or were referred to me by other interviewees. All interviewees have been given pseudonyms.

13. Simon Szreter has recently encouraged medical historians to seek opportunities to seek ways in which to apply their research findings to informing health policy. Simon Szreter, "History, Policy, and the Social History of Medicine," *Social History of Medicine* 22 (2009): 235–44.

14. Maria Theresa Brancaccio, "Education Hyperactivity: The Historical Emergence of a Concept," *Intercultural Education* 11 (2000): 165–77; Conrad, *Identifying Hyperactive Children*; Andrew Lakoff, "Adaptive Will: The Evolution of Attention Deficit Disorder," *Journal of the History of the Behavioral Sciences* 36 (2000): 149–69; Rick Mayes and Adam Rafalovich, "Suffer the Restless Children: The Evolution of ADHD and Paediatric Stimulant Use, 1900–1980," *History of Psychiatry* 18 (2007): 435–57; Adam Rafalovich, "The Conceptual History of Attention Deficit/Hyperactivity Disorder: Idiocy, Imbecility, Encephalitis, and the Child Deviant," *Deviant Behavior* 22 (2001): 93–115; Adam Rafalovich, *Framing ADHD Children: A Critical Examination of the History, Discourse, and Everyday Experience of Attention Deficit/Hyperactivity Disorder* (Lanham, MD: Lexington Books, 2004); Ilina Singh, "Bad Boys, Good Mothers, and the Miracle of Ritalin," *Science in Context* 15 (2002): 577–603; Ilina Singh, "Biology in Context: Social and Cultural Perspectives on ADHD," *Children and Society* 16 (2002): 360–67; Ilina Singh, "Boys Will Be Boys: Fathers' Perspectives on ADHD Symptoms, Diagnosis, and Drug Treatment," *Harvard Review of Psychiatry* 11 (2003): 308–16; Ilina Singh, "Doing Their Jobs: Mothering with Ritalin in a Culture of Mother Blame," *Social Science and Medicine* 59 (2004): 1193–1205; Ilina Singh, "Will the 'Real Boy' Please Behave: Dosing Dilemmas for Parents of Boys with ADHD," *American Journal of Bioethics* 5 (2005): 34–47.

15. For more on the origins of hyperactivity, see Matthew Smith, "The Uses and Abuses of the History of Hyperactivity," in *(De)constructing ADHD: Critical Guidance for Teachers and Teacher Educators*, ed. Linda Graham (New York: Peter Lang, 2010); Matthew Smith, "A Place for Hyperactivity: *Sputnik*, the Cold War 'Brain Race,' and the Origins of Hyperactivity in the United States," in *Locating Health*, ed. Erika Dyck and Christopher Fletcher (London: Pickering and Chatto, 2011); Smith, "Psychiatry Limited."

16. Leo Kanner, *Child Psychiatry*, 1st ed. (Springfield, IL: Charles C. Thomas, 1935); Leo Kanner, *Child Psychiatry*, 2nd ed. (Springfield, IL: Charles C. Thomas, 1949); Leo Kanner, *Child Psychiatry*, 3rd ed. (Springfield, IL: Charles C. Thomas, 1957); Jules Schrager et al., "The Hyperkinetic Child: An Overview of the Issues," *Journal of the American Academy of Child Psychiatry* 5 (1966): 528.

17. National Center for Health Statistics, "Live Births, Birth Rates, and Fertility Rates, by Race: United States, 1909–1994," *Vital Statistics of the United States, 1994*, vol. 1, *Natality* (Washington, DC: U.S: Department of Health and Human Services, 2007), http://www.cdc.gov/nchs/datawh/statab/unpubd/natality/natab94.htm (accessed February 18, 2008).

18. Steven Mintz and Susan Kellogg, *Domestic Revolutions: A Social History of Family Life* (New York: Free Press, 1988), 184–87.

19. Franklin G. Ebaugh, "The Case of the Confused Parent," *American Journal of Psychiatry* 116 (1960): 1136.

20. Barbara Ehrenreich and Deirdre English, *For Her Own Good: 150 Years of the Experts' Advice to Women* (Garden City, NY: Anchor Books, 1979), 228–32; Palmer Hoyt, "What Is Ahead for Our Schools," *Grade Teacher* 76 (1958–1959): 20–21.

21. Claudia Goldin, "America's Graduation from High School: The Evolution and Spread of Secondary Schooling in the Twentieth Century," *Journal of Economic History* 58 (1998): 345–47; H. G. Rickover, *American Education, a National Failure: The Problem of Our Schools and What We Can Learn from England* (New York: E. P. Dutton, 1963), 71.

22. James Bryant Conant, *Slums and Suburbs* (New York: McGraw-Hill, 1961).

23. Eli Ginzberg and Marcia Freedman, "Problems of Educational and Vocational Development in Adolescence," in *The Psychopathology of Adolescence*, ed. Joseph Zubin and Alfred M. Freedman (New York: Grune and Stratton, 1970), 79–81.

24. Barbara Bateman, "Learning Disorders," *Review of Education Research* 36 (1966): 93; James Bryant Conant, *The American High School Today: A First Report to Interested Citizens* (New York: McGraw-Hill, 1959); Ehrenreich and English, *For Her Own Good*, 232–34; Asa S. Knowles, "For the Space Age: Education as an Instrument of National Policy," *Phi Delta Kappa* 39 (1958): 305–10; Rickover, *American Education*, 57; Joel Spring, *The Sorting Machine: National Educational Policy Since 1945* (New York: Longman, 1976), 1–4. For a poetic impression of the impact of Sputnik, see Steven A. Modée, "Post Sputnik Panic," *English Journal* 69 (1980): 56.

25. Capitals in original. Knowles, "For the Space Age," 76.

26. Rickover, *American Education*, 32.

27. Dorothy Barclay, "A Turn for the Wiser," *Pediatrics* 23 (1959): 760.

28. Gregory Rochlin, "Discussion of David E. Reiser's 'Observations of Delinquent Behavior in Very Young Children,'" *Journal of the American Academy of Child Psychiatry* 2 (1963): 66.

29. Kathreine Reeves, "Each in His Own Good Time," *Grade Teacher* 74 (1956–1957): 8. For more examples of how educators and psychiatrists became increasingly concerned with how hyperactive behavior could effect school performance, see Anthony Davids and Jack Sidman, "A Pilot Study: Impulsivity, Time Orientation, and Delayed Gratification in Future Scientists and in Underachieving High School Students," *Exceptional Children* 29 (1963): 170–74; K. Minde, D. Lewin, Gabrielle Weiss, H. Lavigueur, Virginia Douglas, and Elizabeth Sykes, "The Hyperactive Child in Elementary School: A Five-Year, Controlled, Followup," *Exceptional Children* 38 (1971–1972): 215–21.

30. Michael Fitzgerald, "Wolfgang Amadeus Mozart: The Allegro Composer," *Canadian Journal of Diagnosis* 17 (2000): 61–64; Michael Fitzgerald, "Did Lord Byron Have Attention Deficit Hyperactivity Disorder?" *Journal of Medical Biography* 9 (2001): 31–33; Michael Fitzgerald and W. Flannery, "Did Cromwell Have Hyperkinetic

Syndrome?" (paper presented to the Royal College of Psychiatrists, Child and Adolescent Meeting, Harrogate, UK, September 20, 2002); A. Siddiqui and Michael Fitzgerald, "Did Winston Churchill Have Hyperkinetic or Bipolar Disorder?" *European Journal of Child and Adolescent Psychiatry* 12 (2003): 219. For more on the problems of such retrospective diagnoses, see Smith, "Uses and Abuses."

31. Charles Bradley, "The Behavior of Children Receiving Benzedrine," *American Journal of Psychiatry* 94 (1937): 577–85; T. S. Clouston, "Stages of Overexcitability, Hypersenstiveness, and Mental Explosiveness and Their Treatment by the Bromides," *Scottish Medical and Surgical Journal* 4 (1899): 481–90; Franklin G. Ebaugh, "Neuropsychiatric Sequelae of Acute Epidemic Encephalitis in Children," *American Journal of Diseases of Children* 25 (1923): 89–90; George F. Still, "The Goulstonian Lectures on Some Abnormal Psychical Conditions in Children, Lecture 1–2," *Lancet* 159 (1902): 1008–12, 1077–82.

32. M. W. Laufer and E. Denhoff, "Hyperkinetic Behavior Syndrome in Children," *Journal of Pediatrics* 50 (1957): 463–74; M. W. Laufer, E. Denhoff, and G. Solomons, "Hyperkinetic Impulse Disorder in Children's Behavior Problems," *Psychosomatic Medicine* 19 (1957): 38–49.

33. Laufer, Denhoff, and Solomons, "Hyperkinetic Impulse Disorder," 39, 48.

34. Howard Fischer, "Fifty Years Ago in the *Journal of Pediatrics*: Hyperkinetic Behavior Syndrome in Children," *Journal of Pediatrics* 150 (2007): 520.

35. Ilana Löwy, "The Strength of Loose Concepts: Boundary Concepts, Federative Experimental Strategies and Disciplinary Growth: The Case of Immunology," *History of Science* 30 (1992): 371–73.

36. Justin M. Call, "Some Problems and Challenges in the Geography of Child Psychiatry," *Journal of the American Academy of Child Psychiatry* 15 (1976): 156.

37. Laufer, Denhoff, and Solomons, "Hyperkinetic Impulse Disorder," 41.

38. Ibid., 45.

39. Ibid., 41. For theories linking hyperactivity to brain trauma, see E. Kahn and L. H. Cohen, "Organic Drivenness: A Brain-Stem Syndrome and an Experience with Case Reports," *New England Journal of Medicine* 210 (1934): 748–56; Alfred A. Strauss and Heinz Werner, "Disorders of Conceptual Thinking in the Brain-Injured Child," *Journal of Nervous and Mental Disease* 96 (1942): 153–72.

40. For more on the relationship between pharmaceutical companies and the emergence of psychiatric conditions, see David Healy, *The Antidepressant Era* (Cambridge: Harvard University Press, 1997); David Healy, *Let Them Eat Prozac: The Unhealthy Relationship Between the Pharmaceutical Industry and Depression* (New York: New York University Press, 2004); David Herzberg, *Happy Pills in America: From Miltown to Prozac* (Baltimore: Johns Hopkins University Press, 2009); Herb Kutchins and Stuart A. Kirk, *Making Us Crazy: DSM: The Psychiatric Bible and the Creation of Mental Disorders* (New York: Free Press, 1997). For more on the proliferation of mental disorders in the postwar period, see Joan Jacobs Brumberg, *Fasting Girls: The History of Anorexia Nervosa* (Cambridge: Harvard University Press, 1989); Ian Hacking, "Making up People," in *The Science Studies Reader*, ed. Mario Biagioli (New York: Routledge, 1999), 161–71; Edward Shorter, *A History of Psychiatry* (New York: John Wiley, 1997); Allan Young, *The Harmony of Illusions: Inventing Posttraumatic Stress Disorder* (Princeton: Princeton University Press, 1995).

41. Warren Belasco, *Appetite for Change: How the Counterculture Took on the Food Industry* (Ithaca: Cornell, 2007).

Chapter 2

1. Wai Chen, "The Laboratory as Business: Sir Almroth Wright's Vaccine Programme and the Construction of Penicillin," in *The Laboratory Revolution in Medicine*, ed. Andrew Cunningham and Perry Williams (Cambridge: Cambridge University Press, 1992), 245–92; Bruno Latour, *The Pasteurization of France*, trans. Alan Sheridan and John Law (Cambridge: Harvard University Press, 1988); Andrea Rusnock, "Catching Cowpox: The Early Spread of Vaccination, 1798–1810," *Social History of Medicine* 83 (2009): 17–36.

2. Warwick Anderson, Myles Jackson, and Barbara Gutmann Rosenkrantz, "Toward an Unnatural History of Immunology," *Journal of the History of Biology* 27 (1994): 575.

3. Mark Jackson, *Allergy: The History of a Modern Malady* (London: Reaktion, 2006); Gregg Mitman, *Breathing Space: How Allergies Shape Our Lives and Landscapes* (New Haven: Yale University Press, 2007).

4. Feingold, *Why Your Child Is Hyperactive*, 1–3.

5. Ibid., 3.

6. Ibid., 3–4.

7. Ibid., 4–5.

8. Ibid., 5.

9. Ibid., 6.

10. E. Benjamini, Ben F. Feingold, and L. Kartman, "Allergy to Flea Bites. III. The Experimental Induction of Flea Bite Sensitivity in Guinea Pigs by Exposure to Flea Bites and by Antigen Prepared from Whole Flea Extracts of *Ctenocephalides Felis Felis*," *Experimental Parasitology* 10 (1960): 214–22; Feingold, *Why Your Child Is Hyperactive*, 6; Alice D. Friedman, *History of the Kaiser Permanente Medical Care Program* (Regional Oral History Office, Bancroft Library, University of California, Berkeley, 1986), 67, http://www.bancroft.berkeley.edu/ROHO/projects/kaiser/index .html (accessed on February 23, 2009).

11. Feingold, *Why Your Child Is Hyperactive*, 7–8; W. B. Shelley, "Birch Pollen and Aspirin Psoriasis: A Study in Salicylate Hypersensitivity," *JAMA* 189 (1964): 985–88.

12. Emphasis in original. Feingold, *Why Your Child Is Hyperactive*, 9.

13. Feingold, *Why Your Child Is Hyperactive*, 37; Friedman, *History of the Kaiser Permanente Medical Care Program*, 68; interview with Alex Drake, April 1, 2008.

14. Feingold's use of the term hyperkinesis in a book entitled *Why Your Child Is Hyperactive*, might be a subtle example of speaking to both a lay and medical audience. While parents were more familiar with the term hyperactivity, the official psychiatric term, as coined in *DSM-II*, was "hyperkinetic reaction of childhood." American Psychiatric Association: Committee on Nomenclature and Statistics, *Diagnostic and Statistical Manual of Mental Disorders-II* (Washington, DC: American Psychiatric Association, 1968), 50; Feingold, *Why Your Child Is Hyperactive*, 11–12.

15. Feingold, *Why Your Child Is Hyperactive*, 13.

16. Ibid.

17. Feingold, *Introduction to Clinical Allergy* (Springfield, IL: Charles C. Thomas, 1973), 147.

18. Ibid.

19. Clemens von Pirquet quoted in Jackson, *Allergy*, 10.

20. Ibid., 23.

21. Theron G. Randolph and Ralph W. Moss, *An Alternative Approach to Allergies: The New Field of Clinical Ecology Unravels the Environmental Causes of Mental and Physical Ills* (New York: Lippincott and Crowell, 1980), 4.

22. Jackson, *Allergy*, 23.

23. Spain's second point, that it was difficult to use skin tests to diagnose food allergy, referred to the idea shared by Feingold and others that testing for food allergies using extracts of various foods was not only an ineffective way to diagnose but was dangerous, leading at times to fatal reactions. As such, many allergists were reluctant to employ the practice and had to rely on elimination diets to determine the foods to which a patient might be allergic. Walter C. Alvarez, "Puzzling Nervous Storms Due to Food Allergy," *Gastroenterology* 7 (1946): 252; Feingold, *Introduction to Clinical Allergy*, 148–49; W. C. Spain, "Review of *Food Allergy* by Herbert J. Rinkel, Theron G. Randolph, and Michael Zeller," *Quarterly Review of Biology* 28 (1953): 97.

24. Charles D. May, "Food Allergy: A Commentary," *Pediatric Clinics of North America* 22 (1975): 219.

25. Francis C. Lowell and Irving S. Schiller, "Editorial: It Is So—It Ain't So," *Journal of Allergy* 25 (1954): 27.

26. Mark Jackson notes that the hope that tests measuring IgE levels would replace skin testing for allergy was not fulfilled, partly because of technical difficulties but also because it was difficult to establish base IgE levels and correlate rising IgE levels with particular symptoms. Jackson, *Allergy*, 125–26.

27. William G. Crook, "Food Allergy: The Great Masquerader," *Pediatric Clinics of North America* 22 (1975): 229; William G. Crook, "Adverse Reactions to Food Can Cause Hyperkinesis," *American Journal of Diseases of Childhood* 132 (1978): 819–20; William G. Crook, "Diet and Hyperactivity," *Journal of Learning Disabilities* 17 (1984): 66; Jackson, *Allergy*, 201.

28. Theron Randolph quoted in Jackson, *Allergy*, 201.

29. Ben F. Feingold et al., "Psychological Studies of Allergic Women: The Relation between Skin Reactivity and Personality," *Psychosomatic Medicine* 24 (1962): 196.

30. Feingold, *Why Your Child Is Hyperactive*, 14.

31. Emphasis in original. Feingold, *Why Your Child Is Hyperactive*, 156–58.

32. Feingold, *Why Your Child Is Hyperactive*, 162.

33. Warren T. Vaughan quoted in Jackson, *Allergy*, 100–101.

34. Arthur C. Coca, *Familial Nonreaginic Food-Allergy* (Springfield, IL: Charles C. Thomas, 1943), 11.

35. Theron G. Randolph, "Human Ecology and Susceptibility to the Chemical Environment," *Annals of Allergy* 19 (1961): 519.

36. Feingold, *Why Your Child Is Hyperactive*, 15–16.

37. Ibid., 17.

38. Feingold was at the Pirquet Clinic in 1929, the year in which von Pirquet and his wife committed suicide. Feingold left that year to take a teaching position at the Northwestern University School of Medicine in Chicago, although it is unclear if von Pirquet's suicide had anything to do with his decision to leave. Feingold, *Why Your Child Is Hyperactive*, 20.

39. Ibid., 21.

40. Ibid., 21–31.

41. Anderson, Jackson, and Rosenkrantz, "Toward an Unnatural History of Immunology," 575–82.

42. Hans Selye, *Stress without Distress* (Philadelphia: J. B. Lippincott, 1974).
43. Mark Jackson, "The Pursuit of Happiness: The Social and Scientific Origins of Hans Selye's Natural Philosophy of Life," *History of the Human Sciences* 23 (2010).
44. Feingold, *Why Your Child Is Hyperactive*, 1–3.
45. B. Raymond Hoobler, "Some Early Symptoms Suggesting Protein Sensitization in Infancy," *American Journal of Diseases of Children* 12 (1916): 134.
46. W. Ray Shannon, "Neuropathic Manifestations in Infants and Children as a Result of Anaphylactic Reaction to Foods Contained in Their Dietary," *American Journal of Disease of Children* 24 (1922): 89–92.
47. Ibid., 90.
48. George Piness and Hyman Miller, "Allergic Manifestations in Infancy and Childhood," *Archives of Pediatrics* 42 (1925): 560.
49. T. Wood Clarke, "The Relation of Allergy to Character Problems in Children," *Annals of Allergy* 8 (1950): 176; Albert H. Rowe and Albert Rowe Jr., *Food Allergy: Its Manifestations and Control and the Elimination Diets, a Compendium with Important Consideration of Inhalant (Especially Pollen), Drug, and Infectant Allergy*, 2nd ed. (Springfield, IL: Charles C. Thomas, 1972), 339.
50. T. Wood Clarke, "Neuro-Allergy in Childhood," *New York State Journal of Medicine* 42 (1948): 393–97; William G. Crook et al., "Systematic Manifestations Due to Allergy: Report of Fifty Patients and a Review of the Literature of the Subject," *Pediatrics* 27 (1961): 790–99; H. M. Davison, "Cerebral Allergy," *Southern Medical Journal* 42 (1949): 712–16; William Waddell Duke, *Allergy, Asthma, Hay Fever, Urticaria, and Allied Manifestations of Reaction* (London: Henry Klimpton, 1925); Theron G. Randolph, "Allergy as a Causative Factor of Fatigue, Irritability, and Behavior Problems of Children," *Journal of Pediatrics* 31 (1947): 560–72; Herbert J. Rinkel, Theron G. Randolph, and Michael Zeller, *Food Allergy* (Springfield, IL: Charles C. Thomas, 1951); Albert H. Rowe, *Elimination Diets and the Patient's Allergies: A Handbook of Allergy*, 2nd ed. (London: Henry Klimpton, 1944); Rowe and Rowe, *Food Allergy*; Warren Taylor Vaughan, *Allergy: Strangest of All Maladies* (London: Hutchinson's Scientific and Technical Publications, 1942).
51. Unfortunately, it is impossible to say whether Feingold received Clarke's survey. Clarke, "The Relation of Allergy," 176.
52. Ibid., 175.
53. T. Wood Clarke, "Neuro-Allergy in Childhood," 396; Clarke, "The Relation of Allergy," 175.
54. Clarke, "The Relation of Allergy," 176.
55. Ibid., 177, 181–82.
56. Ibid., 182.
57. Clarke, "The Relation of Allergy," 186–87.
58. Ben F. Feingold, "Infection in the Allergic Child," *Annals of Allergy* 8 (1950): 718–33; Ben F. Feingold, "Recognition of Food Additives as a Cause of Symptoms of Allergy," *Annals of Allergy* 26 (1968): 309–13; Ben F. Feingold and Eli Benjamini, "Allergy to Flea Bites: Clinical and Experimental Observations," *Annals of Allergy* 19 (1961): 1275–89; Ben F. Feingold, Eli Benjamini, and M. Shimizu, "Induction of Delayed and Immediate Types of Skin Reactivity in Guinea Pigs by Variation in Dosages of Antigens," *Annals of Allergy* 22 (1964): 543–75.
59. Richard Mackarness, *Not All in the Mind: How Unsuspected Food Allergy Can Affect Your Body and Your Mind* (London: Pan Books, 1976), 27.
60. Ibid.

61. Albert H. Rowe, *Clinical Allergy Due to Foods, Inhalants, Contactants, Fungi, Bacteria, and Other Causes, Manifestations, Diagnosis and Treatment* (London: Bailliére, 1937); Rowe, *Elimination Diets*; Rowe and Rowe, *Food Allergy*; Albert Rowe Jr., Albert H. Rowe, and James E. Young, "Bronchial Asthma Due to Food Allergy Alone in Ninety-Five Patients," *Allergy Abstracts* 24 (1959): 1158.

62. Rowe and Rowe, *Food Allergy*, 339–40.

63. Ibid., 340–41.

64. Friedman, *History of the Kaiser Permanente Medical Care Program*, 60.

65. Alice D. Friedman, "Management with the Elimination Diet," in *Introduction to Clinical Allergy*, ed. Ben F. Feingold (Springfield, IL: Charles C. Thomas, 1973), 162–70.

66. Ben F. Feingold, "Treatment of Allergic Disease of the Bronchi," *JAMA* 146 (1951): 319–23.

67. Interview with Phillip Lopes, February 19, 2007.

68. Feingold, "Treatment of Allergic Disease," 233.

69. Ben F. Feingold et al., "Psychological Variables in Allergic Disease: A Critical Appraisal of Methodology," *Journal of Allergy* 38 (1966): 143–55; Edith H. Freeman et al., "Psychological Variables in Allergic Disorders: A Review," *Psychosomatic Medicine* 26 (1964); Edith H. Freeman et al., "Personality Variables and Allergic Skin Reactivity," *Psychosomatic Medicine* 29 (1967): 312–22.

70. Freeman et al., "Psychological Variables," 555. These comments could also be used to describe the research done to connect food additives and hyperactivity.

71. Ibid., 321.

72. Feingold, *Introduction to Clinical Allergy*, 189.

73. For more on psychosomatic theories of allergy, see Mark Jackson, "'Allergy *con Amore*': Psychosomatic Medicine and the 'Asthmogenic Home' in the Mid-Twentieth Century," in *Health and the Modern Home*, ed. Mark Jackson (New York: Routledge, 2007), 153–74; Carla Keirns, "Better than Nature: The Changing Treatment of Asthma and Hay Fever in the United States, 1910–1945," *Studies in History and Philosophy of Biological and Biomedical Sciences* 34 (2003): 511–31. See also Robert A. Aronowitz, *Making Sense of Illness: Science, Society, and Disease* (Cambridge: Cambridge University Press, 1998), 39–56.

74. Shannon, "Neuropathic Manifestations," 93–94.

75. Albert H. Rowe et al., "Diarrhea Caused by Food Allergy," *Journal of Allergy* 27 (1956): 428–29.

76. Mackarness, *Not All in the Mind*, 36–38, 78–79.

77. Ethan Allan Brown, "American Academy of Allergy: The Changing Picture of Allergy," *Journal of Allergy* 28 (1957): 368.

78. Brown, "American Academy of Allergy," 365–66.

79. Feingold, *Why Your Child Is Hyperactive*, 156.

80. Randolph, "Allergy as a Causative Factor."

81. Interview with Alice Kahn, November 6, 2006.

82. Theron Randolph, "Human Ecology and Susceptibility to the Chemical Environment," *Annals of Allergy* 19 (1961), 518–40, 557–77, 779–99, 908–29; Rinkel, Randolph, and Zeller, *Food Allergy*.

83. Feingold and Benjamini, "Allergy to Flea Bites," 1275–89.

84. Randolph, "Human Ecology," 518.

85. Feingold, *Why Your Child Is Hyperactive*, 159–60.

86. Ben F. Feingold, "The Role of Diet in Behaviour," *Ecology of Disease* 1 (1982): 153.

87. Other contemporary observers, however, did associate Feingold and Randolph's work. A 1974 letter to the editor of the *American Journal of Psychiatry*, for instance, referred to both as providing evidence that chemicals in the food supply could lead to hyperactivity. Charlotte C. Taylor, "Chemical Toxicity and Mental Disorder," *American Journal of Psychiatry* 131 (1974): 609.

88. Fred J. Kittler and Deane G. Baldwin, "The Role of Allergic Factors in the Child with Minimal Brain Dysfunction," *Annals of Allergy* 28 (1970): 203–06; Wilmot F. Schneider, "Psychiatric Evaluation of the Hyperkinetic Child," *Journal of Pediatrics* 26 (1945): 567–68.

89. "Obituary of Arthur Fernandez Coca," *Journal of Allergy* 31 (1960): 384; L. N. Ettelson and Louis Tuft, "The Value of the Coca Pulse-Acceleration Method in Food Allergy," *Journal of Allergy* 32 (1961): 155; interview with Desmond Hawking, May 22, 2007.

90. Doris J. Rapp, *Allergies and the Hyperactive Child* (New York: Simon and Schuster, 1979), 3–12.

91. Interview with Josephine Bannister, March 2, 2007.

92. Letter from Ben. F. Feingold to Beatrice Trum Hunter, April 13, 1979, Beatrice Trum Hunter Collection, box 47.

93. Friedman, *History of the Kaiser Permanente Medical Care Program*, 57.

94. Ibid.

95. Ibid.

96. Phillip Lopes.

97. Ibid.

98. Interview with Stuart Unger, March 23, 2007.

Chapter 3

1. Feingold, "Recognition of Food Additives," 309–13.

2. Interview with Maggie Jeffries, February 17, 2008.

3. Feingold, *Why Your Child Is Hyperactive*, 31; Ben F. Feingold, "A View from the Other Side" (speech to the Newspaper Food Editors and Writers Association, Milwaukee, Wisconsin, June 8, 1977), http://www.feingold.org/pg-aboutus.html (accessed March 4, 2009).

4. "Food Additives Tied to Child Behavior," *Hartford Courant*, June 28, 1973; "Hot Dogs and Hyperkinesis"; Feingold, "A View from the Other Side"; Ron Kotulak, "Find Food Tie to Child Behavior," *Chicago Tribune*, June 27, 1973; Morton Mintz, "Study Links Food Additives to Hyperactive Children," *Washington Post*, October 29, 1973; U.S. Congress, "Food Additives and Hyperactivity in Children," *Congressional Record* 119 (October 30, 1973): S19736–42.

5. Feingold, *Why Your Child Is Hyperactive*, 21.

6. Feingold, "A View from the Other Side," 3.

7. Feingold, *Why Your Child Is Hyperactive*, 36–37.

8. Feingold, "A View from the Other Side."

9. Ibid.

10. Lucinda Franks, "F.D.A., in Shift, Tests Pediatrician's Diet for Hyperactivity," *New York Times*, February 9, 1975.

11. "Food Additives Tied to Child Behavior."

12. Kotulak, "Find Food Tie."

13. "Hot Dogs," 53.

14. Feingold, *Introduction to Clinical Allergy*, 194.

15. Mintz, "Study Links."

16. Feingold, "A View from the Other Side," 5.

17. Ibid., 6.

18. A. G. Schauss, "Nutrition and Behavior: Complex Interdisciplinary Research," *Nutrition and Health* 3 (1984): 20–21.

19. Ben F. Feingold, "A Critique of 'Controversial Medical Treatments of Learning Disabilities,'" *Academic Therapy* 13 (1977): 174; Feingold, "A View from the Other Side," 11.

20. Mintz, "Study Links Food Additives"; Feingold, "A View from the Other Side," 6, 11.

21. Ben F. Feingold, "Food Additives and Child Development," *Hospital Practice* 8 (1973): 11–21.

22. Feingold, "A View from the Other Side," 6.

23. C. Keith Conners, *Food Additives and Hyperactive Children* (New York: Plenum, 1980), 4; Feingold, "A View from the Other Side," 6–7, 11.

24. Ben F. Feingold, "Tonsillectomy in the Allergic Child," *California Medicine* 71 (1949): 341–44; Ben F. Feingold "Treatment of Allergic Disease of the Bronchi," *JAMA* 146 (1951): 319–23; Feingold, "A View from the Other Side," 11; Friedman, *History of the Kaiser Permanente Medical Care Program*, 68; Sidney R. Garfield, "A Report on Permanente's First Ten Years," *Permanente Foundation Medical Bulletin* 10 (1952): 1–11.

25. C. Keith Conners, *Feeding the Brain: How Foods Affect Children* (New York: Plenum, 1989), 159.

26. Milton Rockmore, "Can Food Chemical Additives Have Any Effect on Behavior?" *Hartford Courant*, August 3, 1977.

27. American Academy of Allergy, Asthma, and Immunology (AAAAI), "American Academy of Allergy, Asthma, and Immunology, Records, 1923– (Ongoing)," University of Wisconsin–Madison Libraries, Archive Department, box 161, folder 1.

28. Interview with Stuart Unger.

29. Interview with Kevin Osmond, October 8, 2007.

30. The AMA's history of protecting the reputation of its members from controversy and rooting out quackery is indicated in other ways. The only AMA archive open to historical researchers, for example, is its archive on "Historical Health Fraud and Alternative Medicine," which the AMA describes as "the nation's finest collection on medical quackery" and the "result of nearly seventy years of activity [1906–1975] by the AMA's Department of Investigation." Moreover, the "fraudulence existing today in matters pertaining to medicine and nutrition" was one of the traditional targets of the AMA's Department of Investigation. American Medical Association, "Historical Health Fraud and Alternative Medicine," http://www.ama-assn.org./ama/no-index/about-ama/17954.shtml (accessed March 3, 2009).

31. AAAAI, "AAAAI Records," box 242, folder 10; Pluenneke, "Food Chemicals," 12.

32. Pluenneke, "Food Chemicals," 12.

33. Feingold, "Recognition of Food Additives"; Stephen D. Lockey, "Allergic Reactions Due to F. D. and C. Yellow No. 5, Tartrazine, an Aniline Dye Used as a Coloring and Identifying Agent in Various Steroids," *Annals of Allergy* 17 (1959): 719–21; Guy A. Settipane and F. H. Chafee, "Asthma Caused by F. D. and C. Approved Dyes," *Journal of Allergy* 40 (1967): 65–72; Frederic Speer, "Food Allergies," in *The Allergic Child*, ed. Frederic Speer (New York: Harper and Row, 1963), 106–37.

34. AAAAI, "AAAAI Records," box 243, folder 2.

35. It is also possible be that the editors of *JAMA* simply differed with those organizing the AMA conference with respect to Feingold's theory and whether it should be published. Thanks to Rima Apple for offering this suggestion.

36. Feingold, "A View from the Other Side." The Nutrition Foundation was renamed the International Life Sciences Institute in the 1980s.

37. Ibid.

38. "Study Ties Food Dye to Erratic Behavior," *Chicago Tribune*, October 9, 1977; Feingold, "A View from the Other Side," 9.

39. Feingold, "A View from the Other Side," 10.

40. AAAAI, "AAAAI Records," box 137, folder 2; box 243, folder 1.

41. Ben F. Feingold, "Behavioral Disturbances Linked to the Ingestion of Food Additives," *Delaware Medical Journal* 49 (1977): 89–94; Ben F. Feingold, "Hyperkinesis and Learning Disabilities Linked to the Ingestion of Artificial Food Colors and Flavors" (speech to the American Academy of Pediatrics, New York: November 8, 1977), http://www.feingold.org/pg-aboutus.html (accessed January 28, 2009); Feingold, "The Role of Diet," 153–65.

42. Ben F. Feingold, "Food Additives in Clinical Medicine," *International Journal of Dermatology* 14 (1975): 112–14; Ben F. Feingold, "Hyperkinesis and Learning Disabilities Linked to Artificial Food Flavors and Colors," *American Journal of Nursing* 75 (1975): 797–803; Ben F. Feingold, "Food Additives in Dentistry," *Journal of the American Society for Preventive Dentistry* 7 (1977): 13–15; Feingold, "A Critique"; Ben F. Feingold, "Dietary Management of Juvenile Delinquency," *International Journal of Offender Therapy and Comparative Criminology* 23 (1979): 73–84.

43. Letter from Ben. F. Feingold to Beatrice Trum Hunter, April 7, 1978, Beatrice Trum Hunter Collection, box 47.

44. Interview with Kevin Osmond.

45. Josephine Bannister, December 8, 2007.

46. Feingold, "A Critique," 174.

47. Ibid.; Robert L. Sieben, "Controversial Medical Treatments of Learning Disabilities," *Academic Therapy* 13 (1977): 134–36.

48. Feingold, "A View from the Other Side," 11–12.

49. Ben F. Feingold, letter to Beatrice Trum Hunter, December 26, 1979, Beatrice Trum Hunter Collection, box 47.

50. Sushma Palmer, Judith L. Rapoport, and Patricia O. Quinn, "Food Additives and Hyperactivity," *Clinical Pediatrics* 14 (1975): 959; Stuart Unger.

51. Rick Mayes and Adam Rafalovich, "Suffer the Restless Children: The Evolution of ADHD and Paediatric Stimulant Use, 1900–1980," *History of Psychiatry* 18 (2007): 447.

52. John S. Werry, "Food Additives and Hyperactivity," *Medical Journal of Australia* 2 (1976): 282.

53. Letter from Ben F. Feingold to Beatrice Trum Hunter, December 26, 1979, from the Beatrice Trum Hunter Collection, box 47; Friedman, *History of the Kaiser Permanente Medical Care Program*.

54. Tom Monte, "Feingold Diet: A Precious Commodity to Hyperactive Children?" *Chicago Tribune*, January 5, 1980.

55. Interview with Stuart Unger.

56. Feingold would have actually been eighty years old when Conners wrote this statement in 1980. Conners, *Food Additives and Hyperactive Children*, 12.

57. B. W. Hudson, Ben F. Feingold, and L. Kartman, "Allergy to Flea Bites II: Investigations of Flea Bite Sensitivity in Humans," *Experimental Parasitology* 9 (1960): 264–70.

58. E. Benjamini, Ben F. Feingold, and L. Kartman, "Allergy to Flea Bites. III. The Experimental Induction of Flea Bite Sensitivity in Guinea Pigs by Exposure to Flea Bites and by Antigen Prepared from Whole Flea Extracts of Ctenocephalides Felis Felis," *Experimental Parasitology* 10 (1960): 222.

59. Ben F. Feingold et al., "Psychological Studies of Allergic Women: The Relation between Skin Reactivity and Personality," *Psychosomatic Medicine* 24 (1962): 201.

60. Friedman, *History of the Kaiser Permanente Medical Care Program*, 69.

61. Friedman, *History of the Kaiser Permanente Medical Care Program*, 69; Phillip Lopes, February 19, 2007.

62. Roger Cooter and Stephen Pumfrey, "Separate Spheres and Public Places: Reflections on the History of Science Popularization and Science in Popular Culture," *History of Science* 32 (1994): 250.

63. Ibid., 249–50.

64. Ibid., 250.

65. Russell Viner, "Putting Stress in Life: Hans Selye and the Making of Stress Theory," *Social Studies of Science* 29 (1999): 394.

66. Ibid., 396.

67. Ibid., 399–402.

68. Ibid., 402–5.

Chapter 4

1. J. Ivan Williams and Douglas M. Cram, "Diet in the Management of Hyperkinesis: A Review of the Tests of Feingold's Hypotheses," *Canadian Psychiatric Association Journal* 23 (1978): 242.

2. Ibid.

3. George A. Rogers, "Methylphenidate Interviews in Psychotherapy," *American Journal of Psychiatry* 117 (1960): 549–50.

4. For a variety of other explanations for hyperactivity, see R. T. Brown, "Perceived Family Functioning, Marital Status, and Depression in Parents of Boys with Attention Deficit Disorder," *Journal of Learning Disabilities* 22 (1989): 581–87; Oliver J. David, "Association between Lower Level Lead Concentrations and Hyperactivity in Children," *Environmental Health Perspectives* 7 (1974): 17–25; Judith Duffy, "Hyperactive Children 'Need Exercise, Not Drugs,'" *Sunday Herald*, November 12, 2006; R. M. Gibson, "Hyperkinesis: Revisited," *University of Michigan Medical Center Journal* 34 (1968): 213; L. W. Mayron, "Hyperactivity from Fluorescent Lighting—Fact or Fancy: A Commentary on the Report by O'Leary, Rosenbaum, and Hughes," *Journal of Abnormal Child Psychology* 6 (1978): 291–94; F. A. Mettler, "Morphologic Correlates of Azide-Induced Hyperkinesis and Hypokinesis," *Transactions of the American Neurological Society* 93 (1968): 141–44; K. D. O'Leary, A. Rosembaum, and P. C. Hughes, "Fluorescent Lighting: A Purported Source of Hyperactive Behavior," *Journal of Abnormal Child Psychology* 6 (1978): 285–99; M. W. Sauerhoff and I. A. Michaelson, "Hyperactivity and Brain Catecholamines in Lead-Exposed Developing Rats," *Science* 182 (1973): 1022–24; Peter Schworm, "Can Exercise Help Hyperactivity?" *International Herald Tribune*, May 31, 2006, http://www.iht.com/articles/2006/05/10/news/snalt.php

(accessed March 4, 2009); E. K. Silbergeld and A. M. Goldberg, "Hyperactivity: A Lead-Induced Behavior Disorder," *Environmental Health Perspectives* 7 (1974): 227–32; Tara Stevens and Miriam Mulsow, "There Is No Meaningful Relationship between Television Exposure and Symptoms of Attention-Deficit/Hyperactivity Disorder," *Pediatrics* 117 (2006): 655–72; Taylor, "Chemical Toxicity"; Frederick J. Zimmerman and Dimitri A. Christakis, "Associations between Content Types of Early Media Exposure and Subsequent Attentional Problems," *Pediatrics* 120 (2007): 986–92.

5. Smith, "Psychiatry Limited," 541–59.

6. Although there were other theories during the 1970s that linked chemical exposure to hyperactivity, these failed to become as popular or controversial as Feingold's hypothesis. The link between lead and hyperactivity has recently attracted interest, with researchers emphasizing the importance of identifying the genotype that is sensitive to low-level lead exposure. Joel T. Nigg et al., "Low Blood Levels Associated with Clinically Diagnosed Attention-Deficit/Hyperactivity Disorder and Mediated by Weak Cognitive Control," *Biological Psychiatry* 63 (2008): 325–31.

7. Gerald N. Grob, *From Asylum to Community: Mental Health Policy in Modern America* (Princeton: Princeton University Press, 1991), 100; Nathan Hale, *The Rise and Crisis of Psychoanalysis in the United States* (New York: Oxford University Press, 1995); John J. Leveille, "Jurisdictional Competition and the Psychoanalytic Dominance of American Psychiatry," *Journal of Historical Sociology* 15 (2002): 252; Shorter, *History of Psychiatry*.

8. Eveoleen N. Rexford, "A Developmental Concept of the Problem of Acting Out," *Journal of the American Academy of Child Psychiatry* 2 (1963): 6–21; Charles A. Malone, "Some Observations on Children of Disorganized Families and Problems of Acting Out," *Journal of the American Academy of Child Psychiatry* 2 (1963): 22–23; David E. Reiser, "Observations of Delinquent Behavior in Very Young Children," *Journal of the American Academy of Child Psychiatry* 2 (1963): 50–71.

9. Lakoff, "Adaptive Will," 155.

10. Richard L. Jenkins, "Classification of Behavior Problems of Children," *American Journal of Psychiatry* 125 (1969): 1032–33.

11. Leveille, "Jurisdictional Competition," 252–53.

12. Mark A. Stewart, "Correspondence: Dynamic Orientation," *American Journal of Psychiatry* 117 (1960): 85.

13. This quotation came from a Swedish American psychiatrist who lamented the fact that Swedish psychiatrists were turning away from psychoanalysis in favor of biological approaches. His letter received a curt reply from Olof Kinberg, a Swedish psychiatrist who stated that if psychiatrists were turning away from psychoanalysis, then they should be complimented. Olof Kinberg, "Reply to the Foregoing," *American Journal of Psychiatry* 116 (1959): 84; L. Borje Lofgren, "A Comment on 'Swedish Psychiatry,'" *American Journal of Psychiatry* 116 (1959): 83–84.

14. Reiser, "Observations of Delinquent Behavior," 50, 53, 67; Rexford, "A Developmental Concept," 9–10.

15. J. Weinreb and R. M. Counts, "Impulsivity in Adolescents and Its Therapeutic Management," *Archives of General Psychiatry* 2 (1960): 548–58.

16. Reiser, "Observations of Delinquent Behavior," 53; Rexford, "A Developmental Concept," 10–11; Alexander Thomas et al., "Individuality in Responses of Children to Similar Environmental Situations," *American Journal of Psychiatry* 116 (1960): 798.

17. Esther S. Battle and Beth Lacey, "A Context for Hyperactivity in Children over Time," *Child Development* 43 (1972): 757, 772; Adelaide M. Johnson and S. A. Szurek, "The Genesis of Antisocial Acting Out in Children and Adults," in *Learning and its Disorder: Clinical Approaches to Problems of Childhood*, ed. I. N. Berlin and S. A. Szurek (Palo Alto, CA: Science and Behavior Books, 1965), 136; Rexford, "A Developmental Concept," 11.

18. Feingold, *Why Your Child Is Hyperactive*, 38.

19. Interview with Lesley Freeman, January 28, 2008.

20. Ehrenreich and English, *For Her Own Good*, 217.

21. Jackson, "Allergy Con Amore," 159–65.

22. Ibid.

23. Interview with Lesley Freeman.

24. For more on the take up of antidepressants by women, see Ali Haggett, "Housewives, Neuroses, and the Domestic Environment in Britain, 1945–70," in *Health and the Modern Home*, ed. Mark Jackson (New York: Routledge, 2007), 84–110; Herzberg, *Happy Pills*; Jonathan Michel Metzl, *Prozac on the Couch: Prescribing Gender in the Era of Wonder Drugs* (Durham: Duke University Press, 2003).

25. Henry A. Davidson, "The Image of the Psychiatrist," *American Journal of Psychiatry* 121 (1964): 329–34; Robert H. Felix, "The Image of the Psychiatrist: Past, Present, and Future," *American Journal of Psychiatry* 121 (1964): 319.

26. John S. Werry, "The Use of Psychotropic Drugs in Children," *Journal of the American Academy of Child Psychiatry* 16 (1977): 463.

27. Albert J. Solnit, "Who Deserves Child Psychiatry? A Study in Priorities," *Journal of the American Academy of Child Psychiatry* 5 (1966): 3.

28. Leon Eisenberg, "Discussion of Dr. Solnit's Paper 'Who Deserves Child Psychiatry? A Study in Priorities,'" *Journal of the American Academy of Child Psychiatry* 5 (1966): 20–21.

29. Stella Chess, Alexander Thomas, and Herbert G. Birch, "Behavior Problems Revisited: Findings of an Anteroperspective Study," *Journal of the American Academy of Child Psychiatry* 6 (1967): 330; John P. Spiegel, "Social Change and Unrest: The Responsibility of the Psychiatrist," *American Journal of Psychiatry* 125 (1969): 1581–82; E. A. Grootenboer, "The Relation of Housing to Behavior Disorder," *American Journal of Psychiatry* 119 (1962/1963): 471; Malone, "Some Observations," 22–23.

30. Anonymous quoted in Henry A. Davidson, "Comment: The Reversible Superego," *American Journal of Psychiatry* 120 (1963): 192; S. A. Cermak, F. Stein, and C. Abelson, "Hyperactive Children and an Activity Group Therapy Model," *American Journal of Occupational Therapy* 27 (1973): 311–15.

31. Eisenberg, "Discussion of Dr. Solnit's Paper," 23; Charles Hersch, "The Clinician and the Joint Commission Report: A Dialogue," *Journal of the American Academy of Child Psychiatry* 10 (1971): 411.

32. Harold B. Levy, "Amphetamines in Hyperkinetic Children," *JAMA* 216 (1971): 1865.

33. Eveoleen N. Rexford "Child Psychiatry and Child Analysis in the United States," *Journal of the American Academy of Child Psychiatry* 1 (1962): 381.

34. Anna Freud, *Normality and Pathology in Childhood* (New York: International Universities Press, 1965); Irwin Jay Knopf, *Childhood Psychopathology: A Developmental Approach* (Englewood Cliffs, NJ: Prentice-Hall, 1979), 165–66.

35. Paulina F. Kernberg, "The Problem of Organicity in the Child: Notes on Some Diagnostic Techniques in the Evaluation of Children," *Journal of the American Academy of Child Psychiatry* 8 (1969): 537.

36. Sidney Berman, "Techniques of Treatment of a Form of Juvenile Delinquency, the Antisocial Character Disorder," *Journal of the American Academy of Child Psychiatry* 3 (1964): 24; Leon Eisenberg et al., "The Effectiveness of Psychotherapy Alone and in Conjunction with Perphenazine or Placebo in the Treatment of Neurotic and Hyperkinetic Children," *American Journal of Psychiatry* 116 (1960): 1092; Edmund F. Kal, "Organic versus Functional Diagnoses," *American Journal of Psychiatry* 125 (1969): 1128; Judith Rapoport et al., "Playroom Observations of Hyperactive Children on Medication," *Journal of the American Academy of Child Psychiatry* 10 (1971): 531.

37. American Psychiatric Association, "Position Statement on *Crisis in Child Mental Health: Challenge for the 1970s* Final Report of the Joint Commission on Mental Health of Children," *American Journal of Psychiatry* 125 (1969): 1197–1203.

38. Daniel Blain "The Presidential Address: Novalescence," *American Journal of Psychiatry* 122 (1965): 4; C. H. Hardin Branch, "Presidential Address: Preparedness for Progress," *American Journal of Psychiatry* 120 (1963): 10; Henry W. Brosin, "The Presidential Address: Adaptation to the Unknown," *American Journal of Psychiatry* 125 (1968): 7; Jack R. Ewalt, "Presidential Address," *American Journal of Psychiatry* 121 (1964): 1–8, 980; Raymond W. Waggoner Sr., "The Presidential Address: Cultural Dissonance and Psychiatry," *American Journal of Psychiatry* 127 (1970): 1.

39. "Editorial Statement," *Social Psychiatry* 1 (1966): 1.

40. Sir David Henderson quoted in Joshua Bierer, "Introduction to the Second Volume," *International Journal of Social Psychiatry* 2 (1956): 8.

41. Ibid., 8.

42. B. Lieber, "Letter to the Editor," *International Journal of Social Psychiatry* 2 (1956): 235–37.

43. John F. Kennedy, "Message from the President of the United States Relative to Mental Illness and Mental Retardation," *American Journal of Psychiatry* 120 (1964): 734–35.

44. Ibid., 730.

45. George E. Gardner, "Aggression and Violence: The Enemies of Precision Learning in Children," *American Journal of Psychiatry* 128 (1971): 446; Grootenboer, "The Relation of Housing," 471; Malone, "Some Observations," 22–23.

46. Stella Chess et al., "Interaction of Temperament and Environment in the Production of Behavioral Disturbances in Children," *American Journal of Psychiatry* 120 (1963): 147.

47. Chess, Thomas, and Birch, "Behavior Problems Revisited," 330; Irving N. Berlin, "Some Models for Reversing the Myth of Child Treatment in Community Mental Health Centers," *Journal of the American Academy of Child Psychiatry* 14 (1975): 84.

48. Eisenberg, "Discussion of Dr. Solnit's Paper," 23; Leon Eisenberg quoted in Schrager et al., "The Hyperkinetic Child," 530.

49. Feingold, *Why Your Child Is Hyperactive*, 160.

50. Ibid.

51. Henry A. Brosin, "Response to the Presidential Address," *American Journal of Psychiatry* 124 (1967): 7–8.

52. Brosin, "Presidential Address," 5.

53. John W. Gardner quoted in Brosin, "Presidential Address," 5.

54. David J. Franks, "Ethnic and Social Status Characteristics of Children in EMR and LD Classes," *Exceptional Children* 37 (1970–1971): 537–38.

55. John I. Langdell, "Phenylketonuria: Some Effects of Body Chemistry on Learning," *Journal of the American Academy of Child Psychiatry* 6 (1967): 166.
56. Rapoport et al., "Playroom Observations," 524.
57. John S. Werry, "An Overview of Pediatric Psychopharmacology," *Journal of the American Academy of Child Psychiatry* 21 (1982): 3.
58. Conners and Eisenberg, "The Effects of Methylphenidate," 458.
59. Don Mahler, "Review of the Film: *The Hyperactive Child*," *Exceptional Children* 38 (1971–1972): 161; Schrag and Divoky, *The Myth of the Hyperactive Child*, 80–84.
60. Dorothea M. Ross and Sheila A. Ross, *Hyperactivity: Research, Theory, and Action* (New York: John Wiley, 1976), 99.
61. Singh, "Bad Boys, Good Mothers," 593.
62. Nancy Tomes, "The Great American Medicine Show Revisited," *Bulletin of the History of Medicine* 79 (2005): 635.
63. Singh, "Bad Boys, Good Mothers," 593.
64. Interview with Lesley Freeman.
65. Ibid.
66. Maurice Laufer quoted in Robert Reinhold, "Drugs that Help Control the Unruly Child," *New York Times*, July 5, 1970.
67. Eric Denhoff quoted in Reinhold, "Drugs that Help."
68. "Drugs Seem to Help Hyperactive Children," *JAMA* 214 (1970): 2262; Leighton Y. Huey et al., "Adult Minimal Brain Dysfunction and Schizophrenia," *American Journal of Psychiatry* 134 (1977): 1563–65; Larry B. Silver, "The Playroom Diagnostic Evaluation of Children with Neurologically Based Learning Disabilities," *Journal of the American Academy of Child Psychiatry* 15 (1976): 253; Werry, "The Use of Psychotropic Drugs," 453.
69. Jane E. Brody, "If the Child Seems to Be 'Bad,' He Could Have Hyperkinesis," *New York Times*, December 1, 1976.
70. Interview with Trevor Davidson, December 6, 2007; Maggie Jeffries; interview with Lynn Kitchen, November 5, 2007.
71. Interview with Trevor Davidson.
72. Interview with Gayle Davidson, January 20, 2008.
73. Interview with Rosemarie Kushner, April 8, 2008.
74. Interview with Theresa McKay, February 13, 2008.
75. Interview with Maggie Jeffries.
76. Interview with Sharon Aubrey; interview with Justine Ewing, February 5, 2008; interview with Lesley Freeman.
77. Interview with Sylvia Terry, March 29, 2008.
78. Anonymous, "Correspondence to Oprah Winfrey," July 2005. This letter was written by the mother's sister to Oprah Winfrey in the hopes of getting onto Winfrey's show. They have not been on the show as of yet.
79. Interview with Lesley Freeman.
80. Alexander R. Lucas and Morris Weiss, "Methylphenidate Hallucinosis," *JAMA* 217 (1971): 1081.
81. Philip Firestone et al., "The Effects of Caffeine and Methylphenidate on Hyperactive Children," *Journal of the American Academy of Child Psychiatry* 17 (1978): 445–56; Barry D. Garfinkel, Christopher D. Webster, and Leon Sloman, "Methylphenidate and Caffeine in the Treatment of Children with Minimal Brain Dysfunction," *American Journal of Psychiatry* 131 (1974): 723–28; Robert D. Huestis, L. Eugene Arnold, and

Donald J. Smeltzer, "Caffeine versus Methylphenidate and d-Amphetamine in Minimal Brain Dysfunction: A Double-Blind Comparison," *American Journal of Psychiatry* 132 (1975): 868–70; Frederic T. Zimmerman and Bessie B. Burgemeister, "Action of Methyl-Phenidylacetate (Ritalin) and Reserpine in Behavior Disorders of Children and Adults," *American Journal of Psychiatry* 115 (1959): 323–28.

82. This differs from what Ilina Singh has found in parenting magazines (*Woman's Day* and *Parents*) from 1945 to 1965. None "contained an overtly negative article on the issues surrounding children and psychostimulant medication." She suspects that one reason for this was that such "magazines did not give voice to dissent during this period" and that hyperactivity was perceived as a biological problem requiring a biological solution. Matters had certainly changed by the late 1960s. Singh, "Bad Boys, Good Mothers," 594–95.

83. Robert Reinhold, "Learning Parley Divided on Drugs," *New York Times*, February 6, 1968.

84. Ibid.

85. Reinhold, "Drugs that Help."

86. Robert Reinhold, "Rx for Children's Learning Malady," *New York Times*, July 3, 1970.

87. Jonathan Black, "The Speed that Kills," *New York Times*, June 21, 1970. For more on the history of amphetamines, see Leslie Iverson, *Speed, Ecstasy, Ritalin: The Science of Amphetamines* (Oxford: Oxford University Press, 2008); Nicolas Rasmussen, *On Speed: The Many Lives of Amphetamine* (New York: New York University Press, 2008).

88. Black, "The Speed that Kills."

89. Constance Holden, "Amphetamines: Tighter Controls on the Horizon," *Science* 194 (1976): 1027–28.

90. Black, "The Speed that Kills."

91. Boyce Rensberger, "Doctors Consider Pledge to Curb Amphetamine Prescriptions," *New York Times*, June 18, 1971.

92. "Classroom Pushers," *Time*, February 26, 1973, http://www.time.com/time/magazine/article/0,9171,910580,00.html?promoid=googlep (accessed March 23, 2009).

93. Harold M. Schmeck Jr., "Tighter Controls Asked on Two Drugs," *New York Times*, July 17, 1971. Ritalin is still sold as a street drug today. S. E. McCabe et al., "Non-Medical Use of Prescription Stimulants among U.S. College Students: Prevalence and Correlates from a National Survey," *Addiction* 100 (2005): 96–106.

94. Randall Richard, "Drugs for Children: Miracle or Nightmare?" *Providence Journal* February 8, 1972.

95. "Classroom Pushers."

96. Interview with Sylvia Terry.

97. Lawrence Diller, "The Run on Ritalin: Attention Deficit Disorder and Stimulant Treatment in the 1990s," *Hasting Center Report* 26 (1996): 12; Robert Maynard, "Omaha Pupils Given 'Behavior' Drugs," *Washington Post*, June 29, 1970.

98. Peter Conrad, "The Discovery of Hyperkinesis: Notes on the Medicalization of Deviant Behavior," *Social Problems* 23 (1975): 15.

99. Ibid.

100. Denhoff quoted in "Classroom Pushers"; Reinhold, "Rx for Children's Learning Malady," 27.

101. Feingold, *Why Your Child Is Hyperactive*, 34.

Chapter 5

1. Mackarness, *Not All in the Mind*; Elizabeth M. Whalen and Frederick J. Stare, *Panic in the Pantry: Food Facts, Fads, and Fallacies* (New York: Atheneum, 1975).

2. Jacquin Sanders, "Organic Food: A Growing Market," *Washington Post*, June 28, 1970.

3. Derek J. Oddy, *From Plain Fare to Fusion Food: The British Diet from the 1890s to the 1990s* (Woodbridge: Boydell Press, 2003), ix, 31.

4. Harvey Levenstein, *Revolution at the Table: The Transformation of the American Diet* (Oxford: Oxford University Press, 1988), 39.

5. Federal Food and Drugs Act of 1906 (Wiley Act), Public Law Number 59-384, June 30, 1906; Upton Sinclair, *The Jungle* (Harmondsworth: Penguin, 1974).

6. James Harvey Young, "The Pig that Fell into the Privy: Upton Sinclair's *The Jungle* and the Meat Inspection Amendments of 1906," *Bulletin of the History of Medicine* 59 (1985): 468–70.

7. "Deleterious Food," *Brooklyn Daily Eagle*, September 20, 1885.

8. John A. Jakle, "Roadside Restaurants and Place-Product Packaging," in *Fast Food, Stock Cars, and Rock 'n' Roll*, ed. George O. Carney (London: Rowman and Littlefield, 1995), 97.

9. Levenstein, *Revolution at the Table*, 202.

10. Harvey Levenstein, *Paradox of Plenty: A Social History of Eating in Modern America* (Oxford: Oxford University Press, 1993), 113–14, 134–35.

11. Ibid., 112.

12. Ibid., 130.

13. Nestle, *Food Politics*, 31–33.

14. Ibid., 38–39.

15. Quoted in Richard A. Merrill, "Food Safety Regulation: Reforming the Delaney Clause," *Annual Review of Public Health* 18 (1997): 318.

16. Ibid., 320.

17. Quoted in Charles H. Blank, "The Delaney Clause: Technical Naïveté and Scientific Advocacy in the Formulation of Public Health Policies," *California Law Review* 62 (1974): 1088.

18. Levenstein, *Paradox of Plenty*, 112.

19. Ibid., 133; Christopher Sellers, "Discovering Environmental Cancer: Wilhelm Hueper, Post–World War II Epidemiology, and the Vanishing Clinician's Eye," *American Journal of Public Health* 87 (1997): 1832.

20. Richard D. Lyons, "Congressman Says Actress's Speech Helped Bar Cyclamates," *New York Times*, October 22, 1969.

21. If a pesticide left a residue on produce that was then meant to be consumed, it was considered to be a food additive. Levenstein, *Paradox of Plenty*, 134.

22. Ibid., 134.

23. Beatrice Trum Hunter, *The Mirage of Safety: Food Additives and Federal Policy* (New York: Scribner, 1982), 160.

24. Sellers, "Discovering Environmental Cancer," 1832–33.

25. "The Case of the Useful Carcinogen," *New York Times*, December 7, 1978.

26. Thomas H. Jukes, "Food Additives," *Science* 134 (1961): 798.

27. William H. Rodgers Jr., "The Persistent Problem of the Persistent Pesticides: A Lesson in Environmental Law," *Columbia Law Review* 70 (1970): 593.

28. Levenstein, *Paradox of Plenty*, 134

29. Rodgers, "A Lesson in Environmental Law," 594.

30. Rachel Carson, *Silent Spring* (London: Folio Society, 2000), 209–29; Linda Lear, *Rachel Carson: Witness for Nature* (London: Allen Lane, 1998), 480. Philosopher and physicist Sheldon Krimsky has suggested that although "cancer is certainly not the only adverse health effect of industrial chemicals . . . it has largely eclipsed other diseases and reproductive effects as an object of public concern and scientific research." Sheldon Krimsky, *Hormonal Chaos: The Scientific and Social Origins of the Environmental Endocrine Hypothesis* (Baltimore: Johns Hopkins University Press, 2000), 2.

31. Ernest G. Moore quoted in Lear, *Witness for Nature*, 413.

32. Lear, *Witness for Nature*, 428.

33. Ibid., 426–28.

34. Ibid., 430.

35. "Diet and Hyperactivity: Any Connection?" *Nutrition Reviews* 34 (1976): 151–58.

36. The pages to which the Monsanto parody refers are found in Carson's first chapter, "A Fable for Tomorrow." Carson, *Silent Spring*, 39–40; Monsanto quoted in Lear, *Witness to Nature*, 430.

37. Lear, *Witness to Nature*, 430.

38. Ibid., 428–37.

39. Ibid., 447–52.

40. Hunter was a key influence on Carson's environmental research. A series of letters between Carson and Hunter from the late 1950s and until Carson's death, including an eight-page litany of resources listing the dangers of DDT that Hunter wrote to Carson in 1958, indicate how Hunter helped convince Carson to embark on what would become *Silent Spring*. Beatrice Trum Hunter Collection, Howard Gotlieb Archival Research Center at Boston University. Letter from Beatrice Trum Hunter to Rachel Carson, April 4, 1963, Beatrice Trum Hunter Collection, box 23.

41. Lear, *Witness to Nature*, 448–54.

42. These divisions were reflected, for example, in the comments made by the participants in a Wellcome Witness seminar on the fortieth anniversary of *Silent Spring* in 2002. D. Christie and E. Tansey, *Environmental Toxicology: The Legacy of Silent Spring*, Wellcome Witnesses to Twentieth-Century Medicine, 19 (2004), Wellcome Trust Centre for the History of Medicine at UCL, London, http://www.ucl.ac.uk/silva/histmed/downloads/c20th_group/wit19 (accessed July 23, 2008).

43. Rock Brynner and Trent D. Stephens, *Dark Remedy: The Impact of Thalidomide and Its Revival as a Vital Medicine* (Cambridge, MA: Perseus, 2001), 39–59; Morton Mintz, *The Therapeutic Nightmare* (Boston: Houghton Mifflin, 1965), 248–64.

44. Whelan and Stare, *Panic in the Pantry*, 47.

45. Sandra Blakeslee, "Food Safety a Worry in Era of Additives," *New York Times*, November 9, 1969.

46. ABC Evening News, December 15, 1970, http://www.tvnews.vanderbilt.edu/diglib-fulldisplay.pl?SID=20080613905212402&code=tvn&RC=8753&Row=18 (accessed June 13, 2008); Belasco, *Appetite for Change*, 29–30; CBS Evening News, November 8, 1970, http://www.tvnews.vanderbilt.edu/diglib-fulldisplay.pl?SID=20080613905212402&code=tvn&RC=207475&Row=19 (accessed June 13, 2008).

47. Sanders, "Organic Food."

48. Catherine Carstairs, "Look Younger, Live Longer: Gayelord Hauser and the Campaign for a Healthy Old Age" (paper presented to the Canadian Society for the History of Medicine, Vancouver, Canada, June 1, 2008).

49. Dick Cavett, "When that Guy Died on My Show," *New York Times*, May 3, 2007, http://www.cavett.blogs.nytimes.com/2007/05/03/when-that-guy-died-on-my-show/ (accessed June 12, 2008).

50. Jeannette Smyth, "Stores Do a Healthy Business in Natural Food," *Washington Post*, February 28, 1971.

51. Wade Greene, "Guru of the Organic Food Cult," *New York Times*, June 6, 1971.

52. "Catered Health Foods, for Washingtonians, 'More Curious than Committed,'" *New York Times*, March 6, 1972.

53. Levenstein, *Paradox of Plenty*, 179. For more on the American counterculture and diet, see Belasco, *Appetite for Change*.

54. Levenstein, *Paradox of Plenty*, 170–71.

55. Belasco, *Appetite for Change*, 32–33.

56. Beatrice Trum Hunter, *The Natural Foods Cookbook* (New York: Pyramid, 1961).

57. Arthur Kallet and F. J. Schlink, *100,000,000 Guinea Pigs: Dangers in Everyday Foods, Drugs, and Cosmetics* (New York: Vanguard, 1933), 296–303.

58. Hunter, *The Mirage of Safety*, 8.

59. Beatrice Trum Hunter quoted in Patricia Wells, "An Ire Fed by Fabricated Foods," *New York Times*, June 24, 1978.

60. Ibid.

61. Frances Moore Lappé, *Diet for a Small Planet* (New York: Ballantine, 1991), 8.

62. Lappé, *Diet for a Small Planet*, 3.

63. Smyth, "Stores Do a Healthy Business."

64. Belasco, *Appetite for Change*, 40.

65. Ho Man Kwok, "Chinese Restaurant Syndrome," *New England Journal of Medicine* 278 (1968): 796; Ian Mosby, "'That Won-Ton Soup Headache': The Chinese Restaurant Syndrome, MSG, and the Making of American Food, 1968–1980," *Social History of Medicine* 22 (2009): 134.

66. Jean Hewitt, "Organic Food Fanciers Go to Great Lengths for the Real Thing," *New York Times*, September 7, 1970.

67. Robert A. Wright, "Health Foods: Only a Fad?" *New York Times*, October 15, 1972.

68. Jean Hewitt, "Buying Health Foods Is Easier Now," *New York Times*, June 19, 1971.

69. Smyth, "Stores Do a Healthy Business."

70. Ibid.

71. Ibid.

72. Abraham Ribicoff quoted in Hunter, *Mirage of Safety*, 1.

73. Gaylord Nelson quoted in Hunter, *Mirage of Safety*, 2, 5.

74. Hunter, *Mirage of Safety*, 304–5.

75. Marlene Cimons, "Hyperactivity and Food Additives," *Los Angeles Times*, September 15, 1975.

76. According to Sheldon Krimsky, evidence that the synthetic hormone DES was carcinogenic was one of three key factors that led to the development of the "environmental endocrine hypothesis," a theory that posits "that a diverse group of industrial and agricultural chemicals in contact with humans and wildlife have the capacity to mimic or obstruct hormone function—not simply disrupting the endocrine system like foreign matter in watchworks, but fooling it into accepting new instructions that distort the normal development of the organism." Krimsky's analysis of the social factors that contributed to the development and promotion of this hypothesis bears some parallel to the popularization of Feingold's hypothesis. Krimsky, *Hormonal Chaos*, 2–4.

77. Belasco, *Appetite for Change*, 140.

78. "We've Been Asked How Healthful Is 'Health Food'?" *U.S. News and World Report*, July 21, 1975, 64; Hunter, *Mirage of Safety*, 198–225.

79. Whalen and Stare, *Panic in the Pantry*, 6.

80. Ibid., 154–60.

81. Whalen and Stare, *Panic in the Pantry*, 163.

82. "Why Cyclamates Were Banned," *Lancet* 295 (1970): 1091–92.

83. "Frederick Stare," *The Economist*, April 18, 2002, http://www.economist.com/obituary/displaystory.cfm?story_id=E1_TDRGGRJ (accessed June 17, 2008); D. Mark Hegsted, "Frederick John Stare (1910–2002)," *Journal of Nutrition* 134 (2004): 1007–9.

84. Belasco, *Appetite for Change*, 114. Jean Mayer quoted in Jean Hewitt, "Organic Food Fanciers," 23; interview with Josephine Bannister.

85. Greene, "Guru of the Organic Food Cult," SM54.

86. Belasco, *Appetite for Change*, 1–3.

87. Sandra Blakeslee, "Challenge to Food Tests," *New York Times*, November 10, 1969.

88. Elaine Jarvik, "The Calming of the Hyperactive," *Utah Holiday*, May 1978, 48.

89. AMA quoted in Sandra Blakeslee, "Challenge to Food Tests."

90. George Christakis quoted in Grace Lichtenstein, "'Organic' Food Study Finds Pesticides," *New York Times*, December 2, 1972.

91. Anonymous quoted in Blakeslee, "Challenge to Food Tests."

92. Joshua Lederberg quoted in Harrison Wellford and Samuel Epstein, "The Conflict over the Delaney Clause," *New York Times*, January 13, 1973.

93. Interview with Maggie Jeffries.

94. Interview with Sharon Aubrey, January 29, 2008.

95. Interview with Lesley Freeman.

96. Interview with Ellen Miller, May 20, 2008.

97. Interview with Rosemarie Kushner.

98. Whalen and Stare, *Panic in the Pantry*, 114–15.

99. Greene, "Guru of the Organic Food Cult."

100. Rima D. Apple, *Vitamania: Vitamins in American Culture* (New Brunswick, NJ: Rutgers University Press, 1996); John Burnett, *Plenty and Want: A Social History of Diet in England from 1815 to the Present Day* (London: Scolar Press, 1979); Levenstein, *Revolution at the Table*; Terrence McLaughlin, *A Diet of Tripe: The Chequered History of Food Reform* (London: David and Charles, 1978); David F. Smith and Jim Phillips, "Food Policy and Regulation: A Multiplicity of Actors and Experts," in *Food, Science, Policy, and Regulation in the Twentieth Century*, ed. David F. Smith and Jim Phillips (London: Routledge, 2000), 1.

Chapter 6

1. Anna Colamosca, "Health Foods Prosper Despite High Prices," *New York Times*, November 17, 1974.

2. Ibid.

3. Virginia Berridge and Kelly Loughlin, eds., introduction to *Medicine, the Market, and the Mass Media: Producing Health in the Twentieth Century* (London: Routledge, 2005), 6.

4. Ibid.

5. Clive Seale, *Media and Health* (London: Sage, 2002), 70–75.

6. Martin King and Clare Street, "Mad Cows and Mad Scientists: What Happened to Public Health in the Battle for the Hearts and Minds of the Great British Beef Consumer?" in *Representing Health: Discourses of Health and Illness in the Media,* ed. Martin King and Katherine Watson (New York: Palgrave Macmillan, 2005), 119.

7. Richard D. Lyons, "Saccharin Ban Causes Storm of Complaints," *New York Times,* March 11, 1977.

8. Lesley Diack and David Smith, "The Media and the Management of a Food Crisis: Aberdeen's Typhoid Outbreak in 1964," in *Medicine, the Market, and the Mass Media: Producing Health in the Twentieth Century,* ed. Virginia Berridge and Kelly Loughlin (London: Routledge, 2005), 81–86.

9. Diack and Smith, "Media and Management," 88–89.

10. Warren Belasco, *Appetite for Change,* 154–55.

11. Ibid., 155. As sociologist Erin Steuter has observed, the mass media has grown more resistant to alternative medicine during the last fifteen years, and has increasingly called it "junk science." Erin Steuter, "Pedalling Skepticism: Media Representations of Homeopathy as 'Junk Science,'" *Journal of American and Comparative Culture* 24 (2001): 1–10.

12. Feingold, "A View from the Other Side," 10–11; Harry Nelson, "Hyperactive Children and Diet: Is There a Link?" *Los Angeles Times,* April 19, 1976.

13. Mintz, "Study Links."

14. The "Saturday News Quiz" asked readers, "According to recent studies prompted by the popular and controversial 'Feingold diet,' what substances in food affect the behavior of hyperactive children?" Linda Amster, "Saturday News Quiz," *New York Times,* April 5, 1980.

15. Interview with Ellen Miller.

16. One of the newspapers to report on Feingold's first press conference was apparently so eager to break the story it did not bother to copyedit its story. Feingold was described in the first sentence as a psychologist, only later to be correctly identified as an allergist, and one of his colleagues, Donald German, was incorrectly identified as "Daond" German. "Food Additives Tied to Child Behavior," *Hartford Courant,* June 28, 1973.

17. Marian Burros, "Coloring Food: Who Suffers?" *Washington Post,* January 23, 1975; Colman McCarthy, "Color It Dangerous," *Washington Post,* January 23, 1975.

18. G. Timothy Johnson, "Food Additive Link to Hyperactivity Unproven," *Chicago Tribune,* June 24, 1977; G. Timothy Johnson, "Diet-Hyperactivity Link Still Unproved," *Chicago Tribune,* September 21, 1978.

19. Harry Nelson, "Controversial Theory," *Los Angeles Times,* April 19, 1976, B3, B20; "Can Dye-Hyped Foods Cause Hyperactivity?" *Chicago Tribune,* February 17, 1977, D1.

20. Joan Beck, "Another 'Miracle' Diet Cure that Failed," *Chicago Tribune,* July 11, 1977, C2; Monte, "Feingold Diet."

21. "A Skirmish Involving a Pacifist," *New York Times,* November 17, 1986.

22. McCarthy, "Color It Dangerous."

23. "Children and Artificial Food," *Washington Post,* September 14, 1975.

24. Edward Kennedy quoted in "Children and Artificial Food."

25. See chapter 7.

26. Nicholas von Hoffman, "Concerning Hyperkinesis, Food Additives, and Crime," *Washington Post,* September 11, 1974.

27. Ibid.

28. Ibid.
29. Robert Rodale, "Can Pure Food Be a Reality?" *Hartford Courant*, February 26, 1975.
30. Ibid.
31. Robert Rodale, "Food Additives Sometimes Cause Strange Effects," *Hartford Courant*, May 29, 1974.
32. Ibid.
33. Ibid.
34. Morton Mintz, "'Heroine' of FDA Keeps Bad Drug Off of Market," *Washington Post*, July 15, 1962.
35. Mintz, "Study Links."
36. McCarthy, "Color It Dangerous."
37. U.S. Congress, *Congressional Record*, S19736–42.
38. Macrobiotic diets, or "long life" diets, stress local, whole, and unprocessed foods, with grains consisting of at least 50 percent of caloric intake.
39. The information about Tom Monte can be found on http://www.tommonte.com/about.html (accessed August 14, 2008).
40. Monte, "A Precious Commodity?"
41. Ibid.
42. Ibid.
43. Marlene Cimons, "Hyperactivity and Food Additives."
44. Ibid.
45. Elaine Jarvik, "The Calming," 50.
46. Ibid.
47. Ibid., 49.
48. Frederick Stare, "Placebo Effect No Substitute for Research," *Hartford Courant*, March 27, 1975; Frederick Stare, "Do Additives Make Your Child Hyperactive?" *Hartford Courant*, December 30, 1975.
49. Feingold, "A View from the Other Side," 8–12.
50. Stare, "Placebo Effect."
51. Anne Harrington, ed., introduction to *The Placebo Effect: An Interdisciplinary Exploration* (London: Harvard University Press, 1997), 2–8.
52. Feingold quoted in Monte, "A Precious Commodity?"
53. Feingold, "Treatment of Allergic Disease," *JAMA*, 323; Feingold et al., "Psychological Studies," 195, 198, 201.
54. Harrington, *The Placebo Effect*, 4–5.
55. Lawrence K. Altman, "Physicians Urged to Widen Understanding of Placebo," *New York Times*, July 2, 1975; Boyce Rensberger, "Acupuncture Likened to Placebo," *New York Times*, June 19, 1975.
56. Nutrition Foundation quoted in Al Rossiter Jr., "Feingold Diet Disputed," *United Press International*, October 16, 1980.
57. Morris Lipton, "Can Food Chemical Additives Have Any Effect on Behavior?" *Hartford Courant*, August 3, 1977.
58. "The Importance of Food Coloring," *Los Angeles Times*, June 24, 1976.
59. Ben F. Feingold, "Can Food Chemical Additives Have Any Effect on Behavior?" *Hartford Courant*, August 3, 1977.
60. Feingold, *Why Your Child Is Hyperactive*, 156–68.
61. Johnson was and continues to be ABC Television's medical editor. Johnson, "Food Additive Link."
62. Johnson, "Diet-Hyperactivity Link."

63. Ibid.
64. Although Mayer had worked with Stare, their relationship had not been amiable and contributed to Mayer's departure to the less prestigious Tufts University. According to an interviewee, "It was said that Jean Mayer was so opposed to what Stare was doing so that if he met him in a hallway, he would duck into a room so as not to encounter Stare. He just felt that he was a prostitute. And that was why Mayer went to Tufts, because he realized he would never be able to get up on the ladder at Harvard as long as Stare had the influence there." Historian Harvey Levenstein has substantiated this, stating that Mayer and Stare did not agree on many issues. Given Mayer's impressive wartime record with the French Free Army and the French Resistance, as well as his ability to "stand up to and face down the most persistent of critics," the differences with Stare must have been strong indeed. Interview with Josephine Bannister; Levenstein, *Paradox of Plenty*, 155.
65. Ben F. Feingold, "The Arguments Con," *Washington Post*, September 19, 1974; Jean Mayer, "The Arguments Pro," *Washington Post*, September 19, 1974.
66. Feingold, "The Arguments Con"; Mayer, "The Arguments Pro."
67. Mayer, "The Arguments Pro."
68. Ibid.
69. Feingold, "The Arguments Con."
70. Interview with Josephine Bannister.
71. Interview with Marilyn Anderson, December 10, 2007.
72. Feingold, "The Arguments Con."
73. Jean Mayer and Joanna Dwyer, "Food Additives, Hyperactivity, and Dr. Feingold's Diet," *Washington Post*, August 5, 1976.
74. Mayer and Dwyer, "Dr. Feingold's Diet."
75. Paul L. Adams, "Review of *Hyperactivity: Research, Theory, and Action* by Dorothea M. Ross and Sheila A. Ross," *American Journal of Psychiatry* 134 (1977): 833–34.
76. Mayer and Dwyer, "Dr. Feingold's Diet."
77. Jean Mayer and Joanna Dwyer, "Nutrition," *Washington Post*, November 17, 1977.
78. Mayer and Dwyer, "Dr. Feingold's Diet," F3; Mayer and Dwyer, "Nutrition."
79. Mayer and Dwyer, "Nutrition."
80. Ibid.
81. Jean Mayer and Joanna Dwyer, "Diet Changes Seem to Help," *Chicago Tribune*, November 16, 1978, D34. Other stories about the Feingold diet had headlines that were misleading as to the actual content of the story. One Associated Press article, entitled "Report Sees No Relationship between Hyperactivity, Diet" nevertheless concluded with the words of Sanford Miller, director of the foods division of the FDA, that "the jury is still out on the question." Warren E. Leary, "Report Sees No Relationship between Hyperactivity, Diet," Associated Press, October 16, 1980.
82. Jean Mayer and Joanna Dwyer, "Diet Changes."
83. Mayer and Dwyer, "Diet Changes"; Carey Winfrey, "A Controversial Theory Links Hyperactivity to Nutrition," *New York Times*, January 14, 1980.
84. Winfrey, "Controversial Theory."
85. Jane E. Brody, "How Diet Can Effect Mood and Behavior," *New York Times*, November 17, 1982.
86. Interview with Josephine Bannister.
87. Marion Burros, "Eating Well May Be the Best Revenge: The '70s: A Decade of Concern; Looking Back Through the Consumer '70s," *Washington Post*, December 30, 1979.

88. FAUS, "The Feingold Program," http://www.feingold.org/pg-faq.html (accessed October 9, 2008).

89. Interview with Trevor Davidson; interview with Lynn Kitchen; interview with Wendy Lott, July 24, 2008; interview with David Miller, May 19, 2008.

90. Jean Mayer and Joanna Dwyer, "The Latest Tally on Diets for Hyperactive Kids," *Chicago Tribune*, November 24, 1978.

91. Ibid.

92. Jean Mayer and Jeanne Goldberg, "Hyperactive Children: When the Food Dye Is Cast," *Los Angeles Times*, August 28, 1980; Jean Mayer and Joanna Dwyer, "Diet May Help Hyperactive Children," *Chicago Tribune*, August 9, 1979.

93. Jean Mayer and Jeanne Goldberg, "Weighing the Feingold 'Elimination' Diet on Its Tenth Anniversary," *Los Angeles Times*, September 27, 1984.

94. Jane E. Brody, "Diet Therapy for Behavior Is Criticized as Premature," *New York Times*, December 4, 1984.

95. Ibid.

96. Ibid.

97. Carol Pogash, "The Myth of the 'Twinkie Defense,'" *San Francisco Chronicle*, November 23, 2003.

98. The next chapter demonstrates that the results of Harley's trial were not at all clear-cut, as Harley himself admitted in a letter in response to Beck's article. Beck, "Another Miracle Diet"; J. Preston Harley, "Diet for Hyperactivity," *Chicago Tribune*, August 29, 1977.

99. Beck, "Another Miracle Diet."

100. J. Preston Harley quoted in Rose Dosti, "Study Refutes Additive-Hyperactivity Link," *Los Angeles Times*, April 14, 1977.

101. "Is Diet Making Your Child Hyper?" *Tufts University Diet and Nutrition Letter* 7 (1989): 5; Gregory K. Fritz, "Dietary Intervention for Hyperactive Children Supported in New Study," *Brown University Child Behavior and Development Letter* 5 (1989): 5.

102. Feingold, "A View from the Other Side."

103. Ibid.

104. Dosti, "Study Refutes."

105. Feingold, "A View from the Other Side"; Harley, "Diet for Hyperactivity."

106. Feingold, "A View from the Other Side."

107. David Rosner and Gerald Markowitz, "Industry Challenges to the Principle of Prevention in Public Health: The Precautionary Principle in Historical Perspective," *Public Health Reports* 117 (2002): 508–9. Another dispute is ongoing between the ACSH and CSPI over which organization truly represents the consumers in matters of science and public health. American Council on Science and Health, "CSPI vs. ACSH," http://www.acsh.org/about/pageID.86/default.asp (accessed October 22, 2008); Center for Science in the Public Interest, "Non-Profit Organizations Receiving Corporate Funding," http://www.cspinet.org/integrity/nonprofits/american_council_on_science_and_health.html (accessed October 22, 2008).

108. Al Rossiter Jr., "Does Diet Affect Rambunctious Behavior?" United Press International, January 13, 1982.

109. National Institutes of Health, "Defined Diets and Childhood Hyperactivity," *NIH Consensus Statement Online* 4 (January 13–15, 1982), http://www.consensus.nih.gov/1982/1982DietHyperactivity032html.htm (accessed October 22, 2008).

110. Al Rossiter Jr., "Special Diet May Benefit Hyperactive Children," United Press International, January 15, 1982; Cristine Russell, "Additive-Free Diet Found Not to Curb Hyperactivity," *Washington Post*, January 15, 1982.

111. One exception to this was the controversy over the use of artificial sweeteners, such as saccharin, in soft drinks. "House Passes a Delay of Ban on Saccharin," *New York Times*, July 25, 1979; "Key Scientist Favors Elimination of Saccharin Use within Three Years," *New York Times*, April 12, 1979; "Saccharin Held Free of Risk," *New York Times*, November 8, 1985.

112. Nancy Jenkins, "Health Food and the Change in Eating Habits," *New York Times*, April 4, 1984.

113. Belasco, *Appetite for Change*, 1–3; Levenstein, *Paradox of Plenty*, 237–41.

114. Alexandra Penney, "The Year of the Nutritionist," *New York Times*, July 1, 1979.

115. Levenstein, *Paradox of Plenty*, 241–43.

116. "The Bitter Verdict against Saccharin," *New York Times*, March 11, 1977; "The Case of the Useful Carcinogen."

117. Philip M. Boffey, "Cancer Experts Lean towards Steady Vigilance, but Less Alarm, on Environment," *New York Times*, March 2, 1982.

118. Levenstein, *Paradox of Plenty*, 236.

119. Karen De Witt, "Challenging the Additive Rule," *New York Times*, December 10, 1980; Karen De Witt, "Just a Regulated Day in the Life of an Ordinary Citizen," *New York Times*, April 12, 1981.

Chapter 7

1. Gerald S. Golden, "Nonstandard Therapies in the Developmental Disabilities," *American Journal of Diseases of Children* 134 (1980): 489; Kenneth A. Kavale and Steven R. Forness, "Hyperactivity and Diet Treatment: A Meta-Analysis of the Feingold Hypothesis," *Journal of Learning Disabilities* 16 (1983): 324–30; Jeffrey A. Mattes, "The Feingold Diet: A Current Reappraisal," *Journal of Learning Disabilities* 16 (1983): 319–23; J. A. Mattes and R. Gittelman, "Effects of Artificial Food Colorings in Children with Hyperactive Symptoms," *Archives of General Psychiatry* 38 (1981): 714–18; Steer, "Managing Attention Deficit/Hyperactivity Disorder," 122; Esther H. Wender, "The Food Additive-Free Diet in the Treatment of Behavior Disorders: A Review," *Journal of Developmental and Behavioral Pediatrics* 7 (1986): 35–42.

2. Michael F. Jacobson and David Schardt, *Diet, ADHD, and Behavior: A Quarter Century Review* (Washington, DC: Center for Science in the Public Interest, 1999); FAUS, "Diet and ADHD," http://www.feingold.org/pg-research.html (accessed April 8, 2009).

3. Harry Collins and Trevor Pinch, *Dr. Golem: How to Think about Medicine* (Chicago: University of Chicago Press, 2005), 32–34.

4. David W. Schab and Nhi-Ha T. Trinh, "Do Artificial Food Colors Promote Hyperactivity in Children with Hyperactive Syndromes? A Meta-Analysis of Double-Blind Placebo-Controlled Trials," *Journal of Developmental and Behavioral Pediatrics* 25 (2004): 423–34.

5. Conners, *Food Additives and Hyperactive Children*, 9–10.

6. Ibid., 10.

7. Australian medical interest in the risks chemical exposures posed to human health was spurred in part by immunologist Stephen Boyden's 1972 speech to the Australian Medical Congress, in which he warned about the "chemicalization" of

the environment. Boyden claimed that "the first symptoms of exposure to many toxic chemicals are not physiological, but psychological, and include such symptoms as confusion, personality changes, fatigue, loss of memory and mental dullness." Peter Cook and Joan Woodhill, a child psychiatrist and nutritionist team, cited Boyden's concerns in their paper on the Feingold diet. Stephen Boyden, "The Environment and Human Health," *Medical Journal of Australia* 1 (1972): 1231; Peter S. Cook and Joan M. Woodhill, "The Feingold Dietary Treatment of the Hyperkinetic Syndrome," *Medical Journal of Australia* 2 (1976): 85–89; Louis K. Salzman, "Allergy Testing, Psychological Assessment, and Dietary Treatment of the Hyperactive Child Syndrome," *Medical Journal of Australia* 2 (1976): 248–51. John S. Werry, "Food Additives and Hyperactivity," *Medical Journal of Australia* 2 (1976): 281–82.

8. Helen Tryphonas and Ronald Trites, "Diet and Hyperactivity," *Nutrition Bulletin* 9 (1984): 27–28.

9. National Advisory Committee on Hyperkinesis and Food Additives (NACHFA), *Report to the Nutrition Foundation* (New York: Nutrition Foundation, 1975).

10. NACHFA, *Final Report* (New York: Nutrition Foundation, 1980), appendix, vi.

11. J. C. M. Friend, "The Syndrome of Childhood Hyperactivity," *Medical Journal of Australia* 1 (1977): 822.

12. NACHFA, *Final Report*, appendix, vii–viii.

13. Ibid, vii.

14. Mortimer D. Gross et al., "The Effects of Diets Rich in and Free from Additives on the Behavior of Children with Hyperkinetic and Learning Disorder," *Journal of the American Academy of Child and Adolescent Psychiatry* 26 (1987): 53.

15. FAUS, "Diet and ADHD," http://www.feingold.org/pg-research.html (accessed January 21, 2009).

16. "Feingold's Regimen for Hyperkinesis," *Lancet* 2 (1979): 617.

17. T. J. David, "Reactions to Dietary Tartrazine," *Archives of Disease in Childhood* 62 (1987): 120; F. Levy et al., "Hyperkinesis and Diet: A Double-Blind Crossover Trial with a Tartrazine Challenge," *Medical Journal of Australia* 1 (1978): 61–64.

18. Benjamin F. Feingold quoted in Bernard Rimland, "The Feingold Diet: An Assessment of the Reviews by Mattes, by Kavale and Forness and Others," *Journal of Learning Disabilities* 16 (1983): 331; NACHFA, *Final Report*, 9.

19. NACHFA, *Final Report*, 7–9.

20. Bonnie J. Kaplan, "The Relevance of Food for Children's Cognitive and Behavioural Health," *Canadian Journal of Behavioural Science* 20 (1988): 359–73.

21. Kaplan, "The Relevance of Food," 360.

22. C. H. Goyette et al., "Effects of Artificial Colors on Hyperkinetic Children: A Double-Blind Challenge Study," *Psychopharmacological Bulletin* 14 (1978): 39–40; J. P. Harley, C. G. Matthews, P. Eichman, "Synthetic Food Colors and Hyperactivity in Children: A Double-Blind Challenge Experiment," *Pediatrics* 62 (1978): 976; NACHFA, *Final Report*, 2, 9–10; J. Ivan Williams et al., "Relative Effects of Drugs and Diet on Hyperactive Behaviors: An Experimental Study," *Pediatrics* 61 (1978): 812.

23. Rimland, "The Feingold Diet," 331.

24. NACHFA, *Final Report*, 10.

25. Conners, *Food Additives and Hyperactive Children*, 105; Alexander G. Schauss, "Nutrition and Behaviour: Complex Interdisciplinary Research," *Nutrition and Behavior* 3 (1984): 23; T. J. Sobotka, "Estimates of Average, 90th Percentile and Maximum Daily Intakes of FD & C Artificial Food Colors in One Day's Diets Among

Two Age Groups of Children," *Food and Drug Administration Memorandum*, July 1976.

26. Rimland, "The Feingold Diet," 331.

27. Strangely, both the studies using the lowest dose and the highest dose yielded positive results. Two of the most recent studies, both of which yielded positive results, also used relatively low dosages of between 20 and 25 mg. B. Bateman et al., "The Effects of a Double-Blind, Placebo Controlled, Artificial Food Colourings and Benzoate Preservative Challenge on Hyperactivity in a General Population Sample of Preschool Children," *Archives of Disease in Childhood* 89 (2004): 507; Donna McCann et al., "Food Additives and Hyperactive Behaviour in Three-Year-Old and Eight/Nine-Year-Old Children in the Community: A Randomised, Double-Blinded, Placebo-Controlled Trial," *Lancet* 370 (2007): 1561; Terry L. Rose, "The Functional Relationship between Artificial Food Colors and Hyperactivity," *Journal of Applied Behavior Analysis* 11 (1978): 441; James W. Swanson and Marcel Kinsbourne, "Food Dyes Impair Performance of Hyperactive Children on a Laboratory Learning Test," *Science* 207 (1980): 1485–87.

28. NACHFA, *Final Report*, 10.

29. NACHFA, *Final Report*, 10.

30. Mattes and Gittelman, "Effects of Artificial Food Colorings," 715.

31. Bernard Weiss et al., "Behavioural Responses to Artificial Food Colours," *Science* 207 (1980): 1487–89.

32. NACHFA, *Final Report*, 11.

33. For example, in some studies both the dye and the placebo were disguised in a capsule. J. Egger et al., "Controlled Trial of Oligoantigenic Treatment in the Hyperkinetic Syndrome," *Lancet* 325 (1985): 540; Swanson and Kinsbourne, "Food Dyes Impair Performance."

34. Mattes and Gittelman, "Effects of Artificial Food Colorings," 717.

35. Conners, *Feeding the Brain*, 12.

36. Bateman et al., "Effects of a Double-Blind," 507; I. Pollock, J. O. Warner, "Effects of Artificial Food Colours on Childhood Behaviour," *Archives of Disease in Childhood* 65 (1990): 76. The compliance of test subjects was also a major issue in the trials of the first AIDS drugs. Subjects were often reluctant to be given the placebo, for obvious reasons. Steven Epstein, *Impure Science: AIDS, Activism, and the Politics of Knowledge* (Berkeley: University of California Press, 1996), 194–207.

37. Feingold, "Hyperkinesis and Learning Disabilities"; J. Preston Harley et al., "Hyperkinesis and Food Additives: Testing the Feingold Hypothesis," *Pediatrics* 61 (1978): 821.

38. David, "Reactions to Dietary Tartrazine," 119–22; Gross et al., "The Effects of Diets Rich in and Free from Additives."

39. Gross et al., "The Effects of Diets Rich in and Free from Additives," 54–55.

40. Ibid., 53–55.

41. Later trials have involved hundreds of children. Bateman et al., "Effects of a Double-Blind"; McCann et al., "Food Additives and Hyperactivity."

42. Conners, *Food Additives and Hyperactive Children*, 105–6.

43. Interview with Stuart Unger.

44. Williams and Cram, "Diet in the Management of Hyperkinesis," 243.

45. Interview with Stuart Unger.

46. Bonnie J. Kaplan et al., "Dietary Replacement in Preschool-Aged Hyperactive Boys," *Pediatrics* 83 (1989): 7.

47. Interview with Kristine Johnson, November 5, 2007.

48. Ibid.

49. Ibid.

50. Arnold Brenner, "A Study of the Efficacy of the Feingold Diet on Hyperkinetic Children: Some Favorable Personal Observations," *Clinical Pedicatrics* 16 (1977): 652–56; Cook and Woodhill, "The Feingold Dietary Treatment"; R. C. Hindle and Janelle Priest, "The Management of Hyperkinetic Children: A Trial of Dietary Therapy," *New Zealand Medical Journal* 88 (1978): 43–45.

51. NACHFA, *Final Report*, 2.

52. Kaplan et al., "Dietary Replacement," 17.

53. Interview with Kristine Johnson.

54. Interview with Stuart Unger.

55. L. Eugene Arnold, "Alternative Treatments for Adults with Attention-Deficit Hyperactivity Disorder (ADHD)," *Annals of the New York Academy of Sciences* 931 (2001): 314; K. S. Rowe, "Synthetic Food Colourings and 'Hyperactivity': A Double-Blind Crossover Study," *Australian Paediatric Journal* 24 (1988): 144; Geoffrey Thorley, "Pilot Study to Assess Behavioural and Cognitive Effects of Artificial Food Colours in a Group of Retarded Children," *Developmental Medicine and Child Neurology* 26 (1984): 56; Williams and Cram, "Diet in the Management of Hyperkinesis," 246–47.

56. Mattes, "The Feingold Diet," 321; Rimland, "The Feingold Diet," 332.

57. Harley et al., "Hyperkinesis and Food Additives"; Weiss et al., "Behavioral Responses."

58. The amount of funding was not listed in Harley's published reports, but in Werry, "Food Additives," 282.

59. Harley et al., "Hyperkinesis and Food Additives," 821.

60. Ibid, 826.

61. Ibid., 825.

62. Ibid., 826.

63. Feingold, "Hyperkinesis and Learning Disabilities," 800; Thorley, "Pilot Study," 56; Williams and Cram, "Diet in the Management of Hyperkinesis," 245–46.

64. Conners, *Food Additives and Hyperactive Children*, 39.

65. Mattes, "The Feingold Diet," 319; Bernard Weiss, "Food Additives as a Source of Behavioral Disturbance in Children," *Neurotoxicology* 7 (1986): 200; Werry, "Food Additives," 282; Williams and Cram, "Diet in the Management of Hyperkinesis," 244.

66. Harley et al., "Hyperkinesis and Food Additives," 826.

67. Ibid.

68. Bernard Weiss, "Food Additives and Environmental Chemicals as Sources of Childhood Behavior Disorders," *Journal of the American Academy of Child Psychiatry* 21 (1982): 144–45.

69. Ibid., 145.

70. Weiss, "Food Additives as a Source," 200.

71. Weiss, "Food Additives and Environmental Chemicals," 145–51.

72. Weiss et al., "Behavioral Responses."

73. Ibid., 1487.

74. Ibid., 1488.

75. Ibid.

76. Feingold, "Hyperkinesis and Learning Disabilities," 800; Goyette et al., 39–40; Weiss, "Food Additives as a Source," 151; Williams and Cram, "Diet in the Management of Hyperkinesis," 244–46.

77. Mattes and Gittelman, "Effects of Artificial Food Colorings," 715; NACHFA, *Final Report*, 24.

78. Rimland, "The Feingold Diet," 331; Weiss, "Food Additives as a Source," 144–45.

79. A similarly worded assessment can be found in Gladys Witt Strain, "Nutrition, Brain Function, and Behavior," *Psychiatric Clinics of North America* 4 (1981): 253–68; Weiss, "Food Additives as a Source," 151–52.

80. Mattes, "The Feingold Diet," 322.

81. Interview with Jane Parker, February 3, 2009.

82. Werry, "Food Additives," 282.

83. Council of Australian Food Technology Association, Inc., "Dr. Benjamin Feingold: Hyperactivity," *Food Technology in Australia* 29 (1977): 433.

84. Hindle and Priest, "The Management of Hyperkinetic Children," *New Zealand Medical Journal* 88 (1978): 43–45; R. C. Hindle and Janelle Priest, "Dietary Control of Hyperkinesis," *New Zealand Medical Journal* 88 (1978): 345; Werry, "Food Additives," 282; John S. Werry and M. G. Aman, "Dietary Control of Hyperkinesis," *New Zealand Medical Journal* 88 (1978): 297–98.

85. One particularly animated symposium on the Feingold diet in which Feingold himself participated was published in *Academic Therapy*. Robert Buckely, "Hyperkinetic Aggravation of Learning Disturbance," *Academic Therapy* 13 (1977): 153–60; Allan Cott, "A Reply," *Academic Therapy* 13 (1977): 161–71; Benjamin F. Feingold, "A Critique of 'Controversial Medical Treatments of Learning Disabilities,'" *Academic Therapy* 13 (1977): 173–83; Sieben, "Controversial Medical Treatments," 133–47.

86. "Feingold's Regimen," 617; C. Warren Bierman and Clifton T. Furukawa, "Food Additives and Hyperkinesis: Are There Nuts among the Berries?" *Pediatrics* 61 (1978): 932–33.

87. For an analysis of how the contrasting opinions about sick building syndrome were also shaped by ideological and political factors, see Michelle Murphy, *Sick Building Syndrome and the Problem of Uncertainty: Environmental Politics, Technoscience, and Women Workers* (Durham: Duke University Press, 2006).

88. Weiss, "Food Additives as a Source," 198.

89. Ibid., 204.

90. Morris A. Lipton and James P. Mayo, "Diet and Hyperkinesis: An Update," *Journal of the American Dietetic Association* 83 (1983): 132.

91. Feingold, *Why Your Child Is Hyperactive*, 89–90, 126; Lipton and Mayo, "Diet and Hyperkinesis," 132.

92. Bierman and Furukawa, "Food Additives and Hyperkinesis," 933.

93. Interview with Stuart Unger.

94. Murphy, *Sick Building Syndrome*, 81–110.

95. Feingold, "Role of Diet," 164.

96. Emphasis in original. Conners, *Feeding the Brain*, 175.

97. Most of the historical work on the risk of disease and public health policy has not considered how patients themselves have interpreted such risks, although work on patient activism has provided some insight into this. Michelle Murphy's work on sick building syndrome, for example, shows how patients were concerned about the risks posed by their work environment even when toxicologists were unable to detect what was making workers unwell. Murphy, *Sick Building Syndrome*, 57–110. See also Barbara Ley, *From Pink to Green: Disease Prevention and the Environmental Breast Cancer Movement* (New Brunswick, NJ: Rutgers University

Press, 2009); Steve Kroll-Smith and H. Hugh Floyd, *Bodies in Protest: Environmental Illness and the Struggle over Medical Knowledge* (New York: New York University Press, 1997). For more on how changing notions of risk have affected public health policy, see Ulrich Beck, *Risk Society: Towards a New Modernity* (London: Sage, 1992); Luc Berlivet, "'Association or Causation?' The Debate on the Scientific Status of Risk Factor Epidemiology, 1947–c. 1965," in *Making Health Policy: Networks in Research and Policy after 1945*, ed. Virginia Berridge (Amsterdam: Rodopi, 2005), 39–74; Rosenberg, "Pathologies of Progress"; Rothstein, *Public Health and the Risk Factor*.

98. NACHFA, *Final Report*, 31–34.

99. Wender, "Food Additive-Free Diet," 42.

100. American Council on Science and Health, *Food Additives and Hyperactivity* (Summit, NJ: American Council on Science and Health, 1984).

101. Lipton and Mayo, "Diet and Hyperkinesis," 133.

102. Kenneth A. Kavale and Mark P. Mostert, *The Positive Side of Special Education: Minimizing its Fads, Fancies, and Follies* (Oxford: Scarecrow Education, 2004), 210.

103. Kavale and Forness, "Hyperactivity and Diet Treatment," 325.

104. Feingold's critics, for instance, often charged that his diet was unsafe because it would leave children malnourished. While Feingold did advocate removing several fruits and a few vegetables out of the child's diet in the initial stages of his regimen, he strongly encouraged reintroducing these foods after a couple of months, since he believed children most often reacted only to food additives. As early as 1976, more-over, researchers were reporting that, although the Feingold diet was lower in nutri-ents, particularly vitamin C, it still exceeded the recommended daily allowances (RDAs) set out by the FDA. Moreover, a study in 1980 concluded that "a diet free of artificial colors and artificial flavors does not significantly change the nutrient intakes of children." Nevertheless, many commentators continued to warn about the nutritional deficiencies of the Feingold diet. C. M. Carter et al., "Effects of a Few Food Diet in Attention Deficit Disorder," *Archives of Disease in Childhood* 69 (1993): 568; Conners et al., "Food Additives and Hyperkinesis," 164; David, "Reactions to Dietary Tartrazine," 122; Joanna Dwyer et al., "Nutrient Intakes of Children on the Hyperkinesis Diet," *Journal of the American Dietetic Association* 73 (1980): 515–20; Feingold, *Why Your Child Is Hyperactive*, 170; Wendy Lott; Wender, "Food Additives," 1206.

105. David, "Reactions to Dietary Tartrazine," 112.

106. Conners received funding from both the National Institute of Education and NIMH. Conners, *Food Additives and Hyperactive Children*, xi.

107. Conners et al., "Food Additives and Hyperkinesis," 161.

108. James S. Miller, "The Diet Wasn't Controlled," *Pediatrics* 61 (1978): 326.

109. Ibid., 327.

110. Goyette et al., "Effects of Artificial Colors," 40. A *Newsweek* report, however, stated that the results of this study were negative. Matt Clark et al., "The Curse of Hyperactivity," *Newsweek*, June 23, 1980, 59.

111. Conners, *Food Additives and Hyperactive Children*, 7, 107.

112. Ibid., 111.

113. Conners, *Feeding the Brain*, 3.

114. Ibid., 184

115. Interview with John Bright, January 14, 2009.

116. Ibid.

117. For other examples of how similar factors have affected the outcome of debates in medical history, see Roberta Bivins, *Alternative Medicine? A History* (New York: Oxford University Press, 2007); Erika Dyck, *Psychedelic Psychiatry: LSD from Clinic to Campus* (Baltimore: Johns Hopkins University Press, 2008); Johnson, *Osler's Web: Inside the Labyrinth of the Chronic Fatigue Syndrome Epidemic* (New York: Crown, 1996); Murphy, *Sick Building Syndrome*; Ley, *From Pink to Green*; Jack D. Pressman, *Last Resort: Psychosurgery and the Limits of Medicine* (Cambridge: Cambridge University Press, 1998); Thomas Söderqvist, *Science as Autobiography: The Troubled Life of Niels Jerne*, trans. David Mel Paul (London: Yale University Press, 2003); Alfred I. Tauber, *The Immune Self: Theory or Metaphor?* (Cambridge: Cambridge University Press, 1994).

Chapter 8

1. Interview with Maggie Jeffries.
2. Interview with Lynn Kitchen.
3. Interview with Wendy Lott.
4. Interview with Laura Lamb, April 17, 2008.
5. Interview with Ellen Miller.
6. Interview with Justine Ewing.
7. Interview with Rosemarie Kushner.
8. Interview with Ellen Miller.
9. Interview with David Miller.
10. Interview with Sylvia Terry.
11. Interview with Lesley Freeman.
12. Interview with Trevor Davidson.
13. Interview with Gayle Davidson.
14. Interview with Wendy Lott.
15. Interview with Liz Grossman, February 19, 2008.
16. Interview with Barbara Beck, January 17, 2008.
17. Interview with Lesley Freeman.
18. Interview with Bonnie Thompson, January 28, 2008.
19. Interview with Greg Hewson, February 4, 2009.
20. Interview with Theresa McKay.
21. Interview with Hanna Johnston, February 4, 2008.
22. Interview with Frank Kushner, April 22, 2008; interview with Rosemarie Kushner.
23. Interview with Ellen Miller.
24. Although the Internet has provided parents access to much more information about alternatives to conventional medical treatment, as Rima Apple suggests, the number of choices can be overwhelming. Despite this, research by the Pew Internet and American Life Project suggests that health advice seekers who employ the Internet are quite savvy and are relatively skilled at rejecting web sites that seem too commercial or unprofessional. Rima Apple, *Perfect Motherhood: Science and Childrearing in America* (New Brunswick, NJ: Rutgers University Press, 2006), 140–41; Pew Internet and American Life Project, "Vital Decisions: How Internet Users Decide What Information to Trust When They or Their Loved Ones are Sick," http://www.pewinternet.org/~/media//Files/Reports/2002/PIP_Vital_Decisions_May2002.pdf.pdf (accessed April 14, 2009).
25. Interview with Jennifer Illing, February 12, 2008; interview with Maggie Jeffries; interview with Lynn Kitchen; William H. Koch, *Chiropractic: The Superior*

Alternative (Calgary: Bayeux Arts, 1995), 95; Maura Roan and Jessica Roan, "ADHD and Chiropractic," *Aspire Magazine* (August/September 2007), http://www.aspiremag .net/articles/parenting/childrenshealth/adhdandchiropractic.html (accessed February 23, 2009).

26. Apple, *Perfect Motherhood*, 162–63.
27. Ibid., 134–36.
28. Ibid.
29. Interview with Wendy Lott.
30. Interview with Lynn Kitchen.
31. Interview with Theresa McKay.
32. Interview with Rosemarie Kushner.
33. Interview with Justine Ewing.
34. Interview with David Miller; interview with Ellen Miller; interview with Sylvia Terry.
35. Jane Hersey, *Why Can't My Child Behave?* Williamsburg, VA: Pear Tree Press, 2006), 40.
36. Carter et al.,"Effects of a Few Food Diet," 568.
37. Gross et al., "The Effects of Diets Rich in and Free from Additives," 55.
38. Interview with Darren Aubrey, May 20, 2008. Tomatoes were one of the salicylate fruits and vegetables that were banned on the first stage of the diet. Unfortunately, this interviewee reacted to them and grapes.
39. Interview with Frank Kushner.
40. Interview with Rosemarie Kushner.
41. Interview with Erik Terry, April 1, 2008.
42. Interview with Jason Atwater, February 7, 2008.
43. Interview with David Miller.
44. Ibid.
45. Interview with David Miller; interview with Ellen Miller.
46. Interview with Laura Lamb.
47. Interview with Donna Larkin, February 25, 2008.
48. Interview with Lesley Freeman.
49. Ibid.
50. Marsha Swindler, "Feingold – Swindler Family," unpublished essay written for Azusa Pacific University, 1999.
51. Interview with Donna Larkin.
52. Interview with Laura Lamb.
53. Interview with Justine Ewing.
54. Interview with Sylvia Terry.
55. Interview with Barbara Beck.
56. Ibid.
57. Interview with Rosemarie Kushner.
58. Interview with Ellen Miller.
59. Interview with Maggie Jeffries.
60. Interview with Hanna Johnston.
61. Ibid.
62. Ibid.
63. Interview with Trevor Davidson; interview with Justine Ewing; interview with Hanna Johnston; interview with Bonnie Thompson.
64. Interview with Ellen Miller.

65. Interview with Barbara Beck.
66. Interview with Jennifer Illing.
67. Interview with Hanna Johnston.
68. Susan Ormiston, "Will Heavyweight Krispy Kreme Step on Tim's Toes?," *Marketplace*, March 20, 2002, http://www.archives.cbc.ca/lifestyle/food/clips/15211/ (accessed February 24, 2009).
69. Interview with Theresa McKay.
70. Interview with Justine Ewing.
71. Interview with Rosemarie Kushner.
72. Interview with Donna Larkin.
73. Interview with David Miller.
74. Ibid.
75. Interview with Frank Kushner.
76. Interview with Rosemarie Kushner.
77. Interview with Erik Terry.
78. Interview with Maggie Jeffries.
79. Interview with Lynn Kitchen.
80. Interview with Bonnie Thompson.
81. Interview with Darren Aubrey.
82. Ibid.
83. Ibid.
84. Interview with David Miller.
85. Interview with Justine Ewing.
86. Interview with Lynn Kitchen.
87. Interview with Hanna Johnston.
88. Interview with David Miller.
89. Interview with David Miller; interview with Erik Terry.
90. Interview with Justine Ewing; interview with Hanna Johnston; interview with Lynn Kitchen; interview with Theresa McKay.
91. Interview with Lynn Kitchen.
92. Interview with Jennifer Illing.
93. Interview with David Miller.
94. Interview with Theresa McKay.
95. Interview with Lesley Freeman.
96. Interview with Justine Ewing.
97. Interview with Jennifer Illing.
98. Interview with Sylvia Terry.
99. Interview with Laura Lamb.
100. Interview with John Bright; interview with Gina Zimmerman, February 17, 2009.
101. Interview with Liz Grossman. Other parents also disagreed with the notion that the changes in behavior they witnessed, often lasting over a period of decades, were merely placebo. Interview with Janice Atwater, January 26, 2008; interview with Wendy Lott.
102. Interview with Trevor Davidson.
103. Roy Porter, "The Patient's View: Doing Medical History from Below," *Theory and Society* 14 (1985): 175–98.
104. Interview with Laura Lamb.
105. Interview with Ellen Miller.
106. Apple, *Perfect Motherhood*, 167.

107. Similar approaches have been used in assessing the efficacy of other hyperactivity treatments. See: Peter S. Jenson et al., "Findings from the NIMH Multimodal Treatment Study of ADHD (MTA): Implications and Applications for Primary Care Providers," *Developmental and Behavioral Pediatrics* 22 (2001): 60–73.

Chapter 9

1. Interview with Mark Ridge, March 16, 2009.
2. Bateman et al., "Effects of a Double-Blind," 506–11.
3. Carl I. Cohen et al., "The Future of Community Psychiatry," *Community Mental Health Journal* 39 (2003): 460; Michael Rutter, "Isle of Wight Revisited: Twenty-five Years of Child Psychiatric Epidemiology," in *Annual Progress in Child Psychiatry and Child Development*, ed. Stella Chess and Margaret E. Hertzig (New York: Psychology Press, 1990): 148; Michael Rutter et al., "Research Report: Isle of Wight Studies, 1964–1974," *Psychological Medicine* 6 (1976): 313–32.
4. Bateman et al., "Effects of a Double-Blind," 510–11.
5. Herbert H. Nehrlich, "Feingold Revisited and Acknowledged," *Archives of Disease in Childhood* 89 (2004), http://www.adc.bmj.com.login.ezproxy.library.ualberta.ca/cgi/eletters/89/6/506#927 (accessed March 6, 2009).
6. Emphasis and uppercase in original. Richard B. Mailman, "Where's the Effect?" *Archives of Disease in Childhood* 89 (2004), http://www.adc.bmj.com.login.ezproxy.library.ualberta.ca/cgi/eletters/89/6/506#927 (accessed March 6, 2009).
7. Howard Bauchner, "Food Colourings and Benzoate Preservatives: Do They Change Behaviour?" *Archives of Disease in Childhood* 84 (2004): 499.
8. Batemen et al., "Effects of a Double-blind," 510.
9. Bauchner, "Food Colourings," 499.
10. McCann et al., "Food Additives and Hyperactivity," 1566.
11. Food Standards Agency, "Agency Revises Advice on Certain Artificial Colours," September 11, 2007, http://www.food.gov.uk/news/newsarchive/2007/sep/foodcolours (accessed March 20, 2009); McCann et al., "Food Additives and Hyperactivity," 1566.
12. Interview with Mark Ridge.
13. David Andreatta, "Food Additives Found to Fuel Hyperactivity," *Globe and Mail*, September 6, 2007, http://www.theglobeandmail.com/servlet/story/RTGAM.20070906.whyperkids06/BNStory/specialScienceandHealth/home (accessed March 9, 2009); "Parents Warned of Additives Link," September 6, 2007, http://www.news.bbc.co.uk/1/hi/health/6979976.stm (accessed March 9, 2009); Valerie Elliot, "Food Alert as Every Additive Comes Under Suspicion," *Times*, September 6, 2007, http://www.timesonline.co.uk/tol/news/uk/health/article2395623.ece (accessed March 9, 2009); Krishnan Guru-Murthy, *Channel 4 News*, September 6, 2007; interview with Mark Ridge.
14. Andrew Wadge, "Colours and Hyperactivity," http://www.fsascience.net/2007/09/06/colours_and_hyperactivity (accessed March 9, 2009).
15. Alison Schonwald, "ADHD and Food Additives Revisited," *AAP Grand Rounds* 19 (2008): 17.
16. "Editor's Note," *AAP Grand Rounds* 19 (2008): 17.
17. Philippe A. Eigenmann and Charles A. Haenggeli, "Food Colourings and Preservatives: Allergy and Hyperactivity," *Lancet* 364 (2004): 823–24; Philippe A. Eigenmann and Charles A. Haenggeli, "Food Colourings, Preservatives, and Hyperactivity," *Lancet* 370 (2007): 1525.

18. M. Boris and F. S. Mandel, "Foods and Additives Are Common Causes of the Attention Deficit Hyperactive Disorder in Children," *Annals of Allergy* 72 (1994): 462–68; J. Egger et al., "Controlled Trial of Oligoantigenic Treatment in the Hyperkinetic Syndrome," *Lancet* 325 (1985): 540–45; Bonnie J. Kaplan et al., "Dietary Replacement in Preschool-Aged Hyperactive Boys," *Pediatrics* 83 (1989): 7–17; I. Pollock and J. O. Warner, "Effects of Artificial Food Colours on Childhood Behaviour," *Archives of Disease in Childhood* 65 (1990): 74–77; K. S. Rowe, "Synthetic Food Colourings and 'Hyperactivity': A Double-Blind Crossover Study," *Australian Paediatric Journal* 24 (1988): 143–47; K. S. Rowe and K. J. Rowe, "Synthetic Food Coloring and Behavior: A Dose Response Effect in a Double-Blind, Placebo-Controlled, Repeated-Measures Study," *Journal of Pediatrics* 125 (1994): 691–98.

19. Andreatta, "Food Additives"; Eigenmann and Haenggeli, "Food Colourings," 823; Maggie Fox, "Food Additives May Cause Hyperactivity: Study," September 5, 2007, http://www.reuters.com/article/healthNews/idUSN0520103220070905 (accessed September 7, 2007); Julian Hunt quoted in "Food Watchdog Condemned for 'Totally Inadequate' Response to Harmful Food Additives," *This Is London*, September 6, 2007, http://www.thisislondon.co.uk/news/article-23411169-details/Parents+warned:+additives+in+food+DO+harm+our+children/article.do (accessed March 13, 2009); John Bright; Mailman, "Where's the Effect?"; Gina Zimmerman.

20. Boris and Mandel, "Foods and Additives"; Egger et al., "Controlled Trial"; Kaplan et al., "Dietary Replacement"; Pollock and Warner, "Effects of Artificial Food"; Rowe, "Synthetic Food Colourings"; Rowe and Rowe, "Synthetic Food Coloring."

21. J. L. Rapoport et al., "Urinary Noradrenaline and Playroom Behaviour in Hyperactive Children," *Lancet* 296 (1970): 1141; Mark. A. Stewart, "Urinary Noradrenaline and Playroom Behaviour in Hyperactive Children," *Lancet* 297 (1971): 140.

22. Laufer, Denhoff, and Solomons, "Hyperkinetic Impulse Disorder," 38–49.

23. Steven Box, preface to *The Myth of the Hyperactive Child: And Other Means of Child Control*, by Peter Schrag and Diane Divoky (New York: Penguin Books, 1982), 17.

24. "Minimal Brain Dysfunction," *Lancet* 302 (1973): 487–88; Mark A. Stewart and B. H. Burne, "Minimal Brain Dysfunction," *Lancet* 302 (1973): 852.

25. "Minimal Brain Dysfunction," 488.

26. Emphasis in original. "Hyperactivity," *Lancet* 312 (1978): 561.

27. "Does Hyperactivity Matter?" *Lancet* 327 (1986): 73–74.

28. Morris Zwi, Paul Ramchandani, and Carol Joughin, "Evidence and Belief in ADHD," *BMJ* 321 (2000): 975–76.

29. Geoffrey D. Kewley, "Personal Paper: Attention Deficit Hyperactivity Disorder Is Underdiagnosed and Undertreated in Britain," *BMJ* 316 (1998): 1594–96; Eileen Orford, "Commentary: Diagnosis Needs Tightening," *BMJ* 316 (1998): 1594–96.

30. "Feingold's Regimen"; "Food Additives and Hyperactivity"; "Subclinical Lead Poisoning," *Lancet* 301 (1973): 87; David, Clark, and Voeller, "Lead and Hyperactivity"; Egger et al., "Controlled Trial"; Ann Swain et al., "Salicylates, Olioantigenic Diets, and Behaviour," *Lancet* 326 (1985): 41–42.

31. "Feingold's Regimen"; "Food Additives and Hyperactivity"; Thomas H. Jukes, "Friedrich Wöhler RIP," *Nature* 273 (1978): 421; Thomas H. Jukes, "Language in Action," *Nature* 264 (1976): 602.

32. Hyperactive Children's Support Group, "Our Publications," http://www.hacsg.org.uk/HACSG%20PUBLICATIONS.htm (accessed March 16, 2009).

33. For more on the origins of the British organic food movement, see Michael Brander, *Eve Balfour: Founder of the Soil Association and Voice of the Organic Movement: A Biography* (Haddington: Glenneil Press, 2003); Philip Conford, *Origins of the Organic Movement* (Edinburgh: Floris Books, 2001); Philip Conford, "The Alchemy of Waste: The Impact of Asian Farming on the British Organic Movement," *Rural History* 6 (1995): 103–14; David Matless, "Bodies Made of Grass Made of Earth Made of Bodies: Organism, Diet, and National Health in Mid-Twentieth-Century England," *Journal of Historical Geography* 27 (2003): 355–76; Richard Moore-Colyer, "Towards 'Mother Earth': Jorian Jenks, Organicism, the Right and the British Union of Fascists," *Journal of Contemporary History* 39 (2004): 353–71; Richard Moore-Colyer and Philip Conford, "A 'Secret Society'? The Internal and External Relations of the Kinship in Husbandry," *Rural History* 15 (2004): 189–206.

34. "Millions Turn to Organic Food," *BBC News*, February 8, 2000, http://www.news.bbc.co.uk/1/hi/health/634371.stm (accessed March 13, 2009); "'Growing Fears' over Mad Cow Disease," *BBC News*, October 19, 2000, http://www.news.bbc.co.uk/1/hi/scotland/979103.stm (accessed March 13, 2009); Karen Birchard, "Europe Tackles Consumer Fears over Food Safety," *Lancet* 357 (2001): 1276; Kelly Morris, "A Danger at My Table?" *Lancet* 354 (1999): 1565; Rachel Schurman, "Fighting 'Frankenfoods': Industry Opportunity Structures and the Efficacy of the Anti-Biotech Movement in Western Europe," *Social Problems* 51 (2004): 254.

35. For an insider's perspective on how the media cover food scares, see Nicola Carslaw, "Communicating Risks Linked to Food: The Media's Role," *Trends in Food Science and Technology* 19 (2008): S14–S17. Recent popular explorations of the issue of food safety and processed food include Robert Kenner, *Food, Inc.* (Magnolia Pictures, 2008); Hugh T. Pennington, *When Food Kills: BSE, E. coli, and Disaster Science* (Oxford: Oxford University Press, 2003); Eric Schlosser, *Fast Food Nation: The Dark Side of the All-American Meal* (New York: Houghton Mifflin, 2001); Morgan Spurlock, *Supersize Me* (Kathbur Pictures, 2004).

36. Channel 4, *Jamie's School Dinners*, http://www.channel4.com/life/microsites/J/jamies_school_dinners/index.html (accessed March 13, 2009).

37. Jamie Oliver, http://www.feedmebetter.com/why/junkfood.html (accessed October 10, 2007).

38. "Oliver's School Meal Crusade Goes On," *BBC News*, September 4, 2006, http://www.news.bbc.co.uk/1/hi/uk/5313882.stm (accessed March 13, 2009).

39. Nigel Bunyan, "Jamie Oliver Supports School Lunch Lock-ins," *Daily Telegraph*, September 6, 2007, http://www.telegraph.co.uk/news/main.jhtml;jsessionid=AOOQCMF2RSGZJQFIQMGCFF4AVCBQUIV0?xml=/news/2007/09/06/njamie106.xml (accessed March 13, 2009).

40. "Food Watchdog Condemned."

41. Elliot, "Food Alert."

42. "Food Watchdog Condemned."

43. Interview with Hanna Johnston; interview with Laura Lamb; interview with David Miller; interview with Sylvia Terry.

44. Dan Rutz, "Ritalin Comes under Scrutiny after Cancer Found in Mice," January 14, 1996, http://www.edition.cnn.com/HEALTH/9601/ritalin/index.html (accessed March 20, 2009).

45. "Hyperactivity Drug under Scrutiny," November 18, 1998, http://www.cbc.ca/health/story/1998/11/18/ritalin981118a.html (accessed March 20, 2009).

46. Steve Salvatore, "Group Issues Guidelines for Monitoring Ritalin in Children," November 9, 1998, http://www.edition.cnn.com/HEALTH/9811/09/hearts.ritalin/index.html (accessed March 20, 2009).

47. Fred A. Baughman Jr., *The ADHD Fraud: How Psychiatry Makes "Patients" Out of Normal Children* (Victoria, BC: Trafford Publishing, 2006), 1. Other popular books criticizing the notion of hyperactivity proliferated during the 1990s and 2000s: Peter Breggin, *Talking Back to Ritalin: What Doctors Aren't Telling You about Stimulants for Children* (Monroe, ME: Common Courage Press, 1998); Richard J. DeGrandpre, *Ritalin Nation: Rapid-Fire Culture and the Transformation of Human Consciousness* (New York: W. W. Norton, 1999); Lawrence H. Diller, *Running on Ritalin: A Physician Reflects on Children, Society, and Performance in a Pill* (New York: Bantam Books, 1999).

48. Iverson, *Speed, Ecstasy, Ritalin*, 64; Thomas E. Wilens et al., "Stimulants and Sudden Death: What Is a Physician to Do?" *Pediatrics* 118 (2006): 1215.

49. Steven E. Nissen, "ADHD Drugs and Cardiovascular Risk," *New England Journal of Medicine* 354 (2006): 1447–48.

50. Iverson, *Speed, Ecstasy, Ritalin*, 64.

51. Duffy, "Hyperactive Children 'Need Exercise, Not Drugs,'" 27.

52. Elaine Cassel, "Did Zoloft Make Him Do It?" February 7, 2005, http://www.edition.cnn.com/2005/LAW/02/07/cassel.pittman/index.html (accessed March 20, 2009); Lou Dobbs, "Promote Safety Not Profits," January 14, 2005, http://www.edition.cnn.com/2005/US/01/13/fda.safety/index.html (accessed March 20, 2009).

53. "Anti-Depressants, Little Effect," February 26, 2008, http://www.news.bbc.co.uk/1/hi/health/7263494.stm (accessed March 20, 2009); Irving Kirsch et al., "Initial Severity and Anti-Depressant Benefits: A Meta-Analysis of Data Submitted to the Food and Drug Administration," *PLoS Medicine* 5 (2008): 260.

54. A. J. Wakefield et al., "Ileal-Lymphoid-Nodular Hyperplasia, Non-Specific Colitis, and Pervasive Developmental Disorder in Children," *Lancet* 351 (1998): 637–41.

55. Collins and Pinch, *Dr. Golem*, 186.

56. Interview with Janice Atwater; interview with Lesley Freeman; interview with Jennifer Illing; interview with Lynn Kitchen; interview with Wendy Lott.

57. "Measles Fears Prompt MMR Campaign," August 7, 2008, http://www.news.bbc.co.uk/1/hi/health/7545151.stm (accessed March 23, 2009); Madison Park, "Autism Ruling Fails to Convince Many Vaccine-Link Believers," February 14, 2009, http://www.edition.cnn.com/2009/HEALTH/02/12/court.autism.reactions/index.html (accessed March 23, 2009); Jessica Snyder Sachs, "Vaccines: Separating Facts from Fiction," December 9, 2008, http://www.edition.cnn.com/2008/HEALTH/family/11/05/par.vaccine.kids/index.html (accessed March 23, 2009); Stephen Strauss, "Linking Vaccines, Autism Tantamount to Crying 'Fire' When There Isn't One," March 12, 2009, http://www.cbc.ca/technology/story/2009/03/11/f-strauss-autism-vaccines.html (accessed April 1, 2009).

58. Collins and Pinch, *Dr. Golem*, 192–201.

59. Michael Fitzpatrick, *MMR and Autism: What Parents Need to Know* (New York: Routledge, 2004), 1; Kennedy, "Message from the President," 729.

60. Collins and Pinch, *Dr. Golem*, 185.

61. Tammy Boyce, *Health, Risk, and News: The MMR Vaccine and the Media* (New York: Peter Lang, 2007), 1; Collins and Pinch, *Dr. Golem*, 189; Richard Horton, *MMR: Science and Fiction: Exploring a Vaccine Crisis* (London: Granta, 2004), 1–7.

62. "Diet Can Ease Behaviour Problems," February 13, 2002, http://www.news.bbc.co
.uk/1/hi/health/1816938.stm (accessed March 23, 2009); "The Importance of Not
Being Earnest," November 6, 1998, http://www.news.bbc.co.uk/1/hi/health/208729
.stm (accessed March 23, 2009); Rita Baron-Faust, "Biofeedback Widens Its Role
in Medicine," February 17, 2000, http://www.edition.cnn.com/2000/HEALTH/
alternative/02/17/neuro.feedback.wmd/index.html (accessed March 23, 2009).

63. Linda Ciampa, "Ritalin Abuse Scoring High on College Illegal Drug Circuit,"
January 8, 2001, http://www.edition.cnn.com/2001/HEALTH/children/01/08/
college.ritalin/index.html (accessed March 23, 2009); Anne Harding, "Study: Kids
with Eczema More Likely to Have ADHD," February 18, 2009, http://www
.edition.cnn.com/2009/HEALTH/02/18/healthmag.eczema.adhd/index.html
(accessed March 23, 2009); Iverson, *Speed, Ecstasy, Ritalin*, 71–73, 104–5.

Index

About the Author

Matthew Smith is a Wellcome Trust research fellow at the University of Exeter's Centre for Medical History. He has published work on the history of hyperactivity in *Social History of Medicine*, *Health and the Modern Home* (edited by Mark Jackson), *History and Policy*, and elsewhere. He has received the Roy Porter Prize and the Cadogan Award for his essay writing, and the American Association for the History of Medicine's Pressman-Burroughs Wellcome Award. His current project, funded by the Wellcome Trust, is on the history of food allergy in North America and Britain.

Available titles in the Critical Issues in Health and Medicine series: